PEDIATRIC NEPHROLOGY

VOLUME 6

Current Concepts in
Diagnosis and Management

PEDIATRIC NEPHROLOGY

VOLUME 6

Current Concepts in Diagnosis and Management

Edited by

JOSÉ STRAUSS

University of Miami School of Medicine
Miami, Florida

PLENUM PRESS · NEW YORK AND LONDON

The Library of Congress cataloged the first volume of this title as follows:

Pediatric nephrology. v. 1–
New York, Stratton Intercontinental Medical Book Corp.
1974–
v. ill. 24 cm.
"Current concepts in diagnosis and management."
ISSN 0097–5257
1. Pediatric nephrology–Periodicals.
RJ466.P36 618.9'26'1005 73–94018

ISBN 978-1-4684-8806-7 ISBN 978-1-4684-8804-3 (eBook)
DOI 10.1007/978-1-4684-8804-3

Based on the proceedings of the sixth and seventh Pediatric Nephrology Seminars, sponsored by the Division of Pediatric Nephrology, Department of Pediatrics, and the Division of Continuing Education, University of Miami School of Medicine, held January 2-6, 1979 and January 27-31, 1980, in Bal Harbour, Florida

Softcover reprint of the hardcover 1st edition 1981

A Division of Plenum Publishing Corporation
233 Spring Street, New York, N.Y. 10013

RAWLE M. McINTOSH

Genius in a hurry
making new sense out of old problems
creating directions
at his best, a friend and partner

Consumed too soon

Acknowledgements

The continued support of inquisitive registrants, interested sponsors, and cooperative colleagues made possible the Annual Pediatric Nephrology Seminars 6 and 7 on which this volume is based. The inquisitive registrants included some who come every year to participate in the Seminar and many who came for the first time, confident enough to take the chance that their expenditure of time, effort and money would be adequately rewarded.

The interested sponsors included the following who care enough about continuing medical education to invest in it:

Beach Pharmaceuticals
Burroughs Wellcome Company
CenterChem Products, Inc.
Ciba Pharmaceutical Company
Cordis Dow Corporation
Drake-Willock
Eli Lilly & Company
Hemonetics
Hoechst-Roussel Pharmaceuticals, Inc.
Mead Johnson
Merck, Sharpe & Dohme
Pennwalt Corporation
Pfizer Laboratories, Inc.
Quinton Instrument Company
Roche Laboratories
Ross Laboratories
Schering Corporation
Smith, Kline & French Laboratories
E.R. Squibb & Sons, Inc.
The Upjohn Company

The cooperative colleagues included Seminar 6 and 7 guest and local faculty who took time to prepare for and participate in the sessions and complete papers, Pediatric Nephrology Division staff members who accepted responsibility for the endless details the seminars and book entailed - especially Rex Baker, Pearl Seidler and Estela Garcia, Debbie LaBrie and Louise Strauss.

Finally, I acknowledge the continued approval and moral support of Dr. Emmanuel Papper, Dean, and Dr. Bernard Fogel, Associate Dean, of the University of Miami School of Medicine, and Dr. William Cleveland, Chairman of the Department of Pediatrics.

José Strauss, M.D.

Introduction

Infectious and non-infectious tubulointerstitial nephropathies are old subjects but there is enough confusion and disagreement on terminology and etiopathogenesis to warrant a new look at these problems. We were fortunate in having at the Pediatric Nephrology Seminar 6 and as contributors to this volume, the representatives - or shall I say "originators"? - of each of the three most identifiable positions: Dr. Renee Habib - congenital anomalies, Dr. John Hodson - reflux, and Dr. Robert Heptinstall - infection. Although some tend to hold onto one position and exclude others, in this case there was overlapping of perception. Dr. Habib accepts a role for infection in reflux and for infection in the presence of obstruction; Dr. Hodson accepts infection and congenital anomalies as modifiers; and Dr. Heptinstall takes an overall position which encompasses the three.

Thus the first part of the book emphasizes the complexity of something as seemingly simple as UTI and demonstrates awareness of disagreement even among the pros about meanings, interpretations, and treatment.

Drs. Gustavo Gordillo, Jorge de la Cruz and their associates emphasize the importance of predisposing factors for UTI; Dr. Materson focuses on the workup of the patient, Dr. Zilleruelo on bacteriological aspects, and Dr. Gorman on treatment approaches. Dr. Vaamonde reviews nephrotoxic agents. Finally, Drs. Andres and Noble review the immunological aspects of various tubulointerstitial nephritides.

Part Two, based on Seminar 7, presents a broad review of nutritional and other derangements stemming from chronic renal failure or its treatment. Drs. Christakis, Barness, Metcoff and Gordillo review specific nutritional aspects. Dr. Gruskin associates the problem with antibiotics, aluminum and peritoneal dialysis. Dr. Broyer presents hypertension of renal origin, enteral nutrition and amino acids, Dr, Bourgoignie, remal osteodystropy and Dr. Guido Perez, hyperlipidemia. Finally, Dr. Zilleruelo evaluates water and electrolyte homeostasis, and Dr. Richard, diuretics. These papers, and the discussions in which the above authors and Drs. Miller, Pardo, Peters and Yunis participate, provide a rich, up-to-date exchange on the subjects chosen.

For exposure to points of view not often seen in print plus current information and theories about urinary tract infection, infectious and non-infectious tubulointerstitial nephritis, nutritional and other derangements stemming from chronic renal failure or its treatment, and related research ideas, this volume is indispensable.

José Strauss
December 1980

Contents

III. SYSTEMIC ASPECTS OF RENAL DISEASE

PART ONE

URINARY TRACT INFECTION

INFECTIONS AND NON-INFECTIOUS TUBULOINTERSTITIAL NEPHRITIS

IDENTIFICATION AND DOCUMENTATION OF URINARY TRACT INFECTION

Barry J. Materson, M.D.

Dept. Med., Univ. Miami Sch. Med., and Med. Serv., Miami Veterans Adm. Hosp., Miami, Fla. 33125, USA

Urinary tract infection is one of the most common problems of both pediatric and adult practice. It may either be overt (symptomatic) or covert (asymptomatic). Overt infections may either be self-evident or present with signs and symptoms more typical of other common diseases. Covert infections are discovered either by serendipity or by screening of asymptomatic populations. A working knowledge of populations at risk greatly facilitates diagnostic effort and planning for intelligent screening methods.

MAGNITUDE OF PROBLEM

Incidence of Urinary Tract Infection

The general incidence of urinary tract infection in neonates and children is displayed in Table 1. Urinary tract infection in the newborn is uncommon but, when present, is of hematogenous origin and is associated with signs and symptoms of generalized septicemia (1,2,3). Overt infection in the first month occurs mostly in boys at a frequency of 1.4 per 1000 births (1). Covert infection occurs in 1 to 3.7% of boy neonates and 0.3 to 2.1% of girls and may be diagnostically challenging (4).

Overt infections are not common in children and covert infections in boys are rare (about 0.04%). However, they are more common in girls with an incidence of 0.5 to 2% from 2 months to 13 years. There is an incidence of about 1% in later childhood (1-4).

Thereafter, adolescent boys and men uncommonly have urinary tract infection in the absence of obstruction. Older men experi-

Table 1. Incidence of Urinary Tract Infection

Neonates				
Covert:	Boys 1-3.7%	Girls 0.3-2.1%		
Overt:	Boys 1.4/1000 births (Newborn UTI: Hematogenous origin)			
Children				
Covert:	Boys probably rare (0.04%)	Girls	2 mo-13 yrs 6-13 yrs	0.5-2% 1%
Overt:	Not common			

ence a rising frequency *pari passu* with the development of prostatic hypertrophy. Women are much more susceptible to infection particularly in association with "honeymoon cystitis" and pregnancy (2,5). A substantial risk of infection secondary to bladder catheterization exists at all ages.

Relationship to Correctable Abnormalities

This topic is so chaotic in terms of hard data and so charged with emotion that almost any statement made is likely to be subjected to vigorous attack. Clearly, my viewpoint is that of a nonsurgeon and is likely to conflict with presentations by urologists. The major abnormalities identified by urologists for treatment have been vesical neck obstruction, ureterovesical reflux and distal urethral stenosis.

Vesical neck obstruction was popularized in the 1950 to 1965 era as a cause for urinary tract infection, particularly in girls. Popular opinion held that the prevalence of vesical neck obstruction was high in children with recurring or persistent urinary tract infections and that a surgical approach was appropriate treatment (6,7). Two papers which were published in 1967 demonstrated that vesical neck obstruction was only a rare cause of urinary tract infection (8,9) and enthusiasm for surgical correction waned. Stamey (3) makes the strong point that "...surely from the point of history alone, should not many of those who so strongly believe today that ureteral reflux or distal urethral stenosis is the basis for childhood urinary infections recall the recent enthusiasm for correcting vesical neck 'obstruction'? Indeed, it is of interest that several authorities and staunch advocates of ureteral reflux as the primary cause of urinary infections today believed with equal conviction less than a decade ago that the vesical neck was the major cause."

Vesicoureteral reflux continues to be highly controversial. Stamey's excellent discussion (3) and the papers in a symposium on reflux nephropathy cover the basic issues. Some of the important points are that vesicoureteral reflux in infants can cause some renal scarring in the absence of urinary tract infection (10), that the serious damage appears to occur very early in life and generally is not associated with renal failure, that only severe reflux (22% of the total) is associated with renal damage (13% of kidneys examined), and that the prevalence of reflux decreases rapidly with age (11-13). These data suggest that surgery for reflux alone should be confined to the first two or three years of life.

Distal urethral stenosis is also a controversial issue. I refer the reader to Stamey (3) for the basic discussion. I discuss it further in association with dysuria (*vide infra*).

When children with recurrent or persistent urinary tract infections are studied, roughly 50% will have some type of radiographic abnormality (11-13). Hallett et al. (14) studied 73 boys with documented urinary tract infection prospectively for three years. Radiographic abnormalities were found in 22 (30%) but 6 of those had "pyelonephritic" changes and one had a cyst. The rest were reflux and congenital abnormalities. Three of the boys underwent circumcision and only 2 of the 73 required urinary tract surgery: pyeloplasty for a horseshoe kidney and reimplantation of an obstructed megaureter. *Proteus* species accounted for 59% of the isolated organisms and was thought to originate from the preputial sac and urethra. Recurrence of infection was rare in patients without radiographic abnormalities.

My personal recommendations for workup searching for correctable abnormalities are as follows:

1. Workup patients with recurrent or persistent urinary tract infection only.

2. When structural abnormalities are identified, consider most carefully the natural history of the abnormality (it may be totally benign) and the data that surgical intervention is of value.

Morbidity and Mortality of Urinary Tract Infections

Mortality from urinary tract infection is most likely at the extremes of age: in neonates because it is associated with systemic sepsis and in the elderly where infection is likely to occur behind obstruction and lead to septicemia. Some mortality and morbidity is iatrogenic from procedures and treatment. I see numerous patients who develop acute renal failure from aminoglycoside antimicrobials.

The major questions of morbidity are presented so well by Kunin (2) that I will address but a few selected issues.

Covert bacteriuria in schoolgirls. The important work in this area has been summarized by Kunin (15). However, a large group of children was followed by Savage (16) who drew the following conclusions: "The present data suggest that for the majority of these children therapy is not essential, and that renal change when it does occur is of little or no significance; however, there must be a long period of follow-up before these facts can be substantiated."

Urinary infection in adults. Freedman (17) has reviewed the question of consequences of urinary tract infection in adults. His conclusion was that "...there is very little evidence to point to the ability of bacterial infection of the urinary tract to produce hypertension or renal damage in the absence of actual or potential underlying kidney damage." There are two studies which do suggest that mortality is increased in hypertensive patients with urinary tract infections compared with hypertensive non-infected controls (18), and that there is more hypertension in infected patients with radiographic evidence of renal damage as compared to those without renal damage (19). Freedman makes the major point that bacterial infection superimposed on obstruction or renal papillary damage is a totally different disease of catastrophic potential. The classic U.S. Public Health Service study (20) demonstrated that men who did not have obstructive uropathy or renal parenchymal disease did not develop renal failure over 10 years even with persistent bacteriuria. An important note of caution based on long-term follow-up of a large number of women is posed by Alwall (21) whose data suggest that the final answer is not yet in.

Bacteriuria in pregnancy. This topic has been reviewed nicely by Brumfitt (22). While the data bearing on consequences of urinary tract infection on pregnant women seem to be clear, those on the fetus are less so. His conclusions are that untreated bacteriuria leads to acute pyelonephritis in 30% of women; bacteriuric women tend to be more anemic than controls and that the anemia tended to progress; and that papers published since the 1960's have shown no or relatively weak adverse effects of bacteriuria on the fetus. However, his own data suggest lower birth weights and more frequent prematurity in untreated bacteriuric mothers.

The Screening Controversy

This important issue is based on what one expects to find, its frequency in the population, the consequences of non-detection and the benefits of detection and treatment. Although there is still some debate, pregnant women probably should be screened (22). Kunin (23,24) argues for mass screening in motivated communities and points out that it can be accomplished easily in the private practice setting. McCormick (25) addresses data in support of screening, Rapkin (26) takes a neutral stand, and Arbus (27) argues against it. I believe that screening can be accomplished in the private practice setting but, regardless of the situation, if one screens, one must be prepared to deal intelligently with those patients found to harbor infection.

DYSURIA AS AN INDICATOR OF URINARY TRACT INFECTION

Dysuria, i.e. painful or difficult urination, is generally the most commonly accepted symptom of urinary tract infection. Unfortunately, it is not at all specific and may lead to treatment of a disease which does not exist and expose patients to unnecessary risk. True urinary tract infection can be documented as the cause of dysuria in 75% of men but in only 50% of women with that complaint. It is, therefore, extremely important to be aware of the non-infectious causes of dysuria. These are displayed, in part, in Table 2.

Table 2. Non-infectious Causes of Dysuria

Trauma
Motorcycle or bicycle
Masturbation
Self-instrumentation
Sexual intercourse
Irritation
Vaginal tampons
Vulvovaginitis
Vaginal deodorants
Pantyhose
Bubble baths
Jalapeña peppers
Fever
Urethral caruncle
Psychogenic

Urethral trauma must be carefully considered. Some types are obvious such as direct injury, but others may be extremely difficult to detect because of their clandestine nature. In mysterious cases, a flat plate of the abdomen may reveal a foreign body in the bladder. Radiologists frequently have collections of films showing objects such as a thermometer, a large nail or even a string of beads in the bladder (Fig. 1,2). Vigorous sexual foreplay and intercourse may cause dysuria without infection. Such women will not benefit from antimicrobials.

Dysuria may result from irritative stimuli as diverse as vaginal deodorants and jalapeña peppers. Infection of the vulva or vagina should be ruled out, and urine collection performed with extreme care to avoid contamination. Vaginal and bubble bath soap may contain sensitizers or irritants which cause dysuria. The deodorant can be replaced by simple washing with mild soap and water. Pantyhose may be irritating. Sometimes advising that a patient wear cotton underpants under the pantyhose may be curative. Jalapeña peppers are irritating to mucous membranes other than the

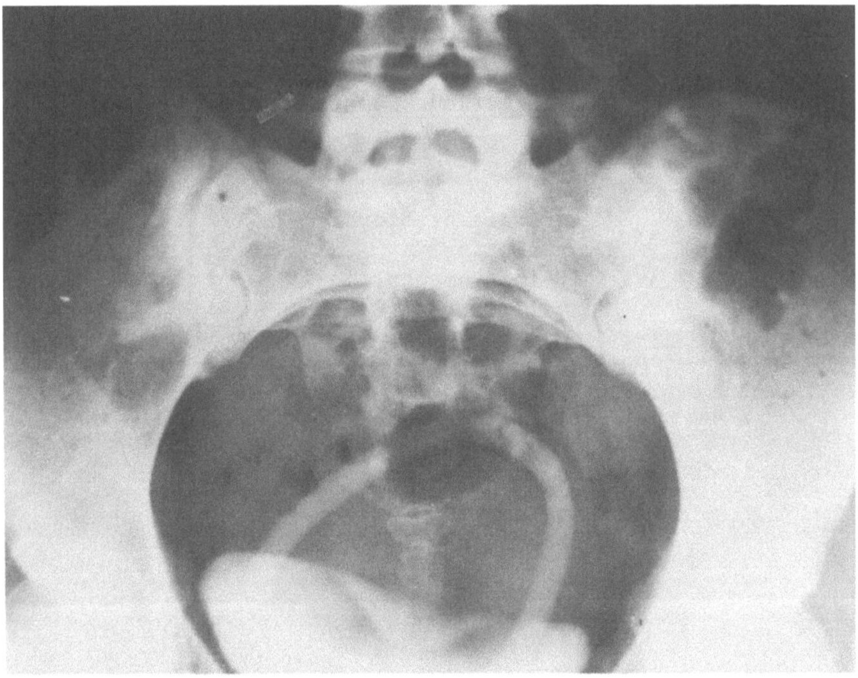

FIG. 1. This pessary caused urinary tract symptoms in the absence of infection, presumably by bladder compression. (Courtesy of Dr. B. Lieberman)

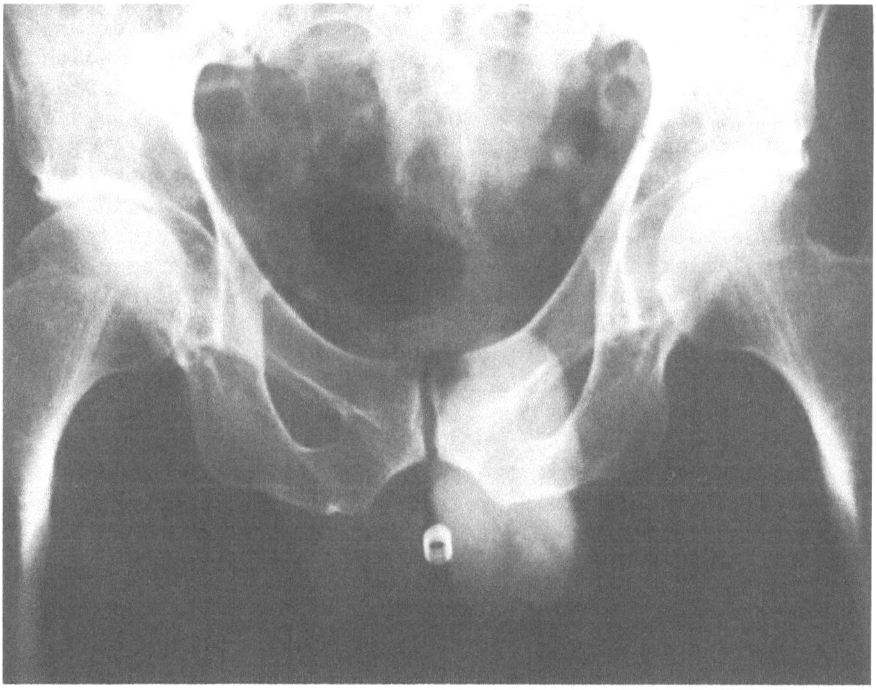

FIG. 2. The metal cylinder is the eraser ferrule of a pencil. The patient had inserted the pencil deeply into his urethra. The pencil broke off and had to be removed surgically. The blood-engorged penis is clearly visible. (Courtesy of Dr. B. Lieberman)

oral mucosa. Avoidance may solve the problem of dysuria. Lest the latter point be misconstrued, let me emphasize that the peppers were eaten. I know of no reports of dysuria due to direct urethral contact with a jalepeña pepper!

Fever from non-urinary tract sources may produce dysuria. If urinary tract infection cannot be documented, it is essential to identify the true source and provide appropriate treatment.

Urethral caruncles tend to be extremely painful. Simple physical examination is diagnostic.

The most difficult cases of dysuria to diagnose and treat are those of psychogenic origin. This remains a diagnosis of exclusion even in patients with obvious psychiatric problems (28).

The so-called urethral syndrome is so controversial that it deserves special comment. Generally, this refers to a symptom complex of burning on urination, feeling of decreased force of stream, frequency and urgency. This is further characterized by occurring almost exclusively in girls and women about 50% of whom have no evidence for urinary tract infection. I have covered the various non-infectious causes above. The controversy is focused upon the urological procedures which are used to "treat" the disorder. These are urethral dilation (29), distal urethroplasty (30), and internal urethotomy. Even an allegedly favorable paper (31) has a 50% failure rate in abacteriuric patients. The concept of distal stenosis as a cause for turbulent flow during micturition and return to laminar flow after dilatation (32,33) has been challenged by work that shows no difference in mean urethral caliber between symptomatic children and controls (34-36). Any tube with an internal diameter of 10F or more should not obstruct flow (37). Good studies (38,39) including a blinded, prospective one (39), have failed to find evidence for obstruction as a cause for urethral syndrome or that urological procedures are superior to medication alone. I do not believe that there are quality data to support a role for urethral interventive procedures in the abacteriuric, dysuric patient. Such patients deserve a careful workup and only after all else fails should urethral dilatation be considered.

One additional rare cause of alleged urinary tract infection should be recalled in unusual or otherwise atypical patients: the Munchausen Syndrome. It is possible for patients to claim urinary tract symptoms and vitiate their urine with blood or pus from other sources. Meadow (40) reports a fascinating case of Munchausen Syndrome by proxy wherein the patient's mother surrepticiously mixed her own vaginal secretions into her daughter's urine specimens and forced the daughter to undergo numerous procedures looking for a non-existent source of infection.

METHODS OF IDENTIFICATION OF URINARY TRACT INFECTION

Index of Suspicion

As with most things in medicine, a high index of suspicion, careful history and thorough physical examination are powerful tools. Knowledge of specific groups at risk *(vide supra)* is helpful for initial assessment.

Newborn infants with overt urinary tract infection tend to present with life-threatening septicemia and endotoxemia (1). The covert infections of infants may present with non-specific signs including fever, unsatisfactory weight gain, gastrointestinal symptoms (including colic) (41), central nervous system symptoms, pallor, cyanosis and gray skin, and even jaundice (2,3).

Common symptoms of urinary tract infection in children include dysuria (56%), frequency, enuresis, abdominal or flank pain and fever. Less common findings are hematuria, abdominal tenderness, vaginitis, vaginal discharge, vomiting and anorexia (42,43).

Some argument has been made (44) for a correlation between allergy and repeated urinary tract infections in children although this remains unconfirmed (45).

Meadow (46) has pointed out that frequency, urgency, perineal soreness and dysuria, enuresis, cloudy urine, discolored urine and smelly urine may be observed in children *without* evidence for urinary tract infection.

One brief word of caution is necessary. The above-mentioned symptoms can be related to urinary tract infection only if subsequent examination of properly collected urine reveals bacteriologic evidence of infection. However, there are organisms which may not be detected by routine bacteriologic methods, and if the index of suspicion is high, more sophisticated methods should be employed (47).

Many algorithms for diagnosis of urinary tract infection have been proposed. Todd (48) presents one for children and adolescents but does not provide validating data. Burger and Wolcott (49) devised an algorithm for their military population using discriminant analysis. Consideration of patients with the combination of dysuria and/or frequency with pyuria, bacteriuria, or a history of a previous positive urine culture identified 87% of those with positive urine cultures (13% false negative), but also 49% of those with negative urine cultures (49% false positive). Their algorithm was designed for use by physician extenders, but as constructed, would provide a safety factor in that all patients would be cultured and a physician consulted for temperature over 100°F, abnormal abdominal examination or CVA tenderness.

Komaroff and colleagues (50) devised an algorithm for urinary tract versus vaginal infection based on findings in 821 women. They found a diagnosis of vaginitis to be twice as likely as a diagnosis of urinary tract infection in a given patient with dysuria. Use of the algorithm permits decision making based on initial evaluation of vaginal discharge and irritation plus internal dysuria and frequency.

The Urine Sediment

Examination of the urine sediment is a time-honored clinical test for abnormalities of the urinary tract. Unfortunately, it is greatly lacking in both sensitivity and specificity. Pyuria is difficult to define because of variations in collection, rate and time of centrifugation, volume in which the sediment is resuspended and size of the sample observed. Pyuria is indicative only of some irritative or inflammatory process and does not necessarily indicate infection. Non-infectious causes include urinary calculi, bladder neoplasms, interstitial nephritis (including that due to analgesic abuse), and effect of recent urological surgery. There is also the possibility of false negative response: infection with *Streptococcus faecalis* is a weak stimulus of pyuria (51) and patients who are immunosuppressed may not be able to have a pyuric reaction to urinary infection. Granulocytopenic patients also lose their ability to mount a pyuric response to infection, especially at absolute granulocyte counts of less than 1000/cu mm (52). Observation of white blood cell casts localizes the source of white cells to the renal parenchyma. Although WBC casts are useful indicators of urinary tract infection in a clinical setting for infection, they are by no means pathognomonic.

Musher et al. (53) used a quantitative approach to the evaluation of pyuria. They counted WBC's in uncentrifuged urine by using a hemocytometer. All of their infected patients save one had greater than 10^4 WBC's/ml while all of those with 10^3 or less were not infected. If one uses uncentrifuged urine and a low power (x10) microscopic field, one WBC per field will represent about 3×10^3 WBC's/ml. In contrast, 10^5 or more WBC's/ml (the mean count in their infected patients was 3.1×10^5) are equivalent to about 30 WBC's per low power field. The hemocytometer method avoids most of the pitfalls of the traditional routine examination, but does require more time and skill.

A rough guide to predict presence of 10^5 or greater colony-forming bacteria on subsequent culture is the observation of one or more bacteria per high power field in an uncentrifuged urine specimen (54). Lewis and Alexander (55) have carried the technique further by examining gram-stained urine smears. When no organisms were observed by oil immersion microscopy in 1,279 stained smears of centrifuged urine, all of the quantitative cultures were negative. When one or more organisms were seen per field, 79% of 900 specimens grew 10^5 or more colonies, 13% were between 10^4 and 10^5 and 8% were less than 10^4. Therefore, no bacteria proved to be a good predictor of negative culture and one or more per field predicted 92% of the cultures with 10^4 or more organisms.

Localization Tests

Localization of the site of urinary tract infection is important in investigative models and in some clinical settings. The general concept is that infections confined to the bladder should be easier to treat (perhaps even with a single injection of an aminoglycoside antimicrobial) (56), would be less likely to cause serious systemic complications and, on occasion, resolve spontaneously. In contrast, upper-tract infections involving the renal parenchyma were assumed to require longer courses of therapy, were a potential risk for sepsis and local abscess as well as renal functional impairment and would not resolve spontaneously. Upper versus lower urinary tract localization studies are of little clinical value in the management of most urinary tract infections since the aim of therapy is eradification of bacteria from all parts of the system. These tests are generally limited to that minority of patients who have otherwise unexplained recurrent infections. Furthermore, urinary tract infections may shift repeatedly from one site to the other so that localization on any given day may be incorrect the next (57). The major localization tests are displayed in Table 3.

Ureteral catheterization. Stamey, Govan and Palmer (58) described a localization test based on comparisons of cultures from the catheterized bladder, urine collected after thorough washing of the bladder and urine collected by catheterization of each ureter. Lower tract infection is defined by bacteria in the catheterized bladder sample but sterile urine from the ureters after bladder washing. A positive culture from one or both ureters denotes upper tract infection. The patient must be well hydrated to minimize the risk of contaminating the upper tract with infected urine from the lower tract. Although this is the "definitive" localization test, false positive upper tract localization is possible and the procedure is obviously interventive.

Antibody titers. Serum antibody response to infecting organisms tends to be more frequent and of greater magnitude in patients with pyelonephritis than cystitis (59). However, this generality does not necessarily obtain for the individual patient. Delay in titer rise will result in a false negative test for pyelonephritis and severe cystitis with tissue invasion may give rise to serum antibodies thus falsely suggesting pyelonephritis (60).

Table 3. Tests for Localization of Urinary Tract Infection

- Ureteral catheterization (Stamey)
- High Ab titers, low concentration (Turck)
- Bladder washout (Fairley)
- Fluorescent antibody coating
- "Three Glass Test" (Meares and Stamey)

Turck, Ronald, and Petersdorf (61) compared bacterial serotypes as indicators of relapse versus reinfection with site of infection as determined by ureteral catheterization. In general, patients who relapsed with the identical serotype tended to have upper tract infections while those who were reinfected with different organisms tended to have lower tract infections.

Renal concentrating ability. Ronald, Cutler, and Turck (62) used bilateral ureteral catheterization as a reference for examining the relationship between site of infection and maximum renal concentrating ability. Patients with lower tract infection concentrated better (913.6 $\pm$ 182.0; range 592-1218 mOsm/kg) than those with upper tract infection (771.7 $\pm$ 122.2; range 545-1002 mOsm/kg). Furthermore, while there was no difference between maximum urine concentration by each kidney in patients with bladder infection, infected kidneys concentrated a mean of 200 mOsm/kg less than the uninfected contralateral kidney. One of their most important observations was that the concentrating defect was reversible with successful treatment. The obvious overlap in data as well as the interventive nature of the procedure prevent this test from being clinically useful.

Bladder washout test. Fairley et al. (63) described and later modified (64) a localization test which does not require ureteral catheterization. The basic procedure is outlined in Table 4. Al-

Table 4. Procedure and Interpretation of the Fairley Test

1. Catheterize bladder (three way Foley) culture urine.

2. Instill 50 ml 0.1% neomycin with two amps elase. Leave for 30 min.

3. Wash bladder with 2 liters sterile water.

4. Collect specimens: IMMEDIATELY
   0-10 min
   10-20 min
   20-30 min

Fairley Test Interpretation

- Bladder only: all washout samples sterile

- Renal: Samples positive > 1,000 per ml
  Often > 10,000 per ml

though this test is interventive in that it requires bladder catheterization, it does not require a special operating room or anesthesia usually associated with ureteral catheterization. In addition, the very procedure of antibiotic instillation may be curative for bladder infections. All of the patients were adult women. The site of infection did not correlate either with symptoms or with serum antibacterial antibody. The Fairley test has become the reference standard for other localization tests instead of bilateral ureteral catheterization.

Antibody-coated bacteria (ACB) test. A non-interventive, risk-free, *in vitro* localization test based on fluorescent antibody-coated bacteria in the urine was developed by Thomas, Shelokov, and Forland (65). They reasoned that even those patients who did not elevate specific serum antibodies to organisms infecting the renal parenchyma, should make enough local antibody to coat the bacteria and be detectable. That is, bacteria originating from a pyelonephritic kidney should be antibody coated while bladder bacteria causing cystitis should not have elicited an immune response and should not be antibody-coated.

The basic technique is as follows (66). Five ml of the patient's urine is centrifuged and the supernatant discarded. The sediment is washed twice with phosphate buffered saline. The washed sediment is then mixed with 0.2 ml fluorescein-conjugated antihuman globulin and incubated for 30 min at 37°C. The mixture is washed twice more with phosphate buffered saline. The final sediment is then smeared onto a slide and examined with a fluorescence microscope. The test is considered positive if at least 25% of the bacterial cells fluoresce.

The bladder washout test has been used to validate the ACB test. Thomas (65) found excellent correlation in that 34 of 35 patients with *clinical* pyelonephritis (only nine had bladder washout) had a positive ACB test while only one of 20 patients with *clinical* cystitis had a positive ACB test. However, four of five patients with bacterial prostatitis had a positive ACB test without evidence of pyelonephritis. This problem of false positivity has been confirmed by Jones (67). Of 18 upper tract infections defined by direct localization, 17 had ACB in the urine while none of the eight lower tract infections was associated with positive ACB. Three patients who had positive ACB had equivocable direct localization tests (68).

The sensitivity and specificity of the ACB tests have been examined by a number of investigators who either support it enthusiastically or raise serious questions of its validity, particularly in the routine clinical setting. Papers are difficult to compare because the controls and even definition of a positive test (69) differ.

Janson and Roberts (70) infected monkeys in such a way that cystitis and pyelonephritis could be controlled. The ACB test was positive in 11 of 11 animals with unilateral pyelonephritis, 2 of 2 with bilateral pyelonephritis and none of the three monkeys with cystitis. Under these very well controlled conditions, correlation was perfect.

A group in Barcelona (71) used clinical definitions for upper and lower tract infections. The ACB test was positive in 35 of 36 patients with pyelonephritis and in none of the 11 with cystitis. They modified the Thomas method so that the urine did not require immediate processing or refrigeration. Curiously, they published this paper *verbatim* elsewhere (72).

One of the inherent problems of the ACB test is observer interpretation. In a study of 253 specimens (73), three independent observers agreed on the first reading 88% of the time. When compared with the majority opinion, the sensitivity of an individual reading was 91% and the specificity 95%.

Jones and Johnson (74) reported their experience with the ACB test under conditions that might obtain in a diagnostic microbiology laboratory. In general the results were reproducible and consistent. Explanations for inconsistencies included the immune response to the infecting bacteria, non-specificity of the antibody coating the bacteria, antibody in prostatic secretions and antibody-coated bacteria contaminating the urine specimens.

Harding et al. (75), using bladder washout as the standard, proved the validity of ACB for lower-tract infections in that ACB was negative in all 14 such patients. However, six of 37 patients with proven upper-tract infection were ACB negative. Of greatest importance was the non-correlation of clinical symptoms with actual site of infection. Rumans and Vosti (76,77) also demonstrated a rather chaotic relationship of positive ACB to clinical symptoms but others (78) have somewhat better correlation.

The ACB test has been studied in different clinical settings. The test appears to be reasonably valid in patients with diabetes mellitus (79), renal transplant patients receiving immunosuppressive agents (80,81), and pregnancy (82). However, questions have been raised about false positives in patients with proteinuria (83) and false negatives in patients with urinary tract cancer (84). None of these studies was rigorously controlled. However, in a study (85) of children using bladder washout as a reference, there were 4 of 12 falsely negative for upper and 10 of 35 falsely positive for lower tract infection. The authors cannot explain why the ACB test correlates so poorly with site of infection in children, but plead that it not be used until more data can be acquired.

In summary, the ACB test has much to offer as a no risk, *in vitro* tool. However, the evidence that it can be of value in a clinical diagnostic setting is incomplete at best and there are no data validating the test in a pediatric population.

The "three glass test". Meares and Stamey (86) described a simple, non-interventive test which may help to localize infection to the urethra, bladder or prostate. Fig. 3 outlines the mechanics of the test. After cleaning and drying the glans, the first 10 ml of urine are collected in a sterile container, a mid-stream clean-catch collection (MSCC) is then made and the patient is instructed to stop his stream. His prostate is then massaged and the expressed prostatic secretions collected. The next 10 ml of voided urine are then collected. Evidence of infection in the first sample only identifies a urethral source. The sample following prostatic massage identifies a prostatic source and MSCC collection suggests bladder and/or upper tract infection. This is an easy test to perform on ambulatory men and permits rapid therapeutic decision making. A similar test which includes a vaginal culture can be done on female patients (Fig. 4) (3).

Other localization tests. A number of other localization tests have been described. Janson and Roberts (70) employed ^{131}I hippur-

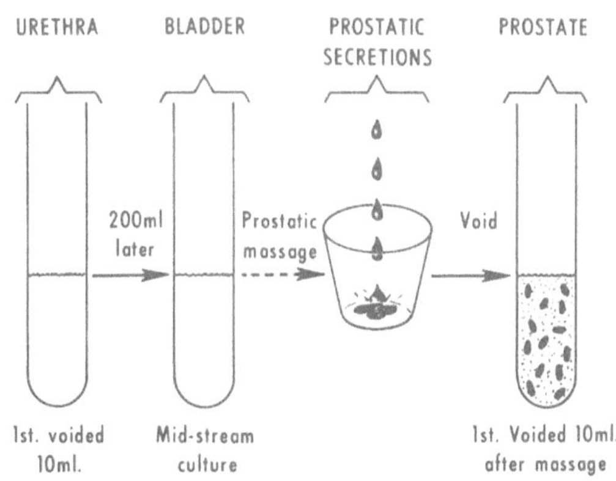

FIG. 3. The "three glass test". (Redrawn and modified from Meares, E.M. and Stamey, T.A.: Bacteriologic localization patterns in bacterial prostatitis and urethritis. Invest. Urol. 5: 492, 1968, with permission).

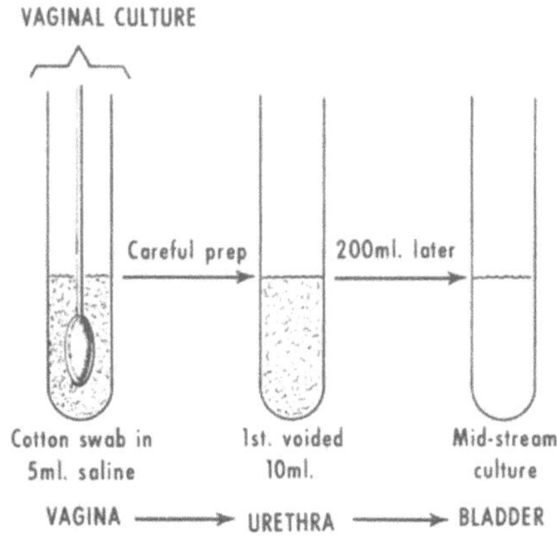

FIG. 4. Simple localization test for urinary tract infection in females. (Redrawn and modified from Stamey, T.A.: Urinary Infections. Baltimore: Williams and Wilkins, 1972, with permission).

an scintiphotos in the hydropenic state plus ^{67}gallium citrate scintiphotos and the ACB test in their experimental monkey model. The three tests combined were highly accurate in differentiating cystitis, ureteritis, pyelonephritis and renal or perinephric abscesses. Hurwitz et al. (87) used ^{67}gallium citrate scintiphotos alone in 73 human patients. Accuracy was 86% with 15% false positives and 13% false negatives. Although intravenous pyelography (IVP) is very useful for identifying anatomic defects (88), it is not useful for localizing sites of infection.

Beta glucuronidase levels have been proposed (89) as an indication of renal parenchymal infection, but this has not been substantiated (90).

Chemical Tests for Urinary Infection

An effective and simple chemical test to replace urinalysis for mass screening for urinary tract infection has been sought for many years. None thus far described is perfect for this purpose although the nitrite test seems to be the best one currently available.

Nitrite (Griess') test. The nitrite test is based on the observation in 1914 by Cruickshank and Moyes that the test for nitrite developed by Griess could be used to test for bacteriuria (91). The test is based on the fact that bacteria reduce nitrate to nitrite. The nitrite reacts with sulfanilic acid and alpha-naphthylamine to form a red azo dye. It should be performed on a first morning specimen. Griess' test is excellent for detection of gram negative enteric bacteria but is poor for staphylococci. Its sensitivity is considered fair and specificity good (23). This test will be discussed in greater detail below because of its commercial availability as a combined culture dip-stick.

Glucose oxidase. Normal people excrete about 2 to 10 mg/dl of glucose in their urine. This test is based on the observation (92) that bacteria will metabolize this small amount of urinary glucose. Therefore, a negative glucose test is positive for infection. It must be performed on the first morning specimen and cannot be used in diabetic patients. False positives range from 0.5 to 3.4% (93). Sensitivity is considered good but specificity fair.

Tetrazolium reduction. This test is based on the ability of bacteria to reduce triphenyltetrazolium to bright red triphenylformazon (94). Although its sensitivity is good, it has poor specificity (88). In addition, it is basically a laboratory test requiring preparation of fresh test solution daily and prolonged incubation.

Catalase test. This test is based on the ability of bacterial catalase to act on hydrogen peroxide to yield oxygen (88). Unfortunately, red and white blood cells and renal tubular cells also contain catalase and the test cannot differentiate between infection and other inflammatory renal disease. Its sensitivity is good, but specificity poor.

Other tests. Giler et al. (95) demonstrated that sterile urine has very low levels of xanthine oxidase but that significant activity occurred in urine with more than 100,000 bacteria per ml. An exception was urine infected with *Staph. aureus* which causes much less or no increase. The authors claim high specificity for the test. The assay for xanthine oxidase is quite complex, but the authors indicated that they were attempting to automate it.

Lamb, Dalton and Wilkins (96) proposed an innovative electrochemical test for bacteriuria. The test measures the change in potential between electrodes in the innoculum and a reference medium. A wide variety of organisms including *Serratia, Acinetobacter (Mima* and *Herellea)*, alpha streptococci and *Candida albicans* were easily detected within 10 hours (94% with 4 hours). There were no false positives. The method could be useful if adapted for mass screening.

Hayward and Jeavons (97) reported a technique amenable to automation which is based on detection of bacterial metabolic products by head-space gas-liquid chromatography. The method has potential, but there are still numerous problems to be solved before it is ready for screening purposes.

Screening Culture Methods

A number of modified culture techniques have been developed both for screening purposes and for permitting culture of urine specimens by patients (or their parents) at home. These are discussed by Gillenwater (88) and Kunin (23). The two which appear to be most reported on in the United States are a "dipslide" and a stick combining a pad culture with a nitrite test strip.

The dipslide (Uricult[R], Medical Technology Corporation, Hackensack, N.J.) consists of a slide coated on one side with a non-specific nutrient agar and on the other with MacConkey's agar which favors enterobacteriaciae. The slide is attached to the cap of a sterile vial into which the slide is inserted. The slide is briefly dipped into the urine sample or placed directly in the urine stream. It is then incubated for 18 to 24 hours at 37°C. Adelman (98) provides a practical description of its use. Asscher et al. (99) argue for more widespread use. The dipslide compares favorably with standard techniques (100) and, if used properly, has a very high sensitivity and specificity (101). Martin and McGuckin (102) sound a note of caution. They suggest that the dipslide is not an effective screen in populations with a high incidence of urinary tract infection. They also suggest that it was necessary for trained laboratory personnel to perform the test for useful accuracy. They do point out that there was some resistence to performing the test on the part of their clinic staff.

A number of features of the chemical tests for bacteriuria have been combined with culture media on a single dipslide (Microstix, Ames Laboratories, Elkhart, Indiana). The plastic strip has a modified nitrite test reaction area (bacteria convert nitrate to nitrite which reacts with p-arsonilic acid to form a diazonium compound which couples with N-1(1-naphthyl) ethelenediamine which turns pink) which indicates the presence of organisms in 30 seconds. There is one culture area which supports the growth of both gram-positive and gram-negative organisms and a second area which selects for gram-negative organisms. The stick is dipped in urine (first morning specimen) for 5 seconds, the nitrite test read in 30 seconds and then incubated at 37°C for 12 hours and read between 12 to 18 or 24 hours. Laboratory confirmation of positive tests was 95.2%, negative cultures 100%, type of organism 100% and antimicrobial sensitivity 90% (103).

Kunin (104) demonstrated how the nitrite portion of the Microstix used alone could be applied to mass screening. The false positive rate was 0.3% but the false negatives were over 12%. One interesting consequence of the screening was that 23 of the 26 girls with documented infection had intravenous urograms performed (two had caliectasis) and 22 had cystograms (three had gross reflux). One girl subsequently had her ureters reimplanted because of gross reflux. Although the authors had no control over the decisions, five girls were subjected to urethral dilatation and five to urethrotomy.

A number of other commercial dipsticks use either the nitrite or glucose method of detecting urinary infection (105,106). They are convenient and have acceptable sensitivity and specificity for screening use.

Radiographic and Radionuclide Methods

Radiographic and radionuclide methods of indentification of urinary tract infections are expensive, interventive, time-consuming and not necessarily accurate. Nevertheless they are critical for detection of anatomic abnormalities, calculi and other lesions which will alter diagnosis, prognosis or therapeutic approach. Friedland (107) has reviewed pediatric urinary tract infection from the viewpoint of a radiologist. Brock et al. have reviewed some of the aspects of radionuclide renography (108) and other methods have already been mentioned in comparison with the fluorescent antibody-coated bacteria localization test *(vide supra)*.

DOCUMENTATION OF URINARY TRACT INFECTION

The ultimate diagnosis of urinary tract infection depends upon laboratory proof of viable colony-forming organisms in the urine. Several problems serve to confuse this issue: improper collection, prolonged time between collection and culture, improper storage of specimens, failure to follow-up with a confirmatory collection leading to both over- and under diagnosis, refusal to accept properly documented counts of less than 10^5 as evidence for infection, and lack of appropriate skills in the microbiology laboratory.

Collection methods will be discussed elsewhere, but the basic principles are crucial. The distal urethral orifice must be scrupulously cleansed to avoid contamination by preputial or perineal flora. This is relatively easy for most men but for women, a certain amount of gymnastic and acrobatic skill is useful. The labia must not be permitted to close once the introitus is cleansed. The disinfectant must be rinsed out thoroughly to avoid false negative cultures. Children, infants and invalids pose special problems for which there must be some practical compromise. However, when the patient is ill or diagnosis is difficult, suprapubic aspiration or careful, aseptic bladder catheterization may be used. Once collected, the specimen must either be cultured within one hour or immediately refrigerated for not longer than 48 hours. Positive cultures should be followed up with a second culture in asymptomatic patients or in symptomatic patients with equivocal culture results. The diagnostic criterion of 10^5 or more organisms per ml was intended to screen out probable contaminated specimens (most true infections have over 10^6 organisms per ml) and thus avoid over diagnosis and concomitant interventive procedures, including unwarranted treatment (109). However, when collection is made by suprapubic aspiration, very low or low counts (10^2 - 10^4) may be clinically significant (110).

The practice of culturing the tip of a Foley catheter upon removal from the bladder has been attacked by Gross et al. (111, 112) and by Uehling and Hasham (113) who were unable to find a good correlation between the catheter tip organism and subsequent infecting organism. These data have been challenged by Burleson et al. who claim good correlation in their select population of transplant patients (114). The correlation appears to be, in large part, a function of the interest of staff in collecting and culturing the tips. Institutions probably need to define whether correlation is good in their own laboratories if they wish to use this technique.

SUMMARY

Urinary tract infection (UTI) is one of the most common problems of both adult and pediatric practice. Early identification and response is essential to detect correctable abnormalities of the urinary tract. Untreated urinary tract infections have morbid consequences for the pregnant woman and her fetus, neonates and children. Screening is cost-effective only when target populations are carefully defined and when the screeners are prepared to follow up infected patients. Dysuria is a poor indicator of UTI. Only 50% of women with dysuria actually have UTI. Documentation of UTI is therefore crucial to avoid mistreatment. Conversely, many UTI's are totally asymptomatic and a high index of suspicion is required.

Urine sediment may give useful clues but is not diagnostic. Of the many chemical tests available, the nitrite (Griess') appears to be the best. "Microstix" combine a semiquantitative culture method with a nitrite test and can be valuable for office practice.

Many tests have been devised to locate the site of UTI. The Fairley bladder washout test has become the research standard and may actually cure cystitis, but is not a routine office practice tool. Examination of the urine sediment for fluorescent antibody-coated bacteria correlates reasonably well with the Fairley test, but is not useful as an office procedure.

The ultimate documentation of UTI remains the demonstration of significant numbers of bacteria in a carefully collected, fresh urine specimen.

REFERENCES

1. Bergstrom, T., Larson, H., Lincoln, K. et al.: Studies of urinary tract infections in infancy and childhood. XII. Eighty consecutive cases with neonatal infection. J. Pediat. 80: 858, 1972.

2. Kunin, C.M.: Detection, Prevention and Management of Urinary Tract Infections, 2nd ed. Philadelphia: Lea and Febiger, 1974.

3. Stamey, T.A.: Urinary Infections. Baltimore: Williams and Wilkins, 1972.

4. Boineau, F.G. and Levy, J.E.: Urinary tract infection in children - an overview. Pediat. Ann. 4: 515, 1975.

5. Kass, E.H.: Bacteriuria and pyelonephritis of pregnancy. Arch. Int. Med. 105: 194, 1960.

6. Marshall, V.F.: Management of the child with urinary infection. New York J. Med. 64: 733, 1964.

7. Spence, H.M., Murphy, J.J., McGovern, J.H. et al.: Urinary tract infections in infants and children. J. Urol. 91: 623, 1964.

8. Harrow, B.R., Sloane, J.A. and Witus, W.S.: A critical examination of bladder neck obstruction in children. J. Urol. 98: 613, 1967.

9. Shopfner, C.E.: Roentgenological evaluation of bladder neck obstruction. Amer. J. Roentgenol. 100: 162, 1967.

10. Hodson, J., Maling, T.M.J., McManamon, P.J. and Lewis, M.G.: Reflux nephropathy. Kidney Int. 8: S-50, 1975.

11. Rolleston, G.L., Shannon, F.T. and Utley, W.L.F.: Follow-up of vesicoureteric reflux in the newborn. Kidney Int. 8: S-59, 1975.

12. Smellie, J., Edwards, D., Hunter, N. et al.: Vesico-ureteric reflux and renal scarring. Kidney Int. 8: S-65, 1975.

13. Scott, J.E.S.: The role of surgery in the management of vesicoureteric reflux. Kidney Int. 8: S-73, 1975.

14. Hallett, R.J., Pead, L. and Maskell, R.: Urinary infection in boys: a three-year prospective study. Lancet 2: 1107, 1976.

15. Kunin, C.M.: Epidemiology and natural history of urinary tract infection in school age children. Pediatr. Clin. N. Am. 18: 509, 1971.

16. Savage, D.C.L.: Natural history of covert bacteriuria in schoolgirls. Kidney Int. 8: S-90, 1975.

17. Freedman, L.R.: Natural history of urinary infection in adults. Kidney Int. 8: S-96, 1975.

18. Shapiro, A.P., Sapira, J.D. and Scheib, E.: Development of bacteriuria in a hypersensitive population: A seven year follow-up study. Abs. Am. Soc. Nephrol. 4: 71, 1970.

19. Kincaid-Smith, P., Fairley, K.F. and Heale, W.F.: Pyelonephritis as a cause of hypertension in man. In Onesti, G., Kim, K. and Moyer, J. (eds.): Hypertension: Mechanisms and Management. New York: Grune and Stratton, 1973, pp. 697-705.

20. Freeman, R.B., Smith, W. Mc., Richardson, J.A. et al.: Long-term therapy for chronic bacteriuria in man. Ann. Int. Med. 83: 133, 1975.

21. Alwall, N.: On controversial and open questions about the course and complications of non-obstructive urinary tract infection in adult women. Acta. Med. Scand. 203: 369, 1978.

22. Brumfitt, W.: The effects of bacteriuria in pregnancy on maternal and fetal health. Kidney Int. 8: S-113, 1975.

23. Kunin, C.M.: Urinary tract infections in children. Hospital Practice 11: 91, 1976.

24. Kunin, C.M.: Urinary tract infections in children (Editorial). Hospital Practice 12: 11, 1977.

25. McCormick, M.C.: The recognition of urinary tract infections in office-based pediatric practice: need for a systematic approach to the use of urine cultures in ambulatory care. Clin. Pediatr. 17: 713, 1978.

26. Rapkin, R.H.: Urinary tract infection in childhood. Pediatr. 60: 508, 1977.

27. Arbus, G.S.: Urinary screening program to detect renal disease in preschool and kindergarden children. CMA Journal 116: 1141, 1977.

28. Rees, D.L.P. and Farhoumand, N.: Psychiatric aspects of recurrent cystitis in women. Br. J. Urol. 49: 651, 1977.

29. Hendry, W.F., Stanton, S.L. and Williams, D.I.: Recurrent urinary infections in girls: Effects of urethral dilatation. Br. J. Urol. 45: 72, 1973.

30. Splatt, A.J. and Weedon, D.: The urethral syndrome: Experience with the Richardson urethroplasty. Br. J. Urol. 49: 173, 1977.

31. Farrar, D.J., Green, N.A. and Ashken, M.H.: An evaluation of Otis urethrotomy in female patients with recurrent urinary tract infections. Br. J. Urol. 45: 610, 1973.

32. Hinman, Jr., F.: Mechanisms for the entry of bacteria and the establishment of urinary tract infection in female children. J. Urol. 96: 546, 1966.

33. Halverstadt, D.B. and Leadbetter, G.W.: Internal urethrotomy and recurrent urinary tract infection in female children: I. Results in the management of infection. J. Urol. 100: 297, 1968.

34. Immergut, M., Culp, D. and Flocks, R.N.: The urethral caliber in normal female children. J. Urol. 97: 693, 1967.

35. Immergut, M.A. and Wahman, G.E.: The urethral caliber of female children with recurrent urinary tract infections. J. Urol. 99: 189, 1968.

36. Graham, J.B., King, L.R., Kropp, K.A. and Uehling, D.T.: The significance of distal urethral narrowing in young girls. J. Urol. 97: 1045, 1967.

37. Tanagho, E.A., Miller, E.R., Lyon, R.P. and Fisher, R.: Spastic striated external sphincter and urinary tract infection in girls. Br. J. Urol. 43: 69, 1971.

38. Rees, D.L.P., Whitfield, H.N., Islam, A.K.M.S. et al.: Urodynamic findings in adult females with frequency and dysuria. Br. J. Urol. 47: 853, 1976.

39. Kaplan, G.W., Sammons, T.A. and King, L.R.: A blind comparison of dilatation, urethrotomy and medication alone in the treatment of urinary tract infection in girls. J. Urol. 109: 917, 1973.

40. Meadow, R.: Munchausen syndrome by proxy: The hinterland of child abuse. Lancet 2: 343, 1977.

41. Du, J.N.H.: Colic as the sole symptom of urinary tract infection in infants. CMA Journal 115: 334, 1976.

42. Margileth, A.M., Pedreira, F.A., Hirschman, G.H. and Coleman, T.H.: Urinary tract bacterial infections: Office diagnosis and management. Peditr. Clin. N. Am. 23: 721, 1976.

43. Redman, J.F.: Keys to the diagnosis of occult urologic disease in children. J. Family Prac. 5: 337, 1977.

44. Horesh, A.J.: Allergy and recurrent urinary tract infections in childhood. II. Ann. Allergy 36: 174, 1976.

45. Unger, D.L.: Letter to the Editor. Ann. Allergy 36: 439, 1976.

46. Meadow, R.: Disorders of micturition, abnormalities of urine, and urinary tract infection. Br. Med. J. 1: 1200, 1976.

47. Fairley, K.F., Becker, G.J., Butler, H.M. et al.: Diagnosis in the difficult case. Kidney Int. 8: S-12, 1975.

48. Todd, J.K.: Urinary tract infections in children and adolescents. Postgrad. Med. 60: 225, 1976.

49. Burger, L.M. and Wolcott, B.W.: A clinical algorithm for urinary tract symptoms. Military Med. 143: 476, 1978.

50. Komaroff, A.L., Pass, T.M., McCue, J.D. et al.: Management strategies for urinary and vaginal infections. Arch. Int. Med. 138: 1069, 1978.

51. Rees, D.L.P.: Urinary tract infection. Clinics in Obst. Gyn. 5: 169, 1978.

52. Sickles, E.G., Greene, W.H. and Wiernik, P.H.: Clinical presentation of infection in granulocytopenic patients. Arch. Int. Med. 135: 715, 1975.

53. Musher, D.M., Thorsteinsson, S.B. and Airola II, V.M.: Quantitative urinalysis: diagnosing urinary tract infection in men. J. Am. Med. Assoc. 236: 2069, 1976.

54. Kass, E.H.: Asymptomatic infection of the urinary tract. Trans. Assoc. Am. Phys. 69: 56, 1956.

55. Lewis, J.F. and Alexander, J.: Microscopy of stained urine smears to determine the need for quantitative culture. J. Clin. Microbiol. 4: 372, 1976.

56. Fang, L.S.T., Tolkoff-Rubin, N.E. and Rubin, R.H.: Localization and management of urinary tract infection. Ann. Rev. Med. 225, 1979.

57. Whitworth, J.A. and Fairley, K.F.: Tests for localization of urinary infections. N. Engl. J. Med. 299: 312, 1978.

58. Stamey, T.A., Govan, D.E. and Palmer, J.M.: The localization and treatment of urinary tract infections: The role of bactericidal urine levels as opposed to serum levels. Med. 44: 1, 1965.

59. Neter, E.: Estimation of *Escherichia coli* antibodies in urinary tract infection: a review and perspective. Kid. Int. 8: S-23, 1975.

60. Darwish, M.E., Staubitz, W.J., Scheuller, E.F. et al.: Antibody response of dogs to experimental infection of bladder pouch. Invest. Urol. 6: 66, 1968.

61. Turck, M., Ronald, A.R. and Petersdorf, R.G.: Relapse and reinfection in chronic bacteriuria: II. The correlation between site of infection and problem of recurrence in chronic bacteriuria. N. Engl. J. Med. 278: 422, 1968.

62. Ronald, A.R., Cutler, R.E. and Turck, M.: Effect of bacteriuria on renal concentrating mechanisms. Ann. Int. Med. 70: 723, 1969.

63. Fairley, K.F., Bond, A.G., Brown, R.B. and Habersberger, P.: Simple test to determine the site of urinary-tract infection. Lancet 2: 427, 1967.

64. Fairley, K.F., Carson, N.E., Gutch, R.C. et al.: Site of infection in acute urinary-tract infection in general practice. Lancet 2: 615, 1971.

65. Thomas, V., Shelokov, A. and Forland, M.: Antibody-coated bacteria in the urine and the site of urinary-tract infection. N. Engl. J. Med. 290: 588, 1974.

66. Thomas, V.L., Forland, M. and Shelokov, A.: Antibody-coated bacteria in urinary tract infection. Kid. Int. 8: S-20, 1975.

67. Jones, S.R.: Prostatitis as a cause of antibody-coated bacteria in the urine. N. Engl. J. Med. 291: 365, 1974.

68. Jones, S.R., Smith, J.W. and Sanford, J.P.: Localization of urinary tract infections by detection of antibody-coated bacteria in urine sediment. N. Engl. J. Med. 290: 591, 1974.

69. Jones, S.R.: Antibody-coated bacteria in urine. N. Engl. J. Med. 295: 1380, 1976.

70. Janson, K.L. and Roberts, J.A.: Non-invasive localization of urinary tract infection. J. Urol. 117: 624, 1977.

71. Pujol, A., Linares, F., Muñoz, J. et al.: A new method for detection and localization of urinary infection: the fluorescence antibody test. Urol. Int. 31: 501, 1976.

72. Pujol, A., Linares, F., Muñoz, J. et al.: A new method for detection and localization of urinary infection: the fluorescence antibody test. Eur. Urol. 2: 145, 1976.

73. Schaberg, D.R., Haley, R.W., Terry, P.M. and McGowan, Jr., J.E.: Reproducibility of interpretation of the test for antibody-coated bacteria in urinary sediment. J. Clin. Microbiol. 6: 359, 1977.

74. Jones, S.R. and Johnson, J.: Further evaluation of the test for detection of antibody-coated bacteria in the urine sediment. J. Clin. Microbiol. 5: 510, 1977.

75. Harding, G.K.M., Marrie, T.J., Ronald, A.R. et al.: Urinary tract infection localization in women. J. Am. Med. Assoc. 240: 1147, 1978.

76. Rumans, L.W. and Vosti, K.L.: The relationship of antibody-coated bacteria to clinical syndromes: as found in unselected populations with bacteriuria. Arch. Int. Med. 138: 1077, 1978.

77. Rumans, L.W. and Vosti, K.L.: Antibody-coated bacteria. J. Am. Med. Assoc. 237: 531, 1977.

78. Thorley, J.D., Barbin, G.K. and Reinarz, J.A.: The prevalence of antibody-coated bacteria in the urine. Am. J. Med. Sci. 275: 75, 1978.

79. Forland, M., Thomas, V. and Shelokov, A.: Urinary tract infections in patients with diabetes mellitus: Studies on antibody coating of bacteria. J. Am. Med. Assoc. 238: 1924, 1977.

80. Keren, D.F., Nightingale, S.D., Hamilton, C.L. et al.: Antibody-coating bacteria as an indicator of the site of urinary tract infection in renal transplant recipients receiving immunosuppressive agents. Am. J. Med. 63: 855, 1977.

81. Riedasch, G., Ritz, E., Dreikorn, K. and Andrassy, K.: Antibody coating of urinary bacteria in transplanted patients. Nephron 20: 267, 1978.

82. Casanova, A., Liñares, J., Edo, A. et al.: Antibody-coated bacteria and pregnancy. Eur. Urol. 4: 103, 1978.

83. Braude, R. and Block, C.: Proteinuria and antibody-coated bacteria in the urine. N. Engl. J. Med. 297: 617, 1977.

84. Forsum, U., Fritjofsson, A., Frodin, L. et al.: A clinical evaluation of a test for antibody-coated bacteria in the urine. Scand. J. Urol. Nephrol. 12: 45, 1978.

85. Hellerstein, S., Kennedy, E., Nussbaum, L. and Rice, K.: Localization of the site of urinary tract infections by means of antibody-coated bacteria in the urinary sediments. J. Pediatr. 92: 188, 1973.

86. Meares, E.M. and Stamey, T.A.: Bacteriologic localization patterns in bacterial prostatitis and urethritis. Invest. Urol. 5: 492, 1968.

87. Hurwitz, S.R., Kessler, W.O., Alazraki, N.P. and Ashburn, W.L.: Gallium-67 imaging to localize urinary-tract infections. Br. J. Radiol. 49: 156, 1976.

88. Gillenwater, J.Y.: Diagnosis of urinary tract infection: appraisal of diagnostic procedures. Kid. Int. 8: S-3, 1975.

89. Bank, N. and Bailine, S.H.: Urinary beta-glucuronidase activity in patients with urinary tract infection. N. Engl. J. Med. 272: 70, 1965.

90. Harris, R.E., Thomas, V.L., Underwood, J.M. and Gandot, F.: A comparison of two indirect methods for localizing the site of urinary tract infection: beta glucuronidase levels and the presence of antibody-coated bacteria. Am. J. Obstet. Gyn. 131: 647, 1978.

91. Skelton, I.J., Hogan, M.M., Stokes, B. and Hurst, J.A.: Urinary tract infections in childhood: the place of the nitrite test. Med. J. Aust. 1: 882, 1977.

92. Schersten, B. and Fritz, H.: Subnormal levels of glucose in urine. J. Am. Med. Assoc. 201: 949, 1967.

93. Schersten, B., Dahlqvist, A., Fritz, H. et al.: Screening for bacteriuria with a test paoer for glucose. J. Am. Med. Assoc. 204: 205, 1968.

94. Simmons, W.A. and Williams, J.D.: A simple test for bacteriuria. Lancet 1: 1377, 1962.

95. Giler, S., Henig, E.F., Urca, I. et al.: Urine xanthine oxidase activity in urinary tract infection. J. Clin. Path. 31: 444, 1978.

96. Lamb, V.A., Dalton, H.P. and Wilkins, J.R.: Electrochemical method for the early detection of urinary tract infections. Am. J. Clin. Path. 66: 91, 1976.

97. Hayward, N.J. and Jeavons, T.H.: Assessment of technique for rapid detection of *Escherichia coli* and *Proteus* species in urine by head-space gas-liquid chromatography. J. Clin. Microbiol. 6: 202, 1977.

98. Adelman, R.D.: The dipslide in diagnosis of urinary tract infections. J. Family Prac. 3: 647, 1976.

99. Asscher, A.W., Davis, R.H. and Mackenzie, R.: Dipslide diagnosis of urinary-tract infection. Lancet 2: 202, 1977.

100. Duerden, B.I. and Moyes, A.: Comparison of laboratory methods in the diagnosis of urinary tract infection. J. Clin. Path. 29: 286, 1976.

101. McAllister, T.A.: The day of the dipslide. Nephron 11: 123, 1973.

102. Martin, M.J. and McGuckin, M.B.: Evaluation of a dipslide in a university outpatient service. J. Urol. 120: 193, 1978.

103. Litvak, A.S., Eadie, E.B. and McRoberts, J.W.: A clinical evaluation of a screening device (Microstix) for urinary tract infections. So. Med. J. 69: 1418, 1976.

104. Kunin, C.M., DeGroot, J.E., Uehling, D. and Ramgopal, V.: Detection of urinary tract infections in 3 to 5 year old girls by mothers using a nitrite indicator strip. Pediatr. 57: 829, 1976.

105. Todd, J.K.: Home follow-up of urinary tract infection: comparison of two non-culture techniques. Am. J. Dis. Child. 131: 860, 1977.

106. Collacott, R.A.: Urinary infection in a remote practice. Practitioner 218: 123, 1977.

107. Friedland, G.W.: Recurrent urinary tract infections in infants and children. Radiol. Clin. N. Am. 15: 19, 1977.

108. Brock, M., Feneley, R.C.L. and Davies, E.R.: Renography as a prognostic index of urinary tract problems in childhood. Br. J. Urol. 49: 261, 1977.

109. Kass, E.H.: Bacteriuria and diagnosis of infection of the urinary tract. Arch. Int. Med. 100: 709, 1957.

110. Slosky, D.A. and Todd, J.K.: Diagnosis of urinary tract infection: the interpretation of colony counts. Clin. Pediatr. 16: 698, 1977.

111. Gross, P.A., Harkavy, L.M., Borden, G.E. and Kerstein, M.: Positive Foley catheter tip cultures: fact or fancy? J. Am. Med. Assoc. 228: 72, 1974.

112. Gross, P.A., Harkavy, L.M., Borden, G.E. and Kerstein, M.: Foley tip cultures are of no value. Geriatrics 29: 111, 1974.

113. Uehling, D.T. and Hasham, A.I.: Significance of catheter tip cultures. Invest. Urol. 15: 57, 1977.

114. Burleson, R.L., Brennan, A.M. and Scruggs, B.G.: Foley catheter tip cultures: a valuable diagnostic aid in the immunosuppressed patient. Am. J. Surg. 133: 723, 1977.

BACTERIOLOGY OF URINARY TRACT INFECTION

Gaston Zilleruelo, M.D., Rafael Galindez, M.D., Helen M. Gorman, M.B.,B.Ch. and José Strauss, M.D.
Div. Pediatr. Nephrol., Dept. Pediatr., Univ. Miami Sch. Med., Miami, Fla. 33101, USA

The diagnosis of urinary tract infection (UTI) in children requires laboratory determination of the invasion and active multiplication of different organisms in the normally sterile urinary tract. Kass in 1956 introduced the concept of significant bacteriuria as a common denominator of all types of UTI (1). Since then, emphasis has been made on the need to use strict criteria for the interpretation of quantitative cultures in order to prevent overdiagnosing or underdiagnosing of UTI. Unnecessary expenses, medications, irradiation from extensive radiological workup, and even urologic surgery, are some of the consequences of overdiagnosing. Progressive renal damage could be the result of not detecting in time a congenital anomaly associated with UTI. This subject will be reviewed here in an attempt to give general guidelines on the role played by bacteriology in UTI.

DIAGNOSIS OF UTI

First of all, bacteriology is used to confirm or reject the clinical diagnosis of UTI. It has been demonstrated that many children with significant bacteriuria may remain asymptomatic (2), and that many children with classic UTI symptoms such as dysuria or frequency may have sterile urinary tracts (3).

Diagnosis of UTI should *always* be based on bacteriologic analysis of the urine, including the *identification* of the etiological agent and its *quantification*. However, urine culture and colony count will be useful only if three basic conditions are fulfilled: a) adequate collection, b) proper handling, and c) proper interpretation of results.

Collection of the urine specimen. There are many methods of urine collection; all of them have their indications and limitations (Table 1). In infants, double chambered urine collectors provide reliable results only when used by trained personnel and with careful observation of the time of micturiction (Zilleruelo et al., unpublished observations). In this age group, percutaneous suprapubic bladder aspiration has been shown to be a safe, easy and useful method of obtaining urine (4,5); this should be the method of choice.

In older children (and particularly in boys) mid-stream clean catch urine collection is quite reliable. Under special circumstances (ureterostomy, ileal conduit), specimens obtained by catheterization provide the necessary information (6). In addition, suprapubic tap or catheterization may be used even in this group to obtain bladder urine.

Handling of urine specimen. The need for proper handling of the urine specimen should be constantly emphasized. Urine is an excellent culture medium for the common pathogens of the urinary tract. If a urine sample containing only 10,000 orgranisms/ml is allowed to stay at room temperature, it will easily reach the significant level of 100,000 organisms/ml after 2 hours. This is due to the fact that reproduction and duplication time of certain bacteria (including E. Coli) is 20-30 minutes. Urine samples must be sent *immediately* to the laboratory. Alternatively, urine may be kept in a refrigerator (at 4°C) for 24-48 hours without any changes (7).

Interpretation of laboratory results. Careful interpretation of urine cultures is essential. In samples obtained by clean catch, $\geq$ 100,000 col/ml urine is a good approximation to diagnose UTI in symptomatic patients. Three consecutive urine cultures with over 100,000 col/ml of the same organism gives a 99% confidence when correlated with catheter specimens (8). Less than 10,000 col/ml usually means contamination from bacteria in the urethra. Intermediate counts of 10,000-100,000 col/ml are suspicious of UTI and culture should be repeated. If the urine specimen is obtained by

Table 1. Methods of Urine Collection

- Pediatric urine collector	Single Double chambered (U-bag)
- Mid-stream clean catch	
- Percutaneous suprapubic bladder aspiration	
- Catheterization	

suprapubic aspiration, growth of any number of bacteria in pure culture should be considered significant. However, it is important to remember that these figures are based on statistical analyses and that they may not be applicable to a particular child. Several reports have called attention to the finding of low bacterial counts in some patients with confirmed UTI (9,10)(Table 2). Conversely, there are cases with false positive results (over 100,000 col/ml without UTI) due to inadequate urine collection or improper handling of the specimen.

The diurnal variation in bacterial counts has been studied by several investigators (Fig. 1)(9,10). The finding of changes in colony counts of patients with UTI at different times of the day suggests that there may be an optimum time of the day for the collection of urine samples for culture. Additional factors to take into consideration may be the amount of water ingested and the use of bacteriostatic solutions such as zephyrol, iodines, etc. for cleansing of the genitalia.

Identification of the etiological agent is as important as its quantification for the diagnosis of UTI. It may modify the initial workup and also will serve as a guide in selecting the antimicrobial agent. It has been established that infection of the urinary tract is most commonly due to bacteria and only rarely caused by other microorganisms such as protozoa, viruses, or fungi.

Table 2. Interpretation of Laboratory Results

If clean catch:
< 10,000 col/ml → contamination
10,000-100,000 col/ml → suspect infection → repeat
3 consecutive urine cultures with same organism > 100,000 col/ml → 99% confidence
If suprapubic bladder aspiration:
Growth of ANY NUMBER of gram negative organisms is significant

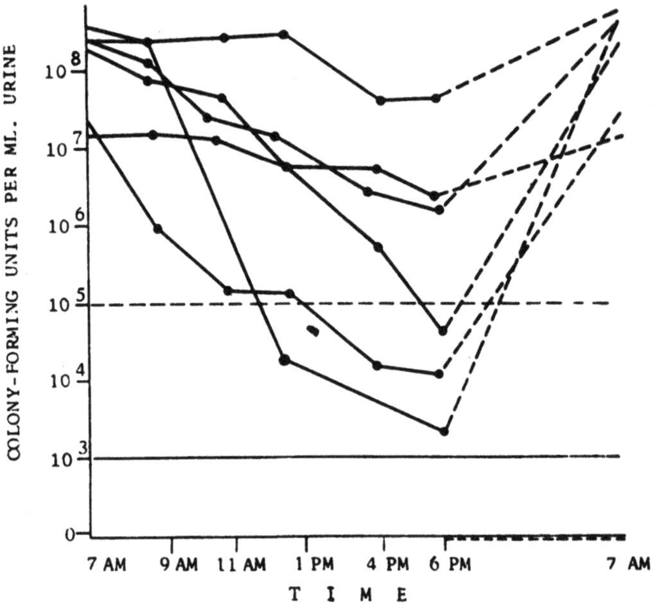

FIG. 1. Influence of the time of urine collection in the colony counts of six patients with documented UTI (note that half of them had low colony counts in the afternoon). Reproduced from Pryles, C. and Lustik, B.: Ped. Clin. of N.A. 18:233, 1971, with permission.

Most UTIs are due to gram negative bacilli found in the gut (Table 3)(11). The most frequent urinary pathogens include E. Coli, Klebsiella, Enterobacter, Proteus sp., Pseudomonas, Enterococcus, and Staphylococcus. Many studies on the prevalence of those agents have demonstrated that E. Coli represents more than 75% of all isolates in children with UTI. However, the relative prevalence of the various species depends on many variables including age and sex of the patients, initial vs recurrent infection, symptomatic vs asymptomatic bacteriuria, UTI uncomplication vs. complication by urological malformations, geographic areas, etc. Therefore, it is not surprising that the prevalence rates are not uniform from one series to another. As an example, in a study of bacteria isolated during the "first" episode of UTI in children of different ages and sexes, there was a high incidence of Klebsiella in neonates (probably explained by blood borne infection) (12). The high frequency of E. Coli infections in girls from one month to 10 years was not different from that in boys of less than 1 year of age. In adolescent girls, however, the incidence of E. Coli dropped to 60% with an increase in staphylococcal infections. In boys from 1 to 16 years the decrease in E. Coli was more significant with an increase in proteus infections and staphylococcus.

Figure 2 shows data obtained from Kunin in his classic studies

Table 3. Etiological Agents

Bacteria		
- Common urinary pathogens	Escherichia Coli Klebsiella Enterobacter Proteus Sp. Salmonella	Gram (-)
	Pseudomonas Enterococci Staphylococcus Aureus	Gram (+)
- Rare urinary pathogens	Serratia marcescens Hemophylus influenza Streptococcus Group B Mycobacterium tuberculosis Anaerobes (bacteroides)	
- L-forms and mycoplasmas		

of schoolgirls with recurrent UTI (13). There was a progressive decline in the number of episodes due to E. Coli with a corresponding increase in those due to other species. In patients with UTI associated with congenital anomalies and treated with multiple courses of antibiotics, E. Coli is rarely found; instead, pseudomonas, indole-positive proteus and enterobacter are the main agents of infection. Other rare pathogens reported occasionally include serratia marcescens, hemophylus influenza, and streptococcus group B (Table 3)(14,15,16). Serratia marcescens, for a long time considered a nonpathogen, has been found to be responsible for outbreaks of nosocomial infections (18). It has been associated mainly with the use of indwelling urethralcatheters, antibiotic therapy and urologic surgery. Mycobacterium tuberculosis may be responsible for infection of the kidney but this diagnosis requires special procedures.

Anaerobic bacteria play a minor role in UTI. In one study, 1.3% of patients with significant bacteriuria had anaerobic bacteria (mainly Bacteroides) confirmed by suprapubic bladder aspiration (17). Most of these patients had significant urologic disease. In routine studies, culture for anaerobes are not indicated. Such studies, however, should be done whenever clinical evidence of infection exists and conventional cultures yield negative results.

The role of L-forms or protoplasts in UTI has not been definitely established. These organisms represent bacteria without a cell wall, thus requiring special culture conditions. Although it does not seem that L-forms account for a significant number of UTI's, they may be present in patients with relapsing infections (19).

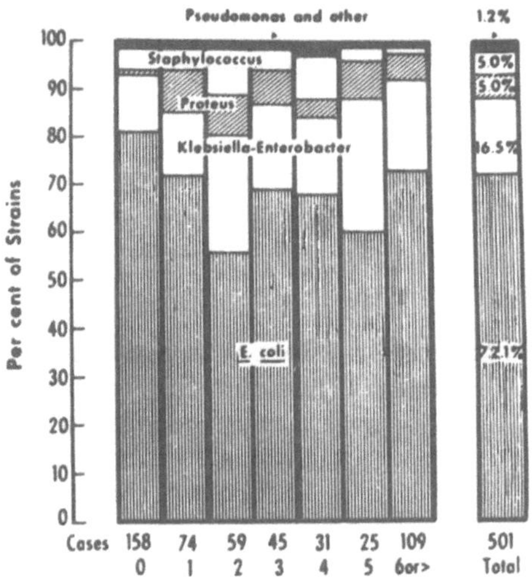

FIG. 2. Distribution of bacteria in each consecutive episode of recurrent UTI in schoolgirls. Reproduced from Kunin, C.M.: J. Inf. Dis. 122: 382, 1970, with permission.

Other nonbacterial etiological agents include (Table 4):

<u>Viruses</u>. They play only a minor role as a cause of UTI although viral urinary excretion by children infected with CMV and rubella is a serious public health problem (20). Viruria is also observed in other entities; adenovirus has been consistently reported as a cause of acute hemorrhagic cystitis (21).

<u>Chlamydia</u>. A unique class of microorganisms characterized as large viruses or small bacteria. They are inhibited by antibiotics, but they are also obligate intracellular parasites. Chlamydia have been found to be responsible for a large spectrum of infectious diseases in man and other animals (22). They have been described as causes of nonspecific infections of the urinary tract (urethritis) in post-puberal patients (23). However, the role of chlamydia in pediatric genito-urinary disease has not been well documented (24).

Table 4. Etiological Agents

Non-bacterial
- Virus (Adenovirus, CMV, Rubella...)
- Chlamydia
- Fungi (Candida Albicans)
- Protozoa

Fungi. They occasionally cause UTI, but are frequently present as contaminants. It has been shown that prolonged hospital stay, antibiotic therapy, and complicated urological diseases with indwelling catheters enhance the patient's susceptibility to candida infections. The incidence of candiduria has increased markedly in hospital practice during the last 10 years. In one study, this increase was from 1.3% to 7-8% of all cultures (25). Not all patients with positive cultures represent a serious problem, and possibly 1/3 improve without specific treatment. The criterium of colony counting is not valid when dealing with a patient with indwelling catheters and candiduria; therefore, other methods for diagnosing UTI have been devised. Under these conditions, renal involvement may be estimated by the presence of elevated serum precipitation antibodies (26).

SENSITIVITY TESTS

Antimicrobial susceptibility tests can be used as guides for therapy in a particular patient or as epidemiological information. Three basic types of in vitro sensitivity tests are available: broth dilution, plate dilution, and disc diffusion (Fig. 3). They are semiquantitative tests and reliability of results depends on their *standardization* and interpretation. Sensitivity test results are usually expressed either as minimal inhibitory concentration (MIC) or minimal bactericidal concentration (MBS) in μg/ml.

The *broth dilution* method is done using 2-fold dilution of a known concentration of an antimicrobial agent. The last tube in the series with no growth is usually the MIC for the organism. This is a reliable test, but too time consuming for routine use. It is reserved for testing of new drugs, standardization of other tests or for unusual organisms.

In the *plate dilution method*, the antibiotic solution is diluted in 2-fold increments and placed in a Petri plate. The bac-

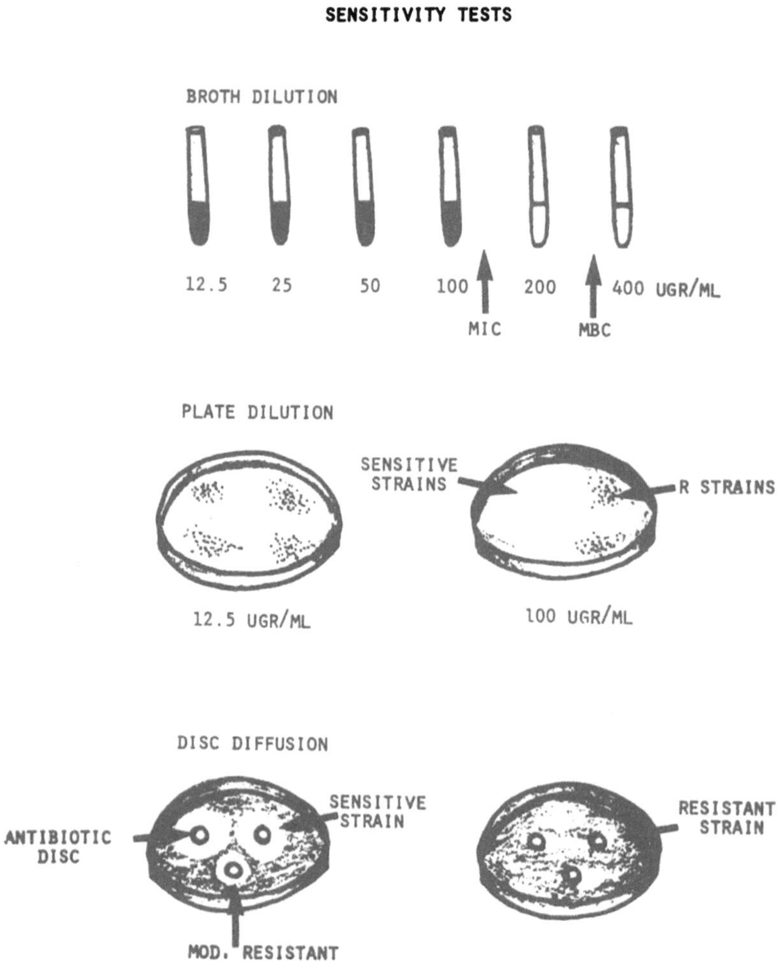

FIG. 3. Schematic representation of antimicrobial susceptibility tests: broth dilution, plate dilution, and disc diffusion.

terium under study is streaked on marked sections of each plate. In this manner, up to 16 organisms may be studied simultaneously. The absence of growth on a given plate represents the MIC for the bacterium.

In the *disc diffusion method*, a paper disc is impregnated with a standard amount of an antimicrobial agent and applied to agar seeded with the bacterium to be tested. Several discs with different antimicrobials may be used. Sensitivity is judged by the size of the clear zone without bacterium growing around the disc, quantified in mm. This is the simplest and most accurate routine method for antibiotic sensitivity available at the present time; it is especially suited for urine cultures. When the disc diffusion method is used, the results are expressed as resistant, intermediate, or susceptible strains according to the antibiotic concentration in blood and urine needed to inhibit a given bacterium. In ordinary therapeutic doses, an antibiotic can be considered effective if the reading corresponds to the intermediate or susceptible zone (11).

Table 5 compares the usual MIC of the most frequent bacteria isolated in UTI with the concentration of antibiotics obtained in urine when they are used in therapeutic doses. With these values, predictable ranges of effectiveness of the drug may be attained. However, it must be remembered that there may be differences between their in vivo and in vitro sensitivities. Many variables may be involved; the most likely ones are: concentration of the antibiotic in different body fluids (urine, blood, tissue), action at different urine pHs, and host defense factors.

Regardless of the method used, the sensitivity tests are important guides for the use of specific drugs in the treatment of UTI. This is especially important in recurrent UTI with unusual organisms, or in the interpretation of repeatedly positive urine cultures that are thought to be due to contamination.

In addition to their use as a guide for treatment of a particular patient, sensitivity tests are also valuable in epidemiological surveys. They allow the development of charts with recommendations of first and second choices of antibiotics for each bacterium isolated in certain geographical areas. Based on this experience it is possible to treat a first episode of an uncomplicated UTI without prior sensitivity testing.

VIRULENCE FACTORS

Host-parasite relationships are essential in the understanding of why UTI is so common and recurs so often. Two factors seem mainly involved: virulence of the infecting microorganism and defense mechanisms of the host. E. Coli is the most commonly found organism; it can be serologically typed into over 150 different 0 or cell wall antigens, and into about 50 capsular (K) and flagellar (H) antigens. It has been found that more than half the E. Coli isolated in either initial or recurrent UTI correspond to a few 0 serotypes such as 0_1, 0_2, 0_{4}-$_{6}$-$_{7}$-$_{18}$-$_{75}$ (20).

In general, it seems that the same serotypes of E. Coli appear in urine as in stool (27). Some surveys, however, have shown different infecting strains in patients with symptomatic "upper" UTI when compared to those patients with lower UTI and asymptomatic

Table 5. Sensitivity to drugs of bacteria causing urinary infections. Res. = resistant to concentrations attainable in urine.

Drug	Concentration attained in urine (μg/ml)	Minimum Inhibitory Concentration (μg/ml)					
		Escherichia coli	Proteus mirabilis	Klebsiella aerogenes	Pseudomonas aeruginosa	Staphylococcus aureus	Streptococcus faecalis
Sulphonamides	1000	1	8	Res.	50	4-16	Res.
Nitrofurantoin	125	16	200	100	Res.	4	25
Ampicillin	250+	8	4	Res.	Res.	0.04	2
Carbenicillin	2000	5	2.5	250	50	0.5-50	25
Cephaloridine	300	4	4	4 to Res.	Res.	0.1-5	16
Kanamycin	300	2	4	2	64	0.5	64
Gentamycin	50	1-4	2-8	1-2	1-8	0.1-1	8-16
Trimethoprim	50	0.4 to Res.	7.5 to Res.	25 to Res.	Res.	4-30	4-125
Nalidixic Acid	200	3.0-7.5	2.5-20	1.6-50	4.0-500	50	500

Reproduced from Barrat, T.M.: Urinary Tract Infection. In Williams, D.I., Barrett, T.M., Eckstein, H.B. et al. (eds.): Urology in Childhood. New York: Springer-Verlag Publishers, 1974, p. 91, with permission.

bacteriuria (ABU) (Table 6)(28). Patients with pyelonephritis had 79.8 % common "O" groups and patients with ABU had a marked increase of rough strains with spontaneous agglutination. The finding of a rough strain usually sensitive to serum bactericidal activity in patients with ABU may suggest a harmless condition in which host and bacteria have adjusted to each other (27).

Other study findings have suggested that the presence of capsular polysacharide K antigen may be of special significance to allow bacterium to invade the kidney. At least 70% of the strains from patients with acute pyelonephritis have some K typable E. Coli (Table 7)(29). In fact, all K typable E. Coli strains should be considered potentially invasive, especially those containing Kl and K12 (30). Earlier studies have shown that K and 0 circulating antibodies are protective against experimental pyelonephritis (31), with K antibodies more efficient than 0 antibodies. Since only 5 E. Coli K antigens account for about 70% of all acute pyelonephritis in children, vaccines containing those antigens have been proposed to be administered to high risk populations (29).

Another interesting finding is the ability of E. Coli to become attached to normal epithelial cells from the urinary tract (31). This adherence to uroepithelial cells is much greater with E. Coli isolated from patients with acute symptomatic UTI than in those isolated from patients with ABU (31). The production of hemolysis and the fermentation of dulcitol are other in vitro studies that seem to correlate well with the ability of E. Coli to produce symptomatic upper UTI (32).

RECURRENT UTI - RELAPSE VS REINFECTION

According to Kunin, following successful treatment, 80% of recurrences of UTI are due to reinfection with a new serologic type

Table 6. Serogroups of E. Coli Isolated in Children with UTI*

	Pyelonephritis (%)	Cystitis (%)	ABU (%)
E. Coli 0-Groups 1,2,4,6,7,16,18,75	79.8	58.7	31.3
Other 0-Groups	18.5	34.8	23.5
Spontaneously Agglutinating	1.7	6.5	45.2

*Data from U. Lindberg et al.: Acta Paediatr. Scand. 64: 432, 1975.

Table 7. Frequency of E. Coli K Antigen*

Source of Isolates	No. of Isolates	K-Antigen (%) K-1	K-12	K-Typable (Total)
Pyelonephritis	118	39	11	70
Cystitis	108	16	3	53
ABU	120	29	0	42
Stools (Controls)	100	26	0	55

*Data from Kaijser, B. et al.: Lancet, 1:663, 1977.

of E. Coli or with new bacteria (11). The major interest in E. Coli serotyping rests on the need to differentiate, following a period of antibacterial treatment, relapses due to inadequate suppression of an organism from reinfection due to a new strain (Fig. 4). Unfortunately, the serotyping of E. Coli is time consuming, involves many steps, and is not used in routine clinical laboratories. Another practical though unreliable approach to differentiate relapse from reinfection may be the bacterial sensitivity to various antimicrobials. An unchanged sensitivity may be due to an unchanged bacterial serotype.

LOCALIZATION OF INFECTION

The pendulum has been moving from the concept that *all UTI* implies renal involvement, to the concept that there may be localized processes which involve either the lower or the upper urinary tract. Identification of the area involved may only be of academic interest; however, the evaluation and therapeutic approaches could be different (33,34).

Several methods have been proposed to establish the area of UTI involvement (Table 8). Some are direct, others are indirect (noninvasive) methods. The result of the so-called direct method of localization must be interpreted with caution. The washout technique either with ureteral (35) or bladder catheterization (36) may give misleading results due to intermittent discharge of bacteria from the kidney or because some bacteria may be carried up from the bladder, either by the catheter or by reflux. Some studies have shown that patients with the clinical diagnosis of pyelonephritis have elevated CRP and serum antibody levels (38). Our own ex-

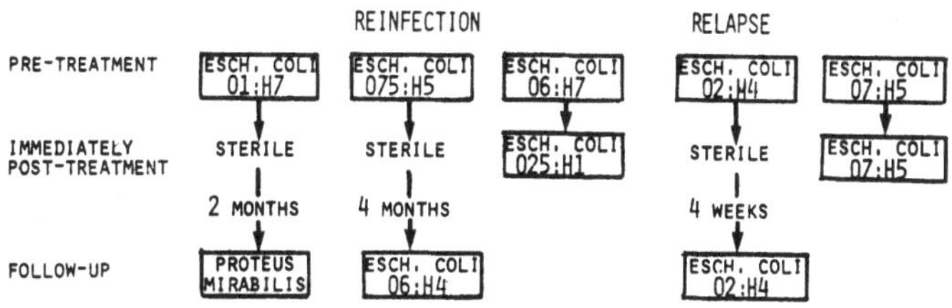

FIG. 4. Differences observed in bacterial cultures after treatment: reinfection (left side of figure) vs relapse (right side of figure). (From Zilleruelo, G. et al., unpublished observations).

perience and that of others suggest a good correlation between an elevated quantitated CRP and a clinically diagnosed upper UTI.

The presence of antibody coated bacteria in urinary sediment has been proposed as a method to diagnose upper UTI (39) (Fig. 5).

Table 8. Localization of Infection

Direct		Indirect
Renal biopsy	Culture Histology Immunofluorescence	Urine antibody coated bacteria Serum antibodies (O antigen)
Ureteric catheterization		Urine concentration ability Urinary enzyme excretion
Bladder wash-out		CRP
		Erythrosedimentation rate
		Prednisolone stimulation test
		Serum autoantibodies to Tamm-Horsfall protein

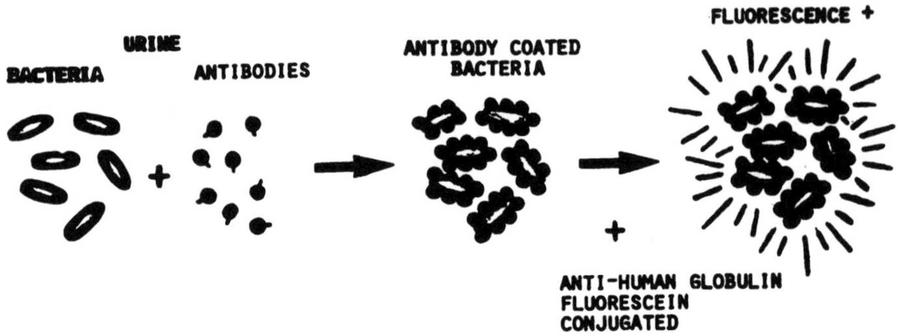

FIG. 5. Schematic representation of an indirect immunofluorescent method for detection of antibody coated bacteria in urinary sediments.

Results are contradictory and possibly depend on the criteria used to make the clinical diagnosis. Some results correlate poorly with bladder washout but correlate well with symptomatic UTI (40,41). Since it is an indirect qualitative measurement of the host antibody response, it probably depends on age, moment of the collection, immunoglobulin response, etc. The measurement of lactic dehydrogenase isoenzymes has been shown to be a reliable method of differentiating upper from lower infection, although there is an important zone of overlapping results (42).

We could say that probably none of these tests alone can provide sufficient information to make a firm diagnosis of localization. A combination of tests and thorough clinical evaluations should always be followed in order to attain reliable information.

In summary, we have discussed several ways through which bacteriology can help in the diagnosis and management of UTI. However, the most important is still the simplest one: the identification and quantification of the etiologic agent through urine culture and colony counting.

REFERENCES

1. Kass, E.H.: Bacteriuria and the diagnosis of infections of the urinary tract. Arch. Intern. Med. 100: 709, 1957.

2. Kunin, C.M., Southall, I. and Paquin, A.J.: Epidemiology of urinary tract infections. N. Engl. J. Med. 263: 817, 1960.

3. Köhler, L., Fritz, H. and Schersten, B.: Health control of the four-year-old child: A study of bacteriuria. Acta. Paediatr. Scand. 61: 289, 1972.

4. Sacharow, L. and Pryles, C.V.: Further experience with the use of percutaneous suprapubic aspiration of the urinary bladder: Bacteriologic studies in 654 infants and children. Pediatrics 43: 1018, 1969.

5. Aronson, A.S., Gustafson, B. and Svenningsen, N.W.: Combined suprapubic aspiration and clean voided urine examination in infants and children. Acta Pediatr. Scand. 62: 396, 1973.

6. Spence, B., Ireland, G.W. and Cass, A.S.: Bacteriuria in intestinal loop urinary diversion in children. J. Urol. 106: 780, 1971.

7. Mon, T.W. and Feldman, H.A.: The enumeration and preservation of bacteria in urine. Am. J. Clin. Pathol. 35: 572, 1961.

8. Kass, E.H.: How and why to treat urinary infections. Hosp. Med. 4:73, 1968.

9. Pryles, C.V. and Lustik, B.: Laboratory diagnosis not urinary tract infection. Pediatr. Clin. N. Am. 18: 233, 1971.

10. Slosky, D.A. and Todd, J.K.: Diagnosis of urinary tract infection. The interpretation of colony counts. Clin. Pediatr. 16: 698, 1977.

11. Kunin, C.M.: Detection, Prevention and Management of Urinary Tract Infections. Philadelphia, Lea & Fabiger, 1979.

12. Winberg, J., Andersen, H.J., Bergström, T. et al.: Epidemiology of symptomatic urinary tract infection in childhood. Acta Paediatr. Scand., Suppl. 252, 9, 1974.

13. Kunin, C.M.: A ten-year study of bacteriuria in schoolgirls: final report of bacteriologic, urologic, and epidemiologic findings. J. Inf. Dis. 122: 382, 1970.

14. Granoff, D.M. and Roskes, S.: Urinary tract infection due to Hemophilus influenzae type B. J. Pediatr. 84: 414, 1974.

15. Madduri, S.D., Mauriello, D.A., Smith, L.G. and Seebode, J.J.: Serratia marcescens and the urologist. J. Urol. 116: 613, 1976.

16. St-Laurent-Gagnon, T. and Weber, M.: Urinary tract streptococcus group B infection in a 6-week-old infant. JAMA 240: 1269, 1978.

17. Segura, J.W., Kelalis, P.P., Martin, W.J. and Smith, L.H.: Anaerobic bacteria in the urinary tract. Mayo Clin. Proc. 47: 30, 1972.

18. Allen, S.D. and Conger, K.B.: Serratia marcescens infection of the urinary tract: a nosocomial infection. J. Urol. 101: 621, 1969.

19. Dominque, G.J. and Schlegel, J.U.: The possible role of microbial L-forms in pyelonephritis. J. Urol. 104: 790, 1970.

20. Neter, E.: The microbiologic aspects of urinary tract infection. In Rubin, M.I. and Barratt, T.M. (eds.): Pediatric Nephrology. Baltimore: Williams & Wilkins Company, 1975, p. 646.

21. Mufson, M.A., Zollar, L.M., Mankad, V.N. and Manalo, D.: Adenovirus infection in acute hemorrhagic cystitis. Am. J. Dis. Child. 121: 281, 1971.

22. Grayston, J. and Wang, S.: New knowledge of chlamydia and the diseases they cause. J. Inf. Dis. 132: 87, 1975.

23. Dunlop, E., Jackson, J., Doragar, S. and Jones, B.: Chlamydial infection in nonspecific urethritis. Br. J. Vener. Dis. 48: 425, 1972.

24. Hieber, J.P.: Infections due to chlamydia. J. Pediatr. 91: 864, 1977.

25. Wise, G.J., Goldberg, P. and Kozinn, P.J.: Genitourinary candidiasis: Diagnosis and Treatment. J. Urol. 139: 778, 1976.

26. Wise, G.J., Ray, B. and Kozinn, P.J.: The serodiagnosis of significant genitourinary candidiasis. J. Urol. 107: 1043, 1972.

27. Hanson, L.A.: Host-Parasite Relationships in Urinary Tract Infections. (Editorial) J. Inf. Dis. 127: 726, 1973.

28. Lindberg, U., Hanson, L.A., Jodal, U. et al.: Asymptomatic bacteriuria in school girls II. Differences in Escherichia Coli causing asymptomatic and symptomatic bacteriuria. Acta Paediatr. Scand. 64: 432, 1975.

29. Kaijser, B., Jodal, U., Hanson, L.A., et al.: Frequency of E. Coli K antigens in urinary tract infections in children. Lancet 1:663, 1977.

30. Kaijser, B.J.: Immunology of Escherichia coli: K antigen and its relation to urinary-tract infection. Inf. Dis. 127: 670, 1973.

31. Svanborg, E., Jodal, U., Hanson, L.A. et al.: Variable adherence to normal human urinary tract epithelial cells of Escherichia Coli strains associated with various forms of urinary tract infection. Lancet 2: 490, 1976.

32. Kalmanson, G.M., Harwick, H.J., Turck, M. and Guze, L.B.: Urinary tract infection: Localization and virulence of Escherichia Coli. Lancet 1: 134, 1975.

33. Ronald, A.R., Boutros, P. and Mourtada, H.: Bacteriuria localization and response to a single dose treatment in women. JAMA 235: 1854, 1976.

34. Rapkin, R.H.: Urinary tract infection in childhood. Pediatr. 60: 508, 1977.

35. Stamey, T., Timothy, M., Millar, M. and Mihora, G.: Recurrent urinary infections in adult women: the role of introital enterobacteria. Calif. Med. 115: 1, 1971.

36. Fairley, K.G., Grounds, A.D., Carson, N.E. et al.: Site of infection in acute urinary-tract infection in general practice. Lancet 2: 615, 1971.

37. Jodal, U., Lindberg, U. and Lincoln, K.: Level diagnosis of symptomatic urinary tract infections in childhood. Acta Paediatr. Scand. 64: 201, 1975.

38. Lindberg, U., Jodal, U., Hanson, L. and Kaijser, B.: Asymptomatic bacteriuria in school girls. IV. Difficulties of level diagnosis and the possible relation to the character of infecting bacteria. Acta Paediatr. Scand. 64: 574, 1975.

39. Thomas, V., Shelokov, A. and Forland, M.: Antibody coated bacteria in the urine and the site of urinary tract infection. N. Eng. J. Med. 290: 588, 1974.

40. Hellerstein, S., Kennedy, E., Nussbaum, L. and Rice, K.: Localization of the site of urinary tract infections by means of antibody coated bacteria in the urinary sediments. J. Pediatr. 92: 188, 1978.

41. Pylkkänen, J.: Antibody coated bacteria in the urine of infants and children with their first two urinary tract infections. Acta Paediatr. Scand. 67: 275, 1978.

42. Carvajal, H.F., Passey, R.B., Berger, M. et al.: Urinary lactic dehydrogenase isoenzyme 5 in the differential diagnosis of kidney and bladder infections. Kidney Int. 8: 176, 1975.

HIGHLIGHTS

PATHOLOGY AND INTERSTITIAL NEPHRITIS

Robert H. Heptinstall, M.D.

Dept. Pathol., John Hopkins Univ. Sch. Med. Baltimore, Maryland 21205, USA

Interstitial nephritis of the primary type is characterized by the appearance of inflammatory cells in the interstitium accompanied by variable degrees of tubular damage but with no primary glomerular change. The interstitium is edematous in the early or acute stages but fibrosis is the rule in the chronic type. The cells are usually of a chronic type - lymphocytes, monocytes, plasma cells and eosinophiles - and these appear at an early stage in the process. In certain forms of glomerulonephritis there is an intense interstitial reaction and this can be referred to as secondary interstitial nephritis.

The acute forms, in which edema is the distinguishing feature from the chronic type, are seen either as part of an infective process or as an adverse reaction to drugs. Polymorphs predominate in the infective types until they are replaced by chronic cells; this occurs by the second week of infection in the experimental model. Chronic cells appear to predominate from the beginning in the drug related types. In the chronic forms there is usually considerable tubular loss accompanied by increase in interstitial fibrosis; chronic inflammatory cells are present in variable numbers and glomeruli may become sclerotic in the more long standing cases.

ACUTE AND CHRONIC URINARY TRACT INFECTION

Jorge de la Cruz-Paris, M.D., Ricardo Muñoz-Arizpe, M.D., and Gustavo Gordillo-Paniagua, M.D.

Dept. Nephrol., Hosp. Lorencita Villegas de Santos Bogotá, Colombia and Dept. Nephrol., Hosp. Infantil de México, México City, Mexico

Urinary tract infection (UTI) remains a public health problem since its incidence is still high in the pediatric age group. In addition, some patients with UTI develop progressive renal parenchymal damage, mainly those cases associated with obstructive uropathy or vesicoureteral reflux (VUR). The prognostic signficance of renal parenchymal damage is emphasized by the fact that in 20 to 50% of uremic children the primary cause of chronic renal failure is chronic pyelonephritis (1,2). In our experience, chronic pyelonephritis is seen only in cases with UTI and obstructive uropathy or VUR, as will be shown below.

Considerations in this chapter are based on data gathered from current literature as well as clinical observations of patients with UTI from two pediatric nephrology wards, one at the Hospital Infantil de México in México City and the other at the Hospital Lorencita Villegas de Santos of Bogotá, Colombia. Etiology of the infectious process, different techniques used to collect urine samples for culturing, interpretation of the urine culture, presence or absence of predisposing factors favoring the infection, and progression to renal parenchymal damage and chronic uremia will be discussed.

Definitions of acute UTI, chronic UTI, pyelonephritis and tubulointerstitial nephritis used here are as follows. Acute UTI, from the clinical viewpoint implies sudden onset of the infectious process within the urinary tract, involving any portion of it. Positive urine cultures are mandatory to reach the diagnosis, but leukocyturia, hematuria and proteinuria also may be present. Acute UTI may be localized in the bladder or lower urinary tract structures, without risking progression to renal parenchymal damage. However, the infecting organisms may reach the kidney either through the bloodstream as in patients with sepsis, or by the ascending pathway through the bladder and ureters in cases of obstructive uropathy or VUR (3). Acute tubulointerstitial nephritis of bacterial origin may develop in the former situation; in the latter, chronic pyelonephritis is more likely to occur. Some cases of UTI with renal parenchymal involvement may develop acute renal failure, but others may show only a transient, slight reduction of renal function (4).

Chronic pyelonephritis implies permanent renal parenchymal damage caused by repeated or constantly present infection. In our experience, all patients with chronic pyelonephritis have obstructive uropathy or VUR, and show slow but progressive renal function impairment. Polyuria and polydipsia appear usually early in the course of the disease due to decreased urinary concentrating capacity. Symptoms of chronic uremia develop later, in variable lengths of time.

Pyelonephritis is a histopathological diagnosis characterized by bacterial invasion of the renal parenchymal tissue, renal pelvis and calyceal system (3). Acute bacterial interstitial nephritis is characterized by the presence of an inflammatory process with microabscess formation within the renal parenchyma, as well as interstitial edema. Polymorphonuclear cells, plasma cells, some lymphocytes and eosinophils may be present, mainly in the interstitium. Tubular involvement is characteristic, with flattening of the epithelium and even destruction of the tubular structures by the inflammatory process.

Chronic interstitial nephritis is characterized by less edema and more fibrosis within the interstitium, as well as the presence of more lymphocytes and plasma cell infiltrates. Tubular atrophy and the presence of tubular casts are common ("thyroid-like appearance"). Most cases show glomerular involvement of variable degree, mainly thickening of the Bowmans' capsule, peri-glomerular fibrosis or hyalinization of the glomerular tuft.

CLINICAL MANIFESTATIONS

Suspicion of UTI arises from the clinical presentation. However, signs and symptoms may not be quite characteristic in newborns and small infants. In them malaise, loss of appetite, failure to thrive, vomiting, diarrhea, jaundice, visceral enlargement and febrile or hypothermic episodes (usually associated with sepsis), may be the clue to the presence of UTI. Sometimes during infancy, but more frequently in pre-school and school age children, urinary symptoms such as dribbling, interrupted voiding, bladder retention, dysuria, frequency and low back pain may indicate the presence of UTI.

DIAGNOSIS

Demonstration of the infection should be based on positive urine cultures. The presence of leukocyturia, WBC casts, and increased leukocyte excretory rate are suggestive, but by no means diagnostic of UTI since non-bacterial renal inflammatory diseases may give similar urinary findings. Gram-stain of the urinary sediment may be helpful, mainly in newborns, small infants and in quite symptomatic patients. In the latter antibiotics ought to be started before urine cultures are reported.

Positive urine cultures are mandatory to reach the diagnosis of UTI. This sounds simple but often difficulties arise in daily clinical practice, mainly regarding reliability of the technique employed to obtain the urine sample and correct interpretation of results. Controversy may arise regarding the bacterial count obtained. According to Kass, significant bacteriuria is present if more than 10^5 col/ml are isolated in a morning, freshly voided specimen obtained by mid-stream voiding technique (5). Results should be interpreted as contamination of the sample if less than 10^3 are present. In-between values are considered doubtful and the culture should be repeated. This criterion is based on a study performed in adults whose urine samples were taken from the first morning voiding sample, thus allowing enough time for bacterial growth in the bladder. Interpretation difficulties may arise since a high water intake could reduce the number of colonies significantly, as pointed out by the same author. Moreover, Cattell studied the effect of fluid loading on bacterial counts in hourly micturition, and showed that bacterial count decreases considerably after fluid loading (6). This situation resembles that of the newborn and small infants who have frequent voidings and diluted urines; it seems reasonable not to apply this criterion to these groups of patients.

METHODS OF URINE COLLECTION

Occasionally interpretation of the urine culture may be difficult since "false positive" results may occur from contamination of the urine sample. Therefore, the technique employed to collect the urine for culturing is important and must be taken into account when interpreting results. Table 1 shows positive urine cultures taken by mid-stream voiding technique and by suprapubic puncture. The importance of the technique used is obvious since 13 positive urine cultures taken by mid-stream technique showed no growth by suprapubic tap. On the other hand, 20 positive results by suprapubic tap were also positive by mid-stream voiding technique. Undoubtedly, suprapubic puncture is the most reliable technique to collect urine for culturing; when the technique has been performed

Table 1. Comparison of Positive Urine Cultures in 33 Cases With Suprapubic and Mid-stream Voiding Techniques

Suprapubic	Mid-stream
20	20*
0	0
0	13

*In 3 cases germs were different from those obtained by SP technique. From Children's Hospital, Bogotá, Division of Nephrology.

properly any bacterial growth should be considered as significant bacteriuria and diagnostic of UTI. However, if midstream voiding technique is used to collect the urine sample, serial cultures are recommended to avoid mistakes in interpreting results. One culture with results different from the other two should be disregarded (Table 2). Serial cultures (three samples) compared well with samples taken by suprapubic tap (Table 3).

INFECTING ORGANISMS

E. Coli was the most frequently isolated bacteria from 167 patients with UTI in Mexico City, as shown in Table 4. Other organisms, such as proteus, pseudomonas and Klebsiella, may be isolated from patients who have undergone urological instrumentation. Gram negative as well as Gram positive bacteria also are frequently isolated from premature and newborn patients, associated mainly with sepsis.

E. Coli also was the most commonly isolated bacteria from patients studied in Bogota (Table 5). A higher incidence of E. Coli was found, almost 93% incidence in the initially diagnosed episode and about 95% in the recurrences. In the latter group this could be explained by the fact that in this series, a more reliable tech-

Table 2. Bacteria Isolated from 22 Urine Cultures

Type of Culture	No. of Cases	E. Coli	Other Bacteria
Single	22	12	10
Serial	10	10	0

From Hospital Infantil de México, Division of Nephrology.

Table 3. Bacteriological Correlation Obtained by Suprapubic Puncture and Serial Mid-stream Voiding Technique in 20 Cases with UTI

	Same Germ	Different Germ
Mid-stream	20	0
Suprapubic	20	0

From Children's Hospital, Bogotá, Division of Nephrology

nique (suprapubic puncture) was used to collect the urine sample. Undoubtedly, E. Coli is the most frequent cause of UTI, independently of the presence or absence of predisposing factors (obstructive uropathy, VU reflux, constipation, vaginitis, etc.). Forty-four patients with intra-urinary tract (intra-UT) predisposing factors were studied in Bogota and followed with repeated bacteriological studies (Table 6). Most of them grew E. Coli in the initially diagnosed episode as well as in the relapses. Other bacteria were less frequently isolated. Only E. Coli was isolated from patients with extra-urinary tract (extra-UT) predisposing factors. Nineteen recurrences were documented with the same organism (Table 7). Twenty-six patients without predisposing factors were followed. Again, E. Coli was isolated in 25 patients and proteus was found in only one case. Recurrences also were due to E. Coli (Table 8).

Table 4. Bacteriological Results of 167 Children with UTI

Bacterial	No. of Cases	%
E. Coli	65	40
Proteus mirabilis	28	17
Klebsiella	25	15
Pseudomonas	20	12
Mixed flora	11	7
Proteus morgagni	5	3
Coagulase neg. Staph.	3	2
Coagulase pos. Staph.	2	1.1
Salmonella	2	1.1
Strep. viridans	1	0.6
Candida alb.	1	0.6
Enterococcus	1	0.6

From Hospital Infantil de México, Division of Pediatric Nephrology.

Table 5. Urine Cultures Obtained by Suprapubic Puncture in Children with UTI

Bacteria	Initial No.	Initial %	Relapses No.	Relapses %
E. Coli	76	92.7	106	94.6
Proteus	3	3.7	2	1.8
Pseudomona	1	1.2	1	0.9
E. Coli + Proteus	1	1.2	2	1.8
E. Coli ± Pseudomona	1	1.2	-	-
Aeromona H.	-	-	1	0.9

From Children's Hospital, Bogotá.

PREDISPOSING FACTORS AND PROGNOSIS

The prognosis of UTI depends mainly upon the presence or absence of predisposing factors, since several patients with UTI associated with urological malformations developed renal parenchymal damage and progressed to chronic uremia. Accordingly, the etiology of chronic renal failure of 211 children seen at the Hospital Infantil de México is shown in Table 9. Other authors have had similar findings (2,7).

The incidence of urological malformations associated with UTI is shown in Table 10. One hundred twenty-seven out of 212 patients showed VU reflux and upper or lower obstructive uropathy. Predisposing factors in relationship with the presence of pyelonephritis and lower UTI also were studied in the Children's Hospital of Bogotá. Sixty-eight out of 100 children showed urological malformations; 47 out of the 78 with lower UTI had predisposing factors,

Table 6. Isolated Bacteria and Predisposing Factors in Children with UTI

Isolated Bacteria*	Intra-UT Predisposing Factor			
	Initial (44)		Relapse (71)	
	No.	%	No.	%
E. Coli	39	86.6	65	91.6
Proteus	2	4.5	2	2.8
Pseudomona	1	2.3	1	1.4
E. Coli + Proteus	1	2.3	2	2.8
E. Coli ± Pseudomona	1	2.3	-	-
Aeromona H.	-	-	1	1.4

*Obtained by suprapubic puncture. From Children's Hospital, Bogotá.

Table 7. Isolated Bacteria and Predisposing Factors in Children with UTI

	Extra-UT Predisposing Factor			
	Initial (12)		Relapse (19)	
Isolated Bacteria*	No.	%	No.	%
E. Coli	12	100	19	100
Proteus	-	-	-	-
Pseudomona	-	-	-	-
E. Coli + Proteus	-	-	-	-
E. Coli + Pseudomona	-	-	-	-
Aeromona H.	-	-	-	-

*Obtained by suprapubic puncture. From Children's Hospital, Bogotá.

whereas 21 out of 22 with pyelonephritis showed predisposing factors associated with infection (Table 11).

Also important is whether a predisposing factor is localized inside the urinary tract (VU reflux or obstructive uropathy), or outside (constipation, vaginitis). Regarding this, 100 children with UTI were studied in Bogotá; 76.5% had intra-UT predisposing factors and 23.5% showed predisposing factors outside the urinary tract (Table 12). Only patients with intra-UT predisposing factors showed chronic infection, while a few cases with extra-UT predisposing factors or without predisposing factors, showed recurrences. None of them went into chronic infection or chronic uremia; all eventually cured.

Table 8. Isolated Bacteria and Predisposing Factors in Children with UTI

	No Predisposing Factor			
	Initial (26)		Relapse (22)	
Isolated Bacteria*	No.	%	No.	%
E. Coli	25	96.1	22	100
Proteus	1	3.9	-	-
Pseudomona	-	-	-	-
E. Coli + Proteus	-	-	-	-
E. Coli + Pseudomona	-	-	-	-
Aeromona H.	-	-	-	-

*Obtained by suprapubic puncture. From Children's Hospital, Bogotá.

Table 9. Etiology of Chronic Uremia in Children from Three Different Studies

Diagnosis	Hospital Infantil de México (1) 211 Cases %	Habib et al. (2) 270 Cases %	Holliday et al. (7) 53 Cases %
Glomerulopathies	56.5	26	45
Obstructive Uropathy and UTI	19.5	21	15
Renal Hypoplasia	5.5	22	10
Hereditary Nephropathies	5.0	23	13
Vascular Nephropathies	0.5	4	4
Miscellaneous	13.0	4	13

From Gordillo-Paniagua, G. et al. Nefrologia Pediatrica. Asoc. Med. Hosp. Inf. Mex. 418, 1976.

SITE OF INFECTION

Another puzzling problem is the location of the infection. Clinical signs and symptoms of UTI are non-specific in many patients. Moreover, some patients with UTI are asymptomatic. Diverse procedures have been devised to provide a reliable diagnostic approach. X-ray studies are not reliable procedures to diagnose UTI or to localize the infection site. X-rays may disclose renal parenchymal alterations (changes in kidney size, scarring, etc.), but their real usefulness is to demonstrate the presence or absence of obstructive uropathies and/or VU reflux accompanying UTI (predisposing factors). Activity of urinary enzymes such as catalase (8), lactic dehydrogenase (9), and betaglucuronidase (10) also have been assessed to localize the site of infection; they are excreted in large quantities upon the presence of renal parenchymal damage, in contrast to infections localized in the lower urinary tract. About a decade ago, Fairley et al. (11) devised

Table 10. Urologic Malformations in 127 Children with UTI

Renal parenchymal alterations	8
Upper urinary tract alterations	101
Lower urinary tract alterations	68
Vesico-ureteral reflux	35
Total	212

From Hospital Infantil de México, Division of Nephrology.

Table 11. Predisposing Factors and Localization of the Infection in 100 Children with UTI

Site	No. Cases	PF
Lower UTI	78	47
Pyelonephritis	22	21
Total	100	68

From Children's Hospital, Bogotá, Division of Nephrology.

the bladder washout technique in order to culture urine coming directly from the kidneys; more recently, indirect methods of measuring serum antibodies to Tamm-Horsfall protein and to the infecting organism (different strains of E. Coli) have been assessed in clinical research (12,13). Again, controversial results lead to the opinion that none of these techniques is one hundred percent reliable, nor in most cases, practical in daily clinical practice. Since the original report of Thomas et al. (14), numerous others seem to confirm the validity of a simple, non-invasive technique to detect antibody-coated bacteria in urinary sediment which appears to correlate well with the site of infection. The suggested technique consists of treating washed urine sediment with fluorescein-conjugated antihuman globulin of horse origin. Positive fluorescence of antibody-coated bacteria is shown when the infecting organisms are located within the renal parenchyma, whereas negative results indicate the presence of cystitis (15). However, other clinical situations (prostatitis), may make the test positive (16).

Other more invasive radioisotopic techniques have been used to detect alterations in renal uptake of isotopes within cortex and medulla (67-gallium citrate) in cases of acute pyelonephritis (18,19). All of these techniques are non-specific to localize the site of infection.

Table 12. Predisposing Factors in 100 Children with Urinary Tract Infection

PF	No. Cases	%
Intra-UT	52	76.5
Extra-UT	16	23.5

From Children's Hospital, Bogotá, Division of Nephrology.

Assessment of renal function is another important matter. Clark et al. (17) studied correlations between site of infection and maximal concentrating ability in patients with bacteriuria. This renal function parameter may be altered early in the presence of an infectious process involving renal parenchyma. Other indexes of renal function may be altered during the course of the disease. However, none of them are specific regarding the presence or absence of infection, nor the site of infection if present. However, assessment of renal function may be viewed from another angle. Since chronic UTI may lead to far advanced renal failure, frequent assessment of renal function becomes quite important. At times, doubt arises regarding whether or not a surgical correction should be carried out, mainly in the initial urological assessment (for instance, in patients with mild or moderate VU reflux). Besides the urological assessment, renal function evaluation can be helpful in deciding upon conservative or surgical management. Routine studies such as maximal concentrating capacity after fluid intake restriction, fractional excretion of sodium and renal failure index, are easily available.

TREATMENT

Antibiotics and surgical procedures used properly and early in the course of the disease can prevent renal parenchymal damage and progression to renal failure. The choice of treatment with antibiotics depends upon in-vitro and in-vivo sensitivity of the isolated bacteria. Bacterial sensitivity or resistance, on the other hand, may vary according to geographical circumstances. Self-prescription and antibiotic abuse may change bacterial sensitivity in some areas. Thus we recommend periodic local bacterial sensitivity assessment.

Bolus treatment with a single antibiotic has been recommended in uncomplicated cases of UTI (20,21). Long term treatment may be indicated in some patients with urological malformations if conservative approach has been chosen, or in some of those for whom surgical management has to be delayed (22).

In addition to treatment with antibiotics, an intravenous pyelogram and urethrocystogram are recommended to rule out obstructive uropathy and/or VU reflux, once the diagnosis of UTI has been reached. This clinical approach stands regardless of age, sex, and whether or not the infection is a recurrence or first episode. Further diagnostic studies and management of UTI should be planned on an individual basis.

REFERENCES

1. Gordillo-Paniagua, G., Mota-Hernández, F., and Velasquez-Jones, L.: Nefrologia Pediátrica. Ed. Med. Hosp. Inf. Mex. 418, 1976.

2. Habib, R., Broyer, M. and Benmaiz, H.: Chronic renal failure in children. Nephron 11: 209, 1973.

3. Heptinstall, R.H.: Pathology of the Kidney. Boston: Little, Brown and Co., 1974, vol. 2, p. 837.

4. Gordillo-Paniagua, G., Alcalá-Carbajal, O., Mota-Hernández, F. Bacterial invasion of the kidney. In Strauss, J. (ed.): Pediatric Nephrology: Epidemiology, Evaluation, and Therapy. New York: Stratton Intercontinental Medical Book Corp., 1976, vol. 2, p. 197.

5. Kass, E.H.: Asymptomatic infections of the urinary tract. Trans. Assoc. Am. Phys. 69: 56, 1956.

6. Cattell, W.R.: Urinary tract infection. In Hendry, W.F.: Recent Advances in Urology. New York: Churchill-Livingston, 1976, p. 75.

7. Holliday, M.A., Potter, D.E. and Dobrin, R.S.: Treatment of renal failure in children. Pediatr. Clin. North Am. 18: 613, 1971.

8. Gillenwater, J.Y.: Diagnosis of urinary tract infection. Appraisal of diagnostic procedures. Kidney Int. 8: 3, 1975.

9. Schmidt, D.J.: Significance of total urinary lactic dehydrogenase activity in urinary tract diseases. J. Urol. 96: 950, 1966.

10. Bank, N. and Balline, S.H.: Urinary betaglucuronidase activity in patients with urinary tract infection. N. Engl. J. Med. 272: 70, 1965.

11. Fairley, K.F.: Localization of urinary tract infection. Lancet 1: 1212, 1969.

12. Clark, H., Ronald, A.R. and Turck, M.: Serum antibody response in renal versus bladder bacteriuria. J. Infect. Dis. 123: 539, 1971.

13. Vosti, K.L. and Remington, J.S.: Host-parasite interaction in patients with infections due to Escherichia Coli. III. Physiochemical characterization of O-specific antibodies in serum and urine. J. Lab. Clin. Med. 72: 71, 1968.

14. Thomas, V., Shelokov, A. and Forland, M.: Antibody-coated bacteria in the urine and the site of urinary-tract infection. N. Engl. J. Med. 290: 588, 1974.

15. Smith, J., Jones, S. and Kaijser, B.: Significance of antibody coated bacteria in urinary sediment in experimental pyelonephritis. J. Inf. Dis. 133: 577, 1977.

16. Gonick, P., Falkner, B., Schwartz, A. and Praisier, R.: Bacteriuria in the catheterized patient cystitis or pyelonephritis? JAMA 233: 253, 1975.

17. Clark, H., Ronald, A.R. and Cutler, R.E.: The correlation between site of infection and maximal concentrating ability in bacteriuria. J. Inf. Dis. 121: 588, 1970.

18. Frankel, R.S., Rickman, S.G. and Levinson, S.M.: Renal localization of 67-gallium citrate. Radiol. 114: 393, 1975.

19. Davis, E.R., Roberts, M. and Royland, J.: The renal scintigram in pyelonephritis. Clin. Radiol. 23: 370, 1972.

20. Balley, R.R. and Abbott, G.: Treatment of urinary tract infection with a single dose of amoxicillin. Nephron 18: 316, 1977.

21. Fang, L.S., Tolkoff-Rubin, N. and Rubin, R.H.: Efficacy of single dose and conventional amoxicillin therapy in urinary tract infection localized by the antibody-coated bacteria technic. N. Engl. J. Med. 298: 413, 1978.

22. Sleekman, R.A.: Trimethoprim-Sulphametoxazole vs. ampicillin in chronic urinary tract infection. JAMA 233: 427, 1975.

PANEL DISCUSSION

Moderator: José Strauss, M.D.

Div. Pediatr. Nephrol., Dept. Pediatr., Univ. Miami Sch. Med., Miami, Fla. 33101, USA

QUESTION: Some of the panelists mentioned that the hypersensitivity reaction caused tubulointerstitial changes. Is it that all the patients who have hypersensitivity reaction to penicillin or antibiotics have "a touch" of renal failure or is it that there are some kinds of predisposing factors which make that patient "special" as compared to others?

RESPONSE: I'm not really sure. The reason I deferred to my colleague here is that I didn't understand the question. I understood part of it. Part of the question was, is the clinical presentation or the renal manifestation the same in all these cases? I don't think that this is necessarily true. What I think is fairly common (and ought to be) is that we do get some elevation in the serum urea nitrogen but probably only a minority do go along to develop a very severe form of renal failure. Another very common feature that I should have mentioned, and this is particularly true in the methicillin group, is hematuria. If you look at the recorded cases of methicillin hypersensitivity, hematuria probably is the single most common feature one encounters.

The other part of the question was: are there certain people likely to be more susceptible than others? I think that would be a very difficult thing to test. Clearly, if you have been exposed to a certain drug and you are highly sensitive to it, then you are going to react adversely. I saw a very dramatic example of this. This was a man who was being treated for some sort of convulsions with Dilantin. Some evidence came forward that he was sensitive to this drug. I can't remember what the circumstances were but in the end he was taken off Dilantin. Several years later he came into a hospital where he was not known and was put on Dilantin again. Within about 48 hours he ran into very big renal problems. I'm not sure really if that answers your question. If it is that are there certain people who are more likely to have this trouble than others, I really can't answer that.

RESPONSE: I don't think that anybody has studied the problem. There are no kidney biopsies which could answer this question. I think that it is very difficult to give you an answer.

RESPONSE: From the clinical point of view, we have seen several cases with this type of problem. We have a wide variation of etiological agents and also a great deal of variation in the renal functional deterioration. There are some very slight manifestations of reduced GFR and others with acute renal failure. Also, there are many cases with hematuria or proteinuria but without acute renal failure. We were unable to find any predisposing factors in those cases.

RESPONSE: You are asking if there are predisposing factors. I believe that, from the clinical point of view rather than from the laboratory point of view, probably it is difficult to predict which patients will progress to chornic renal failure and which will recover. In my experience, there are some patients who have hypersensitivity to methicillin who develop a very mild, transient tubulointerstitial nephritis and others who develop a very severe, chronic, progressive tubulointerstitial nephritis and chronic renal failure. I think that your question should be phrased in terms of what is the predisposition of the patient to develop strong, very severe hypersensitivity reactions. If it is an immunological condition, certainly you have to go back to the genetic predisposition to hypersensitivity reactions. The problem is that we cannot evaluate these antibodies. We cannot evaluate the level of pre-existing antibodies. We cannot systematically screen the patient for the presence of antibodies which are difficult to detect. These are antibodies which result as a consequence of an active system. RNA is a chemical substance which binds to some proteins, perhaps a tubular basement membrane component, perhaps plasma proteins which we don't know very well. So, we have no way to screen these patients. In the very few patients in whom it was possible to make the screening, we knew from previous episodes that the patients made antibodies to methicillin. If we give methicillin again, we are going to produce a very severe tubulointerstitial reaction. If we take a biopsy exactly at that moment - when the urinary findings and the clinical symptoms appear - we can see,by the renal biopsy evidence of massive mast cell and basophilic degranulation - a phenomenon similar to the massive changes of immediate type hypersensitivity. The outcome of this type of disease certainly depends upon the severity of the lesion and the possibility of healing. If we have a patient who has repeated episodes of inflammatory reactions he is certainly going to develop interstitial fibrosis, tubular atrophy, progressive loss of nephrons, and, in the long range, he is going to develop chronic renal failure. We know this on the basis of a few observations and we don't know the whole story. There are only a few renal biopsies and we usually take a biopsy when it's too late and we don't see the phenomenon of mast cell degranulation or presence of antibodies to GBM. We can imagine what will happen but, really, we have no solid proof.

QUESTION: In the tubulointerstitial nephritis due to hypersensitivity reaction to different drugs, is there a different histopathological reaction in each case?

Also, is there any particular segment of the tubule that is more sensitive to the adverse reaction?

RESPONSE: In answer to the second part of your question, with quite a few of the drugs, if you read the various accounts on this, it would appear that the distal part of the tubule seems to be more susceptible than the proximal. But I am just giving this information on the basis of recorded cases. As you know, certain people are good pathologists but they are not exactly precise in describing just where the lesion is. Of course it is very often difficult to tell which particular segment you are seeing being damaged. But the answer is that where this has been precisely pointed out in a paper, it is more the distal part of the nephron rather than the proximal convoluted tubule.

As for the first part of your question, "are there any specific histologic findings from one agent to another?", in my own experience, I don't think there is. If you, for example, were to give me a biopsy and say, "alright, what is the agent that caused this?", I would not be able to tell. I think you would have some idea, though, as to whether you were dealing with a hypersensitivity reaction or a direct action on the tubules. I think probably eosinophils would be much more commonly part of the reaction if it were hypersensitivity but this is not a very common feature of the gentamycin or keflin type of case. I think there would be a more predominant tubular damage although this again would not be absolute because the currently accepted concept is that with drugs like methicillin the damage occurs through the tubular basement membrane which obviously would be affecting the tubular cells. One of the members of this Panel has done quite a lot of experimental work on this; I wonder if he has seen any sort of patterns coming out of all this?

RESPONSE: It is the hypersensitivity reaction which is mediated through antibodies to tubular basement membrane, though I think really that it occurs in the minority of cases. The drug reaction which we usually use in the laboratory is experimental hypersensitivity tubulointerstitial nephritis; it does not have demonstrable antitubular basement membrane (anti-TBM) antibodies. If there are antibodies against tubular basement membrane, it is usually the proximal convoluted tubule which is involved. The reason is not clear but the antigens which are responsible for this immune response are present, in both experimental animals and in humans, mainly in the proximal convoluted tubule.

COMMENT: That certainly seems to be true with the sickle cell anemia and trait patients who were studied by Strauss, Pardo and Kramer in Miami together with McIntosh and Ozawa in Denver. Even though the sickle cell anemia cases were all from Miami and the trait case was from Denver, all cases exhibited histological, electron microscopic, immunofluorescent and immunological changes.

COMMENT: The patients with sickle cell anemia developed immune-complex glomerulonephritis; the antibodies were against antigens localized in the brush border of the proximal convoluted tubules. If these patients had developed an antibody against tubular basement membrane we would have had combined damage to the tubular basement membrane probably due to some cross reactivity. But that was not the case. In Hyman's experimental nephritis, a disease which is produced by circulating immune-complexes of brush border antigens and their antibodies, sometimes there are antibodies against tubular basement membrane.

QUESTION: We work with children and very often we see hematuria and the clinical picture of methicillin-induced nephropathy. We don't usually biopsy them. My question is: is there any relation between the severity of the clinical picture, biochemical changes, and renal lesions? Should we biopsy all of them or which patients should be biopsied? How long do you follow them?

RESPONSE: I would not advise to biopsy most of the cases because of simple hematuria or proteinuria. The cases I have biopsied are those who have had acute renal failure or nephrotic syndrome or something like that.

COMMENT: I don't know anything about methicillin-induced nephropathy but I am very surprised by the results of our colleagues that show that some of the cases have antitubular basement membrane antibodies and some have not. I really don't know why there are those two types of patterns. Of course, in the sense of being able to evaluate the prognosis and things like that, I'm not sure that the biopsy is going to be very useful; but, in order to understand what is going on in this type of reaction to methicillin, I think it should be done. The presence of antitubular basement membrane antibodies is not that frequent in human pathology that we can forget about all the other things we have to learn about. We must find a good experimental way of producing antitubular basement membrane antibodies.

COMMENT: We must be very careful to point out that probably the anti-TBM finding would account for only a certain number of the methicillin cases. I think it's really a complete mystery why so few do have positive immunofluorescence around the tubules. There was quite a large series that came out where they had 7 cases of methicillin hypersensitivity. Immunofluorescence was done in each of them and it was negative in the tubules. Then, later on, they finally came up with this other case in which there was positive immunofluorescence. But on this score I have some ideas. After giving adjuvant as tubular basement membrane to guinea pigs, there is an initial reaction which is rather violent and which could be called acute interstitial nephritis; at this time, linear fluorescence around the tubules can be demonstrated. But, if you leave these animals, then you are no longer able to demonstrate the linear fluorescence nor the presence of circulating antibodies. I just wonder if this possibly could not explain some of the cases in man. Maybe it's the time at which they are being biopsied. I don't think you can, but I think it would be a thought. Perhaps you'd like to comment about how quickly in your experimental model you lose the ability to demonstrate positive linear immunofluorescence around the tubules, and the presence of circulating antibodies.

COMMENT: Well, it's a difficult question which I certainly cannot answer in detail but I can summarize what we know on the basis of experimental pathology. We know that there are only some animals which belong to certain subspecies which develop anti-TBM antibodies. So we need a genetic predisposition which is the result of the presence or absence of the appropriate antigen in tubular basement membrane. You can show the presence or absence of these antigens very nicely by using the experiment of renal transplantation. The second factor is the presence or absence of functional T helper cells; without these cells you do not develop anti-TBM or anti-GBM antibodies. So, there are several components which explain why probably only certain individuals develop antibodies to glomerular and tubular basement membranes.

There is also the question of persistence. How long do the antibodies persist in the circulation? Well, antibodies to glomerular and tubular basement membranes persist in circulation for a relatively short period of time because there is so much antigen available that all the antibodies which are produced are bound to to the basement membrane and the antigen. Thus they may be quickly removed from the circulation. Severity of the damage depends on the amount of antibodies which are produced and the type of mediator which various animals are able to provide in order to develop the inflammatory injury, such as complement, polymorphonuclear lymphocytes, and other types of cells like macrophages. Severity of the disease is proportional to the amount of antibodies produced and remaining in circulation. So, that is why it is so important that we use plasmapheresis or plasma exchange in these patients. If you can remove the antibody quickly you have much better chances of saving the tubules; this is very difficult to do because you first have to make the diagnosis with a kidney biopsy. I agree that the renal biopsy is extremely important in these patients. If you find anti-GBM or anti-TBM disease you are entitled to start extensive plasmapheresis; this is the only treatment at present. In the future, we may have a column of material coated with the GBM or TBM antigens through which the patient's serum is passed in order to remove the antibody. This system is not yet available but perhaps it will be in the near future. Dr. McIntosh was working on this column in Denver at the time of his death.

Finally, regarding the disappearance of linear stains of tubular and glomerular basement membranes, we know very little about persistent disappearance in humans. Anti-TBM disease in man is extremely rare. In our own experience, it is about .0006%. We have seen one patient whom we reported. But in animals, going back to the guinea pig which is the classical model, the linear staining quickly disappears and disappears because the macrophages, the cells which participate in the development of the disease, phagocitize and destroy the TBM. So, disappearance of linear staining is the consequence of destruction of the TBM. If this happens in man, we really don't know, but certainly in man there are very few macrophages and giant cells; in guinea pigs with this disease, there are extraordinarily large numbers of macrophage, epithelioid, and giant cells, all actively involved.

MODERATOR: I wonder if, in our wild thoughts/hypotheses, we couldn't think of other factors which may be associated with the development of anti-tubular basement membrane antibodies or their deposition in tubular basement membrane. In a case which was presented here a couple of years ago and which came out in one of our books, we had a patient with heart failure and then cardiac arrest. I wonder whether poor perfusion could produce a certain damage to tubular basement membrane which could lead to the deposition. Is that possible? Is there anything else that would explain why in some cases there is deposition and in others not?

RESPONSE: The question is difficult because it involves the usual problem that we have to consider every time we have an autoimmune disease. The first hypothesis is that we have tolerance and that this tolerance is broken at a certain point when there is mutation of lymphocytes; this is a very unlikely possibility. The second hypothesis is that at a certain point, there is an increase in antigen which is introduced into the circulation or an antigen which is immunochemically different and therefore is not recognized as self, is released into the circulation. The third hypothesis is that some exogenous factor which by chance cross-reacts with the autologous antigen is introduced from the outside.

So, we have these three hypotheses developed in the last twenty years. The first hypothesis (mutation of lymphocytes) was discussed many years ago and is no longer considered likely, especially to explain autoimmune hemolytic anemia. The second hypothesis (increased amount of antigen perhaps of basement membrane) is a very challenging and interesting hypothesis. If we consider that the disease is not a disease of the basement membrane, but is a disease of the cells which manufacture or produce basement membrane, we can imagine that for some reason that we don't know, they start producing increased amounts of basement membrane or a basement membrane which is qualitatively different and then there is obviously an antibody response. For the third hypothesis (exogenous antigen), so far there are only a few leads. For instance, the influenza type A2 found during an epidemic in the first world war, may be associated with anti-TBM or anti-GBM disease. Certainly I think that the most recent data show that at least for the lung involvement, the frequency and severity of lung pathology is not proportional to the level of antibodies present in the circulation. Perhaps there is some co-factor that we don't know which could damage the lungs such as hydrocarbons. For instance, animals exposed to minimal amounts of mercury chloride develop antibodies to GBM and TBM, (especially TBM) for reasons still unknown. We don't know which is the antigen(s), probably a component of the collagen present in glomerular and tubular basement membranes (especially tubular). The staining is linear and lasts for several weeks and then while the disease progresses, more is released into the circulation, antigen-antibody complexes circulate and complexes are formed in situ with the collagen mass antigen. So, perhaps chemicals or agents of pollution may be those co-factors.

QUESTION: We as pediatricians often use gentamycin particularly against septicemia in small infants. We wonder if there is any dose-related toxicity or if there is any time that the toxicity wouldn't appear, especially since some groups recommend higher doses per kilogram of body weight for small children. My specific questions are: is there any dose which is time related to toxicity? Have you seen a difference in toxicity depending on the age of the patients?

RESPONSE: I think this is very challenging for any pediatric pathologist. The only thing I can say about that is that certainly experimentally this is very, very much dose related. I can't give you any idea of what dosage you should use but certainly all the work pretty well shows that the higher the dose of any of these agents that were listed as having a tubular effect, the more likely they are to cause tubular damage. But on the actual human side of it, for giving of certain doses, I'm really not in a position to answer. Some of the clinicians here may be able to do so.

RESPONSE: We have studied this a few years ago but have not yet published this work. There were 120 patients, all newborn and premature babies treated with kanamycin and gentamycin. The two agents were not given together; it was one or the other. We had about 37 cases which developed urinary findings, including microscopic hematuria and red cell casts. Only 5 patients had elevation of BUN and serum creatinine; they were very sick patients with sepsis and with dehydration. We gave the recommended doses. So after that study we believe that the damage is not dose-related because even with the recommended doses you can get functional and maybe histological changes. We did not biopsy any of them; they all recovered.

RESPONSE: I am a very firm believer in the concept of the sensitized kidney. I think it goes along exactly with what my colleague was saying. The kidney is sensitized by some other ongoing process. For example, dehydration, depletion, hypertension, another drug, or a combination of an aminoglycoside with a diuretic. The clinical setting in large part is going to be a determinate as well as dose and duration. That makes it very difficult to separate these factors out in human patients as opposed to experimental models where it can be separated out, so that there is a predictor of those patients who are likely to get into difficulty with aminoglycoside antibiotics. The other side of the coin, however, is very important and I think it is one which has to be kept in mind when dealing particularly with critically ill patients. That is that if one is so concerned with what will happen with the kidney one can forget about the necessity for having a bacteriotoxic or bactericidal dose of any antimicrobial agent. It certainly does not do the patient any good to attempt to have the kidneys function when the patient is either in deep shock due to gram negative sepsis or when the patient is nearly dead. It is essential that blood levels be followed and in critically ill patients that laboratory determination of the effectiveness of the antibiotic be carried out in vitro.

QUESTION: One of the the panelists presented a couple of slides where he had a scheme for the workup of patients. One of them had like a grade II abnormal upper tract and no reflux but he recommended urological studies and then kidney biopsy. Is it worthwhile? Maybe I just didn't read between the lines.

REPONSE: You are referring to the patient with the recurrent UTI. The workup depends on the clinical situation. If we see recurrences or even if we think we are going to lose the patient from our clinic because the mother is not reliable, we do an IVP and we do a voiding cystourethrogram.

QUESTION: But if it is normal, and the patient has recurrent UTIs then you would suggest doing kidney biopsy and urological workup?

RESPONSE: No.

QUESTION: You would just follow them?

RESPONSE: That's right. Once we have a normal IVP and normal VCU, we don't do anything else.

QUESTION: When would you recommend radiological workup in children with UTI?

RESPONSE: Since we are extremely interested in knowing if the patient has an obstructive uropathy, I prefer doing the urological workup after the first episode of UTI.

QUESTION: Over the last two years we have been following gentamycin levels in terms of the pharmacokinetics of the drug. We found that the metabolism of the drug differs a great deal depending on body size of infants and the degree of clinical illness. Very catabolic children showing a high fever and manifesting a major response to sepsis often require large doses of gentamycin to maintain serum levels which we consider in the therapeutic range - between 4 and 8 μg/ml. Trying to monitor this by blood levels, it has been our clinical impression - I don't have any really hard numbers in yet - that we markedly reduced the incidence of nephrotoxicity. There is the implication that following drug levels is at least as reliable a way of monitoring gentamycin toxicity in the absence of lisozymuria or other urinary changes as all the other methods being used. We find that on a meter square basis the blood levels are much more reliable than using a fixed milligram per kilogram dosage which ranges in small children from 1 to almost 3 mg/kg/dose of gentamycin. There is a tremendous variation in terms of the blood levels that one gets.

RESPONSE: I think this is an extremely important concept. It is the blood level that is the critical factor both in terms of nephrotoxicity and in terms of killing the organism. The rules of 9 and rules of 8 that have been elaborated based on pharmacokinetic studies have been adequately shown not to correlate very well with the blood levels. Trying to predict a blood level using one of the rules based on creatinine frequently is the source of major error either by overshooting and thereby putting the patient at risk for nephrotoxicity, or undershooting and thereby putting the patient at risk for continued progress of infection.

QUESTION: What about urinary levels? What role does this play? Is there a correlation with renal damage?

RESPONSE: I can't tell you from personal investigation or experience. We have had our infectious disease people attempt to determine urinary levels for us. They have done this and I know it can be done but I can't really answer your question specifically as to whether or not they correlate with nephrotoxicity. What we were looking for specifically was whether we were getting enough gentamycin in the urine for the antibiotic to kill the urinary bacteria.

QUESTION: Are the antibiotic urine levels more meaningful than serum levels in terms of the killing power of urinary bacteria?

RESPONSE: Again the question that we always ask in chemotherapy of any kind is: is the drug which is being administered to the patient getting to the target tissue? If one gives a drug that has extremely high serum levels but does not get into the urine to reach the germ that one is trying to attack, one has a problem, especially if the drug is toxic at those levels. This is a critical point. Most antibiotics which we use are given at normal renal function and will get into the urine. But antimicrobials which are excreted mainly through the kidneys will not get in the urine in adequate amounts when the renal function is abnormally low. Such an example are the nitrofurantoins. In addition, toxic problems are increased.

COMMENT: In terms of gentamycin, it has been shown that concentrations in the urine are quite larger (up to 50 times) than the concentration in the serum. Gentamycin is actually concentrated in the renal cortex and that's why the potential risk for the nephrotoxicity. In terms of bacteriology, we have to correlate always the level that we are obtaining in a fluid or a tissue with the minimal inhibitory concentration for the bacteria we are treating; it's the ratio of the level on that fluid versus the MIC of the bacteria in question that is really important. In general, it is 2 to 4 times higher levels that need to be reached in the final fluid as compared to the MIC in μg/ml.

QUESTION: I would like to ask a question concerning the etiology of interstitial nephritis. One of the panelists mentioned new bacterial mechanisms. I was wondering about viral mechanisms. We recently had an 18-year-old patient with infectious mononucleosis and two weeks later had acute interstitial nephritis without glomerular involvement and went into acute renal failure. I would appreciate comments on this, please.

RESPONSE: I can't really comment on it terribly intelligently. I have also seen a case of mononucleosis with interstitial reaction. I suppose viruses can do this. I don't think that's enough to comment on it.

COMMENT: We have the example of the cytomegalovirus which can produce a very typical interstitial nephritis, too. I've seen cases of herpes and varicella with kidney involvement. I think that all these viruses can very well produce interstitial nephritis. The problem is that you can recognize herpes-varicella virus and cytomegalovirus because you have specific cells but there are probably other viral infections that can cause exactly the same thing and you cannot identify what type it is because you don't have the specific cells.

QUESTION: Was there a biopsy on your case of mononucleosis? Was it a pure interstitial nephritis, without glomeruli involved?

RESPONSE: Unfortunately, we had only a few glomeruli in our specimen but there was no involvement of the glomeruli we had.

QUESTION: To go back to the question asked before, I'd like to give a specific answer to the question - hopefully to elucidate some further comment from the panel. Any child that has a normal IVP and a normal cystogram and has recurrent UTIs, does he/she need to have a cystometrogram and cystoscopy? Unfortunately in these children (most specifically little girls), we are going to miss pathology if we don't do a good examination of the female genitalia. All of us know how difficult that is to do on an awake little girl on most occasions. Secondly, urethral pathology, such as stenosis, may be missed. I realize that among a lot of people that's very controversial; however, one uses calibration to determine size of the urethra to be expected in a female if that diagnosis can be arrived at or excluded. Such aspects as neurogenic bladder, incomplete emptying of the bladder, urethral polyps and so forth will be missed if these children are not cystoscoped.

MODERATOR: Any further comment?

QUESTION: In order to make the diagnosis of neurogenic bladder, do you need a cystoscopy or can you make that diagnosis from a post-voiding cystogram?

RESPONSE: I think the diagnosis can be made by post-voiding residual urine and cystometrogram. A cystoscopy helps one to determine questionable cases of neurogenic bladder. But in the more severe ones it determines such changes as trabeculation, whether or not there's spasm of the bladder and so forth. We could go next into the use of urodynamics but I don't think we want to get into that at this point.

COMMENT: I think one of the dominant driving forces for clinicians in taking care of patients should be fear. Fear goes in two directions. One, fear of doing harm by excessive procedures. Second, fear also of doing harm by not looking for something that might be there. This comes under a nebulous and mysterious umbrella of "clinical insulation and clinical experience". I think, in general, if the base studies are negative and urinary tract infection continues to recur, then this is the time when cystoscopy should be done. I don't think they ought to be done routinely on every patient. I don't think that is what was being suggested. Dr. Strauss was interested in stirring up some controversy in the panel. That really hasn't happened too much, but I've been delighted with some of the controversy that's appeared in the audience. I walked into a full scale battle during the coffee break. One of the nephrologists in the audience said, "I never catheterize anyone to obtain a specimen for culture", countered by one of the urologists who stated, "I catheterize everybody to look for urinary tract infections, and get urine cultures...". On that basis of "agreement", there is tremendous discrepancy in what is believed as being right. There probably is no "right". What has to be done, though, is to approach patients intelligently, in a way which will yield data without doing any harm to the individual patient.

At this point, I would like to comment on catheterization in general. We haven't really talked about prevention of urinary tract infection. I did allude to the catheter as a source of infection. The data are extremely clear on catheterization. I think that the minimum one can expect from routine catheterization no matter how carefully done, is about a 1% incidence of infection. This can be a little less frequent when people are trained to do it themselves. For example, paraplegics can catheterize themselves as often as three or four times a day and have an extremely low incidence of infection. Catheter teams, GU technicians, can be trained to catheterize patients pre-operatively; obstetrical services, urological services, or spinal cord injuries services, can greatly minimize the incidence of catheter-induced infection. Obviously, patients who are going for gynecological surgery, certain kinds of urologic surgery, have got to have an indwelling catheter placed if for no other reason than localization. The catheter need not stay in there forever. Somebody has got to decide when (post-operatively) it's best for it to come out. Somebody has to connect it to closed drainage. Somebody in the hospital has got to make certain that the closed drainage is *never* broken. Somebody has got to train the nurses not to break the closed drainage for the purpose of obtaining urine for culture and sensitivity. The most blatant example is the patient in whom urinary sugar and acetone is ordered every four hours because the patient is diabetic. And every four hours the connection is broken in order to obtain urine, and thereby virtually assuring that pseudomonas or some other nasty beast will quickly find its way in. There are now closed catheters drainage systems manufactured with access ports on them so that with proper aseptic techniques, urine can be withdrawn from them without breaking the sterility of the system. So I make a strong and impassioned plea:

1. To catheterize only patients who absolutely require it;
2. To maintain the most rigid aseptic techniques possible;
3. To make certain that a closed drainage system has appropriate air locks built into it;
4. That the catheter collection bag is hooked in some way to the side of the bed or bedrail so that it's below the level of the patient, but yet does not drag on the floor; and
5. That the individual who is transported to radiology, usually to get the IVP or the cystometrogram or some other specific study, not have his bag placed on top of him or, even worse, underneath the mattress on the journey, in order to avoid creating positive pressure reinfusion of his urine.

COMMENT: I was just sitting back here chalking down a few figures. I have estimated very conservatively in our pediatric-urology clinic that we have catheterized a minimum of 5,000 little girls. I firmly agree with what anyone says about catheterizing little boys. I think there are virtually no indications to catheterize a little boy. Occasionally one might have a specific indication. But as far as catheterizing little girls, if this is taught well, as it is to our clinic personnel, it is virtually a noninfective process. Of these 5,000 girls that I am quoting, I cannot recall, albeit in a retrospective fashion, a single instance of induction of urinary tract infection. Obviously, one may comment that we could have missed one; certainly we could have. If we have an in-patient in our hospital, we do not let the nurses on the floor catheterize her. We bring her down to the clinic to our well-trained personnel, for a sterile catheterization. We don't have anything against floor nurses. I think that with these techniques it's a very acceptable method of obtaining urine. Let me add that we've seen problems with suprapubic taps; but I will not argue that they should be done away with totally in favor of catheterization. On the other hand, I think that suprapubic punctures in good hands are likewise excellent methods. As far as problems that I have seen, one was perforation of the intestine which required surgical correction. The second was the needle hitting a large bladder blood vessel which led to a massive hematoma in the wall of the bladder.

COMMENT: I would like to emphasize that all these procedures can result in risk of complications depending on the experience of the person who is doing the procedure. I would like to ask a question to the urologist: how do you know that the urinary bladder catheterization did not produce infection? Did you get a urine culture after each catheter specimen?

RESPONSE: No little girl who was uninfected returned in a short period with infection. I certainly agree that this was not an adequate scientific study but pass it along as a clinical observation. If a child had come back in a short period of time with a urinary tract infection, one thing that would have to be said is that it could have been from the catheterization. This didn't happen.

COMMENT-QUESTION: In our hospital we follow every catheterization with two urine cultures - one at 48 hours and one at 96 hours. We do find actually that our rate of infection is 8%. This is in good hands. The people who do it are specially trained to work with spinal cord injuries. These are silent infections and they don't go away. You can go back and get that checked ten days later and still find E. Coli. I think there are "hidden" infections that we do cause by instrument manipulation. I am all for prevention. I'd like to make one other comment. All of us believe the rule that every kid with a first urinary tract infection should have an IVP. In this manner we will be doing an IVP on 10% of all females before they reach age 12. That's a figure that's always bothered me. As I'm getting older, another figure that bothers me is, most of my patients with positive yields that have severe pathology are not my kids who come with a first urinary tract infection or what I think is a first urinary tract infection but the kid who I come across by accident because in clinic he/she has either asymptomatic bacteriuria or has been picked up as having high diastolic blood pressures for his/her age. When we work these youngsters up, we get an immensely higher yield of pathology than we do on a six-year-old little girl or a four-year-old who comes in with fever, pyuria, or a urinary tract infection. So, I really wonder if this is the right way to approach it. If every kid needs to be examined, maybe we ought to go look more at ultrasound and less invasive techniques than IVPs. If you talk about fallout, there's certainly more fallout from doing IVPs than there is from anything else we've talked about. My other question is to the people who discussed acute and chronic urinary tract infections - do you have any incidence or figures on hypertension in youngsters you were dealing with?

RESPONSE: The first comment is very interesting. I think it depends upon where you are working. For example, we work with a very particular group of patients in our hospital - very low socioeconomic level. We lose many of these patients at followup. We don't know if these patients have the first or the 20th urinary tract infection. We say "this is the first UTI we have diagnosed;" but, we don't know what happened before. If we have any doubt about losing the patient, we probably will do an IVP. Sometimes it happens that we have the first symptomatic urinary tract infection in a reliable patient. There were no symptoms before, we do an IVP and find hydronephrosis. This is disturbing and difficult to explain. Due to all these special circumstances, we do perform an IVP and VCU with the first diagnosed infection. Regarding the question on hypertensive findings, we have not detected hypertension in these patients except when they go into chronic renal failure (CRF) or terminal renal failure (ESRD). I would say that this hypertension is related to hypervolemia which is due to the renal failure and not due to what has been called renal scarring and high renin hypertension. We didn't see that in any of our patients.

COMMENT: About indication for radiological workup, there has been much controversy, especially in regard to females. In males I would say that everybody agrees that they should have an IVP and VCU with the first episode documenting UTI. In the recurrent female, among schoolage children, certainly there is a very high incidence of missed IVPs in the groups studied. But also you must note that 10-12% of schoolage females with recurrent UTI had renal scarring already and approximately 25% of them had vesicoureteral reflux. So, we still are having some yield from that population. But what we are missing probably is the first three or four years of life when we should be more aware of the possibility of UTI; at that age, unexplained fever is usually labelled upper respiratory tract infection.

MODERATOR: I should say about the hypertension, that I believe it does happen in the absence of organic changes. I believe there is a functional hypertension (if you would accept that term) due to temporary obstruction. I can recall two patients who had obstructive problems which were corrected and the hypertension went away without any persistent clinical findings. There was a good study from Houston in terms of blood flow changes in dogs with constriction of the ureter; cortical blood flow decreases markedly. Recently we had a girl from Latin America who had had repeated UTI and severe constipation (impaction). She was hypertensive at that time. We prescribed stool softeners to eliminate one contributing factor for the UTI. A week later she came back and her blood pressure was normal. That is anecdotal, but I believe there is something to that.

COMMENT: I believe that IVP and VCU should be done always following the first urinary tract infection episode. Gradually, as the criteria for diagnosis become more strict, when suprapubic punctures are performed regularly and the "UTIs" are *real UTIs*, out of 100 patients (80 girls) up to 52% of the patients had congenital anomalies (organic obstruction or VU reflux) of the GU tract. Those patients had ready access to good medical followup and belonged to socioeconomic groups higher than the average population. I believe that the series which have only few GU tract anomalies include a large number of *false UTIs* because of loose criteria for the diagnosis.

MODERATOR: It may depend on the referral system also. We find that our incidence of chronic renal failure with obstructive uropathies is about 40% in Miami as opposed to about 20% as reported from Paris, Mexico City and San Francisco.

COMMENT: I would like to make just two comments. One is that in studying end-stage renal disease, that is, all the nephrectomies performed for transplantation in our department, I can tell you that in 25 years of renal pathology, I have never seen, never, a case of chronic pyelonephritis without either obstructive or predisposing cause. I don't understand why the American's (as a European I can say that - I don't undertand what happens on the other side of the Atlantic Ocean) are so excited about studying all these asymptomatic urinary tract infections. My point of view is that the only interest in urinary tract infection is that it allows the discovery of some abnormalities of the urinary tract. Apart from that, I personally would not even be interested in urinary tract infection. That's my point of view and you are not obligated to share it, of course. The more I study the problem kidney under my microscope, the more I feel that, when I said several years ago that pyelonephritis does not exist, I was right. What I meant was pyelonephritis does not exist in the absence of predisposing causes. The second comment is as follows: taking all the nephrectomies performed in patients who were to be transplanted, I was extremely surprised to find 18% of cases of nephronophthisis, or as it is called in this country, medullary cystic disease. My question is, why didn't the speaker mention nephronophthisis among the different patterns of chronic interstitial nephritis? Having been involved in renal pathology for so many years, I know how many people have been ignoring completely the problem of nephronophthisis from a pathology point of view. So I think that maybe that is one of the explanations of the discrepancies among the different reported causes of chronic renal failure. Why are you so excited about urinary tract infection? Is it because you think that it's going to lead to chronic renal failure? If you think that it's not going to lead to chronic renal failure, you become less interested. Regarding all the data published concerning the incidence of chronic pyelonephritis in end stage renal disease, if you tell people that 30% had chronic pyelonephritis of course it becomes a very important problem. But I think that most of the people who have been referring to a high incidence of chronic pyelonephritis in the absence of urinary tract malformation maybe were misinterpreting one of the big causes of chronic renal failure in children which is represented by a typical pattern of what can be called chronic interstitial nephritis. Then, why didn't you mention it?

RESPONSE: I didn't mention it because if I gave all the causes it would go down to the bottom of the screen. I quite agree with you that it is an entity that we recognize. We give it a different name. Nephronophthisis never made very much sense to me but perhaps medullary cystic kidney doesn't make much sense either. I do accept the addition and if I prepared a slide with every cause on it, people would complain because they couldn't read it in the back.

On the other question: "why do people worry about urinary tract infection?" They worry because some people have a different view from you. They feel that this is a significant contribution towards production of end stage kidneys. I don't want to take this up now. A more appropriate time will be when you can deal with the other speaker who will be sitting on the other side of you to present a different point of view. I think it's only fair that he be here to present that point of view. Now, you talk about nephrectomies as being an indication of end stage renal disease. I'm not altogether sure that I agree with that. This is, you must remember, a very selective group. I think that if you are going to work out the causes of end stage renal disease purely on the basis of nephrectomy, you are going to get a very biased group. Let me just tell you that we recently, the last year, looked through the diagnoses that we have made in the nephrectomy specimens that came to us prior to transplantation. I can't remember the exact figures but I think there were approximately 80 patients and I believe eight of those had chronic pyelonephritis that we were prepared to accept as chronic pyelonephritis. You know that I am very conservative. No doubt this is going to be a very small figure compared with what some people diagnose. I can't remember the breakdown of those eight but it was that either five were obstructive and three were not obstructive or the other way around. But we do see them. You can't accuse me of the sort of things that you are suggesting because we did a study a good many years ago in which we looked at the records of 3,500 autopsies of adults and children and we found only eight cases of what we would call chronic nonobstructive pyelonephritis among that group, which is an incidence of about .2-.3%. This figure is considerably lower, if you cast your mind back to some of the exorbitant figures quoted by other people which were around 15% or 20%. So, to go back to your comments and your remarks or criticisms (whatever you like to call them) we do recognize medullary cystic disease or nephronophthisis. I think of this group of eight we had only one or possibly two at the most who may be called that.

QUESTION: But it was mainly adults?

RESPONSE: This was mainly adults. We have a relatively small number of pediatric cases in a general hospital. So the figures, the autopsy ones, were mainly adults. By the same token, the nephrectomy ones too would be predominantly adults, but it would include some children.

COMMENT: Of course, because most of the children with nephronophthisis are dead by the age of 15 or 16 years, you won't see them in an adult population. Although this disease exists also in the adult population, but most of them are dead before they reach that age. That's why it's such a very important problem of pediatric nephrology. It's not a criticism by the way, that

I was making to you. I think that in pediatrics it is very important to mention this as a cause of chronic interstitial nephritis because I am sure that if people are aware of that, the incidence of chronic pyelonephritis is going to diminish considerably. Now, with the nonobstructive pyelonephritis you were talking about, I include also reflux. When I say no abnormalities I don't see reflux as being an abnormality or a favoring cause.

RESPONSE: It functions as an abnormality. But I thought you were talking of organic changes demonstrable to a urologist or a pathologist at autopsy. Of course reflux is an abnormality but it is not an organic abnormality.

REFLUX NEPHROPATHY

John Hodson, M.D., F.R.C.P. (Lond.), F.R.C.R.

Diagnostic Radiol., Yale Univ. School of Medicine
and Yale New Haven Hospital
New Haven, Conn. 06504 USA

"Reflux Nephropathy" is a term coined to encompass the spectrum of kidney disease forms in which vesico-ureteral reflux plays a major etiologic role; a group that has morbic anatomical changes with varying but distinctive features. Urinary infection and raised pressure within the urinary tract are commonly associated, but the ways in which those three etiologic factors combine to produce the differing disease entities is not yet established. The renal damage tends to commence at a very early age; and its more severe complications, severe hypertension and renal failure, are well documented from as young as five years onwards, the bulk of the clinical impact being between the ages of 10 and 30 years. Because the essence of the disease is severe focal fibrosis which strangles the parenchyma it enmeshes and which is largely unaffected by treatment once it has become established, the only hopeful method of approach, as in the case of cystic fibrosis, lies in early diagnosis and prevention rather than later amelioration or cure. Classification, exact definition and pursuit of the natural history of related phenomena are the present requirements so that a true and unbiased view of the whole disease complex may be obtained, for its full understanding and the development of optimal therapeutic approaches. This chapter is a summary of most of the presently appreciated aspects of what is rapidly becoming recognized as a major, possibly preventable, disease process of young people.

Revised and updated with permission from W.B. Saunders, Publisher, and Dr. Fredrich L. Coe, Editor of Volume 62, No. 6, Medical Clinics of North America, November, 1978.

HISTORICAL BACKGROUND

The renal entity of "chronic atrophic pyelonephritis" gradually emerged from a series of clinical and pathological descriptions dating from 1880 (74,80) and extending through to the 1930's (29,81). The gross specimens described varied according to whether they resulted from surgery or from autopsy, the latter often being complicated by added changes resulting from terminal renal failure, or from associated severe hypertension. The specimens were, in the main, coarsely scarred with thickening of the walls of the pelvis and calices, like those removed surgically from children and young adults in more recent years. In most cases there was a history of recurrent urinary infections dating back to early childhood. But in some no such story was elicited, and the same situation obtains today, namely, a minor but significant proportion of cases with the same general gross kidney pathology but with no history of infection.

The close association of chronic atrophic pyelonephritis with vesicoureteric reflux was first documented in 1960 (29), and has since been confirmed by numerous observers (9,34,65,69,83). Furthermore, it soon became evident that the radiographic appearances of the kidney damage were so characteristic, particularly in children, that they formed a sound basis for diagnosis (Fig. 1), and radiology is now used, not only as a means of diagnosis, but of monitoring the progress of the disease and the effects of treatment.

However, further experience also showed that focal scars with concomitant caliectasis commonly situated in the polar regions of the kidneys, and with normal papillae elsewhere, was only one variety of the damage associated with reflux, and that the more severe varieties of the latter produced changes, affecting *all* papillae, more closely resembling those of severe post-obstructive atrophy (35,73)(Fig. 2). Probably at least part of the wide spectrum of renal damage, comprising various forms of "dysplasia," found in kidneys in male infants with posterior urethral valves and vesicoureteric reflux, should also be included in this category (82). Again, in the last few years, the association of reflux with severe focal changes previously known either as "segmental hypoplasia" (8, 24) or the "Ask-Upmark kidney" (8,13,7) has been increasingly reported. The considerable significance of this lies in the fact that it was previously thought that this variety of renal damage, because in some cases no nephron elements are found in the focal lesions, was congenital in origin. But such lesions have now been seen to develop in what were previously normal, or only slightly damaged, kidneys (11,37), and similar lesions have been produced experimentally in the pig as a result of reflux (42).

Two other clinical groups must be mentioned: healthy subjects between the ages of 10 and 30 years, again with no relevant previous

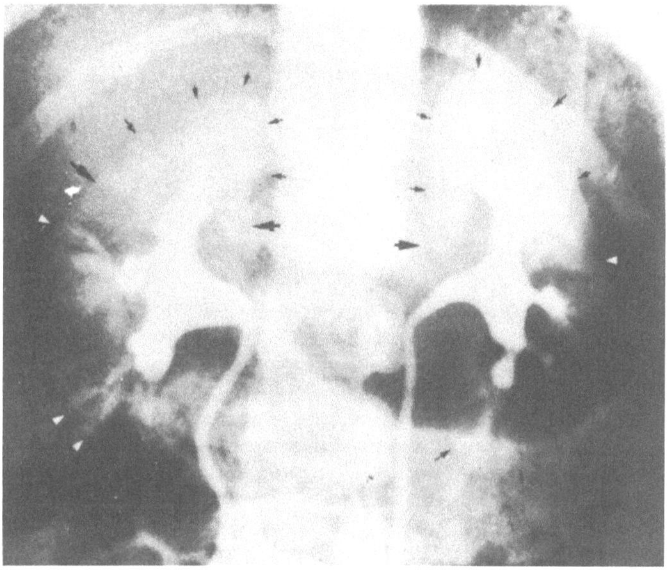

FIG. 1. Cystogram: Intrarenal reflux into human kidneys (girl, aged 8 years) mainly in both upper polar regions, the right midzone, and in wisps in the lower poles (arrows). The renal parenchyma is still normal and the upper tracts undilated. Is this a procedural artifact? Or has intrarenal reflux been present since early childhood? (From Hodson, C.J., Maling, T.M.J., McManamon, P.J., et al.: The pathogenesis of reflux nephropathy. Br. J. Radiol., Suppl. 13, 1975. Reproduced with permission).

history, who are identified by albuminuria or mild hypertension on routine examination, and in whom severe reflux and advanced bilateral renal damage are demonstrated in the later clinical work-up; and secondly, the numerically smaller group (12 to 25 years old) which presents with knock-knees or other evidence of "renal glomerular osteodystrophy" (the mixture of rickets, or osteomalacia, hyperparathyroidism, and bone sclerosis which results from slowly progressive renal glomerular failure over a period of several years). In this group, too, the renal damage is associated with severe reflux. Finally, the now well-established fact that this disease is sometimes familial must be mentioned. The details of inheritance are as yet incompletely worked out, and how commonly it occurs in families is as yet unknown (16,21,47,58,86).

It thus appears entirely logical that this widely protean collection of clinically differing manifestations should be linked by a generic term identifying what appears to be the single common etiological denominator, namely, vesicoureteric reflux. "Reflux Nephro-

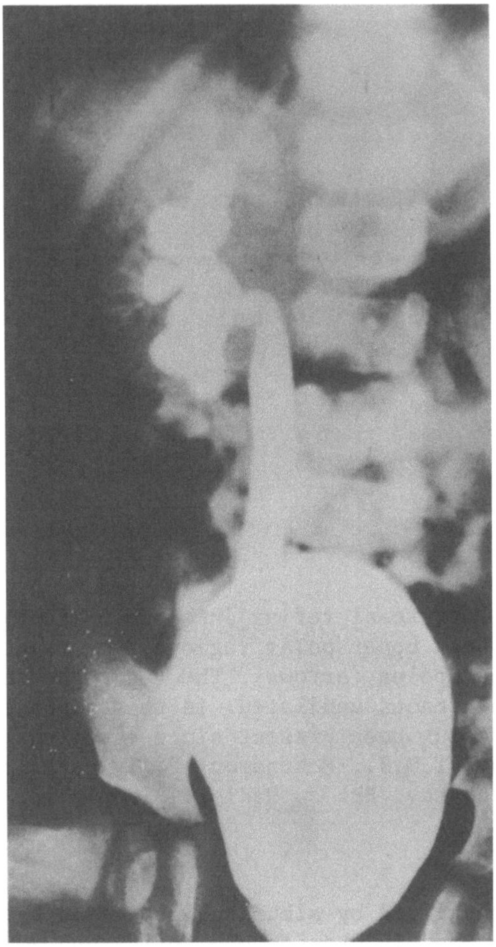

FIG. 2. Cystogram: Scattered intrarenal reflux into all zones of the right kidney of a 2-year-old girl. Here the calices and ureter show marked dilatation with early generalized narrowing of the renal substance. (From Hodson, C.J., Maling, T.M.J., McManamon, P.J., et al.: The pathogenesis of reflux nephropathy. Br. J. Radiol. Suppl. 13, 1975. Reproduced with permission).

pathy" was coined by Ross Bailey in his excellent survey of the subject and has since been receiving increasing acceptance throughout the world.

But this step forward, considerable as it is, is similar to saying "these are not individual stars, but units of a galaxy" and only serves to highlight the vast amount of work that has yet to be done to fill in the gaps so that the problem may be studied as a whole. In other words, hitherto, because such a long period of years, and therefore of clinical subdivision into neonates, children, adolescents, and young adults, is involved, the natural history of reflux nephropathy has been understressed and considered in detail rather than as a whole. It is time attention was specifically directed toward its prevention which, in turn, means its early detection.

STATISTICS

Against the complacency often expressed with regard to this disease must be set two facts. Surveys of "symptomless" schoolgirls comprising over 50,000 individuals have revealed a prevalence of reflux nephropathy of about 1 to 250 (45,53,57,68,70,84). About 10 percent of these have a bad prognosis. Of children with renal failure undergoing dialysis and transplantation (a costly and melancholy business), 20 to 30 percent have this etiology - the wide span of estimated etiology reflecting the lack of firm criteria for its diagnosis (60).

HUMAN PATHOLOGY

It is fair to say that although the diagnosis of classical "chronic atrophic" pyelonephritis presents little difficulty, as its macroscopic features are so characteristic, and that the Ask-Upmark lesion is the same, no hard and fast criteria have been established for diagnosing the more diffuse type of renal damage mentioned previously and which often causes renal failure. This may stem partly from the general tendency to neglect the findings in the lower urinary tract, namely the dilated, often thick-walled, ureters; the abnormal appearance of the ureteric orifices in the bladder, on which increasing diagnostic emphasis is being laid at cystoscopy (51,79, 59), and sometimes hypertrophy of the bladder as well.

Following the paper of Weiss and Parker (81), it was considered that the diagnosis of "chronic pyelonephritis" could be made from histology alone and even from renal biopsy. For a time this simplified approach was accepted, with resulting confusion. Now there has been a reversal of this attitude and it is recognized that many of the previously accepted histologic criteria are nonspecific. Heptinstall's timely article on "The enigma of pyelonephritis" (12) pinpointed the problem, shattered the authority of simple histologic diagnosis, and left the matter in something of a vacuum. Lack of microscopic specificity is not confined to kidney disease and it may well be that, as Heptinstall suggests, it will be necessary to consider all available data, including history, clinical findings, radiology and macroscopic appearances before a conclusive diagnosis can be achieved; particularly any type of evidence which points to present or past vesicoureteric reflux. Until this situation is clarified, such important facts as the incidence of reflux nephropathy as a cause for end-stage kidney disease in adults will remain undetermined.

Another pathologic problem is the cause of hypertension in young people with reflux nephropathy. Two papers dealing with hypertension found an incidence of reflux nephropathy in 17.4 percent of patients under the age of 40 years (12) and in 14 percent of children under the age of 15 years (23). As well, 20 percent of Smellie's cases with scarring under the age of 10 had hypertension (73). Kincaid-Smith suggested that the cause was ischemia in both the scarred and non-scarred areas secondary to arterial changes (41). The possible causes of the latter remain, however, speculative. This concept has received support recently from the growing number of published cases in which high segmental renal vein renin levels have been found in such cases (19,36-38,67,72) with relief or cure of the hypertension from segmental resection of the diseased areas, or from nephrectomy. It is also pertinent that hypertension, with similar arterial lesions, has been reproduced in the experimental pig model (42).

The matter of associated glomerulopathy is another unsolved facet of this disease, and its onset appears to herald a grave prognosis (39,40). Whether it is due to ischemia and hypertension (39) or to the persistence of atypical bacterial forms (17,87), or is a manifestation of an autoimmune process (50) or the result of reflux itself (as suggested by its occurrence in transplanted kidneys subjected to reflux (54)), or all of these things, is yet to be established. Its presence is often indicated clinically by the onset of proteinuria.

Two further features deserve mention in this brief summary. One is the apparent inexorable contraction of the fibrosis in these scars once it has reached a certain stage. When it is considered that a large piece of tissue 3 cm in thickness may contract down to a final depth of only 2 mm, the process is truly remarkable. One cannot help feeling that, whatever may cause the initial fibrosis, ischemia must play a large part in the total disappearance of the parenchyma in such large masses of tissue, although the scars are said to have vessels supplying them (63).

The second is the extensive fibrosis that occurs *outside* the parenchyma proper, particularly when infection is present. Outside the kidney, fibrosis often extends out into the perinephric fat and round the hilar structures. The lymph nodes draining the area are often enlarged. Inside the kidney, fibrosis commonly extends widely between the "internal capsule" and the parenchyma proper, running up into the perivascular spaces. In doing so it invests and compresses vascular structures, both arteries and veins, and it would be improbable that this effect is negligible. The sinus fat is also involved, though to a lesser extent. Fibrosis also extends throughout the walls of the calices, their stems, the renal pelvis and ureters, and in the suburethelial tissues throughout. It is usually assumed that this fibrosis is the result of infection and much of it may well be, but it may also be due to mature urine being forced out by high pressure reflux into the interstitium and perirenal tissues and producing the fibrogenic reaction which usually accompanies its extravasation outside its natural channels. The same phenomena are seen following simple severe obstruction.

In this context, recent experimental work is of considerable interest. By innoculating rats with their own urine, Hoyer demonstrated the development of interstitial nephritis together with high titres of IgG antibodies to Tamm-Horsfall Protein (THP) (31-32). More recently, Mayrer, et al., have produced interstitial nephritis in rabbits by repeated IV inoculations with autologous rabbit's urine (55). They have also demonstrated a cell-mediated immune reaction in these animals which is specific to THP (56). These are initial but complementary findings which may have an important bearing on the whole question of interstitial fibrosis developing in obstructed, or reflux-affected kidneys. Fasth et al. have demonstrated raised antibodies to THP in various clinical conditions in girls with the association of reflux and infection (18).

INDUCED PATHOLOGY IN PIGS

Having had the opportunity, supported by a grant from the British Medical Research Council (27), of observing the effect of complete ureteric obstruction for varying periods of time on the pig's kidney (the *only* experimental animal - including primates* - whose kidney simulates that of man by possessing multiple papillae), it was impressive to note how different these were from those associated with vesicoureteric reflux in children. But it was not until the coincidental observation of the phenomenon of "intrarenal reflux" (focal pyelotubular backflow deep into kidney) during cystography in children in 1968 and, shortly afterwards, the same thing in a piglet whose urethra had been partially obstructed, that a possible explanation of the difference between the effects on the kidney of reflux and of obstruction presented itself, particularly as the same piglet became infected and produced a focal scar in the identical region in which the intrarenal reflux had been demonstrated (30). As well, the intrarenal reflux in the children's cystograms occurred in the polar regions, into parenchymal zones which closely corresponded in extent to those involved in severe polar scarrings (Figs 1 and 2).

---

*With the notable exception of the spider monkey.

Eventually the opportunity came to try out the thesis that intrarenal reflux was a major factor in the pathogenesis of "pyelonephritic scarring," (this time under the auspices of the Canadian Medical Research Council) and an extensive experimental 6 year program was inaugurated. The results of the main program have been published (30), but the results of the long-term follow-up are still in process of preparation. Both may be summarized as follows.

Vesicoureteric reflux resulting from simply rendering the vesicoureteric orifice incompetent was of minor degree and never succeeded in distending the upper urinary tract (the musculature of the pig's bladder being a feeble thing). After six months the kidneys in these uninfected pigs still appeared macroscopically normal.

More forceful bladder contractions were then produced by causing bladder-wall hypertrophy, by controlled progressive urethral obstruction, and the more severe grades of reflux followed, together with focal intrarenal reflux. But, and this must be emphasized, the latter occurred only as a result of bladder pressures greatly increased above the normal levels (Figs. 3 and 4).

It was found that persistent *high pressure* intrarenal reflux of this type produced scars *in the absence of bacteriuria*. Whether viral infection could have complicated the issue is not known, but this appears unlikely. When bacterial infection occurred, or was deliberately induced, the scarring process was intensified.

All the pathologic manifestations of the kidney damage found in children were produced in all their details at various times in this series. Ten animals became hypertensive. Scars varying in age from 6 weeks (Fig. 5) to 4 years (Fig. 7) were obtained. In the latter, the renal parenchyma was reduced to a depth of only 2 mm over the whole of a polar region and contained no nephronic elements, only the remains of tortuous vessels of arcuate size. These severe scars thus resembled the lesions of the Ask-Upmark kidney (Fig. 6).

Intrarenal reflux occurred mainly in the polar regions where it was associated with composite papillae. It always occurred into the same papillae. In severe high-pressure cases, however, it involved *all* papillae eventually, producing a radiographic appearance similar to obstructive nephropathy, but differing noticeably in its pathology, as much more severe focal fibrosis developed where intrarenal reflux had been demonstrated than elsewhere. This severe high pressure situation was produced in 10 animals and was not studied over a prolonged period, so that its late results are as yet unknown. However, one animal developed renal failure over a period of 5 months (Fig. 8).

The early histologic changes in the scars resulting from persistent, *high pressure*, intrarenal reflux were very similar to those

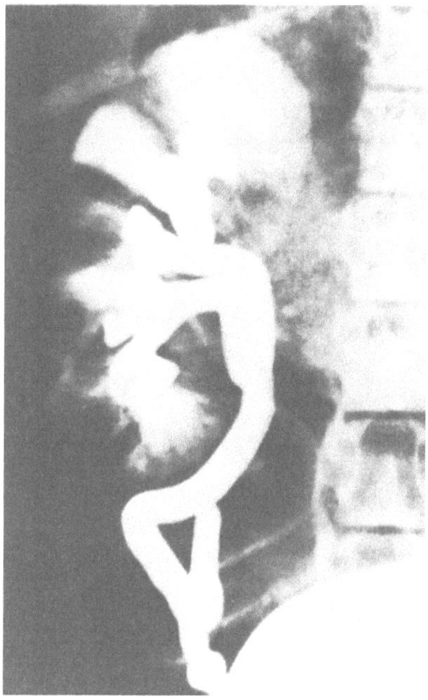

FIG. 3. Cystogram: Extensive intrarenal reflux in a pig with dilatation and tortuosity of the ureter and high bladder voiding pressure (artifically induced). Note mainly polar distribution. Infection under these circumstances will introduce bacteria deep into the kidney and "lobar nephronia" result. (From Hodson, C.J., Maling, T.M.J., McManamon, P.J., et al.: The pathogenesis of reflux nephropathy. Br. J. Radiol., Suppl. 13, 1975. Reproduced with permission).

of severe obstructive nephropathy. The changes in infected animals were similar to those described in chronic pyelonephritis in man, except that "thyroid-like" areas were minimal.

RELATIONSHIP BETWEEN EXPERIMENTAL AND CLINICAL REFLUX NEPHROPATHY

Following this fresh insight into the problem, the association between intrarenal reflux and focal renal scarring (typical reflux nephropathy) was demonstrated in children, all of whom were below the age of 5 years (64). The rarity of demonstrating intrarenal reflux after this age has since been stressed (71,73), although it has even been demonstrated occasionally in adults (4). Intrarenal reflux has also been observed in children with radiographically normal kidneys and undilated upper urinary tracts using pressures of 30 cm of contrast medium at cystography (43). Whether scars will always form later in such cases is not yet known (Fig. 1).

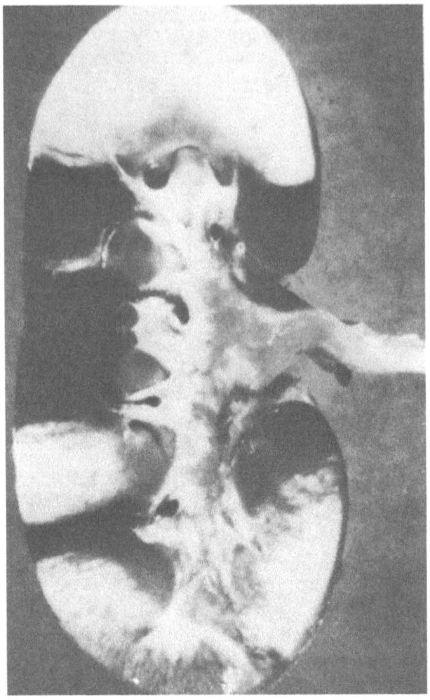

FIG. 4. "Acute lobar nephronia." The large acute lesions of acute bacterial inflammation from infected reflux in the pig. It is the subsequent contraction of these gross lesions which gives rise to the large, focal scars. Note again the mainly polar distribution. (From Margulis, A.R. and Gooding, C.A., eds.: Diagnostic Radiology, 1978. University of California, San Francisco, 1978. By permission.)

The reason for the mainly polar distribution of intrarenal reflux has also since been explained by the elegant anatomic studies of Ransley and Risdon (62,63), who showed that its occurrence related to the nature of the orifices of the ducts of Bellini both in pigs and in children. They showed these to be slit-like in simple single papillae, but to consist of widely gaping openings in the central depressions of composite papillae which commonly occur in the polar regions. Subsequently Tamminen (75) has confirmed these observations, and furthermore has shown that the dimensions of these orifices are the same in the human neonate as in the adult. Funston and Gremin (22) have also shown a direct relationship between age and the pressures required to produce intrarenal reflux in fresh human autopsy kidneys during the first year of life.

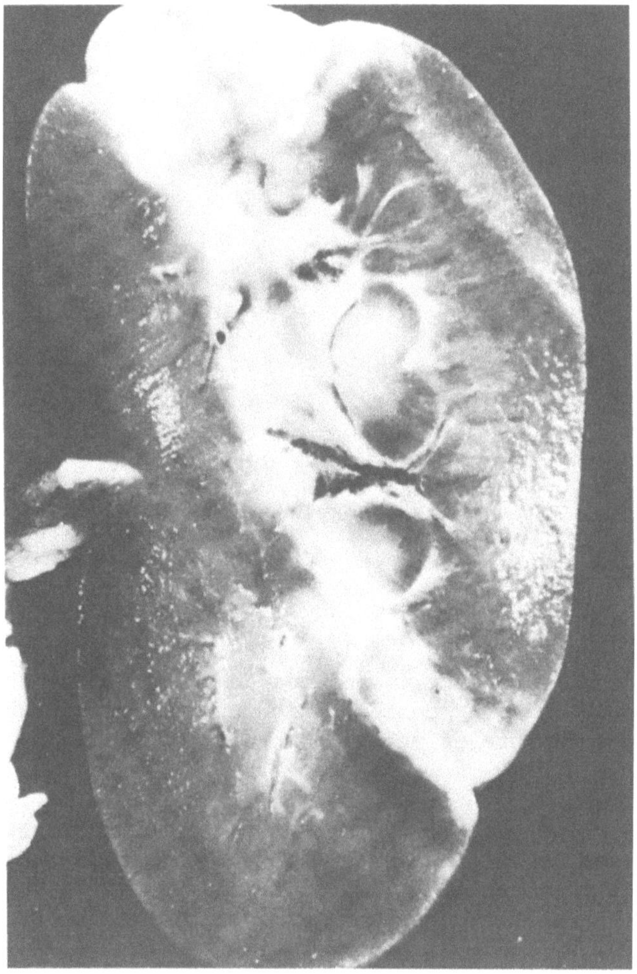

FIG. 5. Early focal scar contraction. The affected tissue is reduced to well over half its normal volume. This scar is about 2 months old. Contraction will now continue inevitable to the final 2 mm, parenchymal thickness. (From Margulis, A.R. and Gooding, C.A., eds.: Diagnostic Radiology, 1978. University of California, San Francisco. By permission.)

CONCLUSIONS FROM THESE OBSERVATIONS

It thus appears that intrarenal reflux occurs only into certain types of papillae (except in a high-pressure situation), and that the younger the kidney the more prone it is to intrarenal reflux and the lower the pressure required to produce it. Indeed, it appears probable that only a slight increase of pressure above the normal is required in the neonatal human kidney.

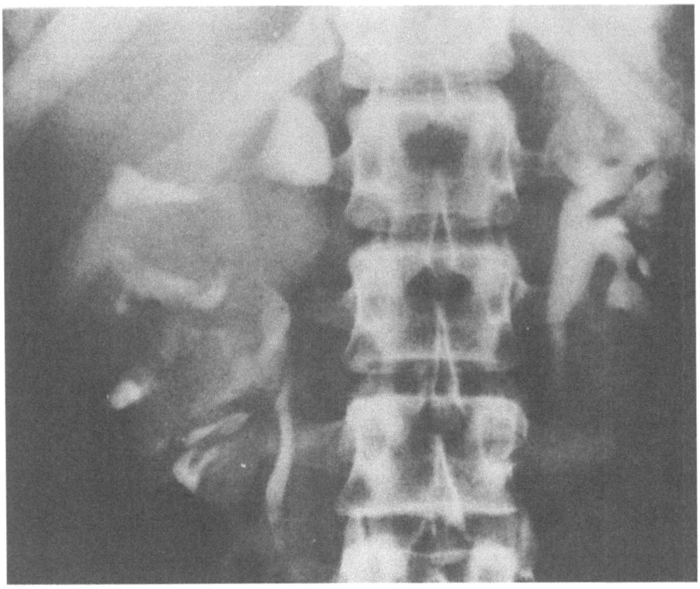

FIG. 6. The Ask-Upmark kidney. Excretion urogram in a 12 year old boy with severe hypertension. The left kidney is grossly scarred and the right renal substance is reduced to 2 to 3 mm in several lobes. Note the astonishing concentration of contrast in spite of severe damage - a feature of reflux nephropathy.

These cumulative observations also appear to highlight the immense significance of the few cystometric observations that have been carried out in infected bladders in children (2,76). The consensus of these is that the presence of cystitis may give rise to bladder pressures well above 100 cm of water. If at the same time reflux is also present the stage is set for the production of intrarenal reflux of infected urine. It is not likely that many such measurements will be made in young children while infection is still present, because of the ethics involved, but until we have firm information on this point the potential hazard of cystitis in the very young will remain conjectural, and a bogey which will haunt all those concerned with these matters.

THE SCARRING PROCESS IN MAN

In vivo human radiographic evidence accumulated over 25 years has taught us a lot about the scarring of reflux nephropathy, although there is much still to be discovered. The following observations are proferred both to provide information and to reflect some of the many aspects of this complex which are still under discussion.

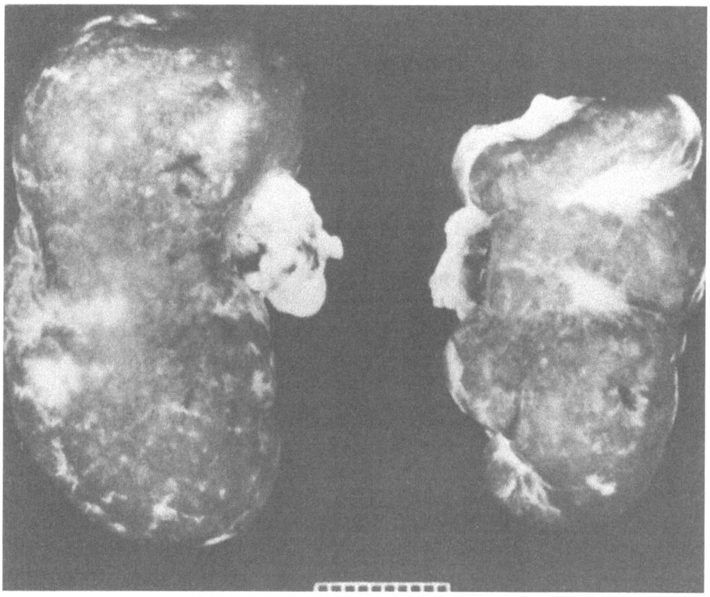

FIG. 7. End-stage scarring in a pig 4 years after production of infected reflux. The scar now contains no nephronic elements, only the remains of the previous arterial system. Animal hypertensive. Note polar, and midzone "slit scars." (From Margulis, A.R. and Gooding, C.A., eds.: Diagnostic Radiology, 1978. University of California, San Francisco. By permission.)

The Early Scar

This is commonly first seen at or before the age of 2 years (15,61,65). At this age the parenchyma of the human kidney is relatively very much thicker than in the adult (28) (Fig. 9), and it is of similar thickness in all four polar regions. The early scar can thus be readily identified by the reduction in parenchymal thickness of one or more poles compared with others (Fig. 9). Likewise, early generalized papillary damage can be distinguished by comparison with the opposite side. Because these simple facts are not understood many early cases are being missed in spite of adequate radiographs.

Will the early scar inevitably contract down to a 2 to 3 mm residual thickness? This is a matter it may be impossible to answer by radiography, as the contraction of the scar fibrosis draws across adjacent normal tissue to overlie and mask the scarred area. In the majority of cases however, the answer appears to be "yes," as only rarely are half-contracted scars seen in adults. Furthermore scarring is seen to continue to contract after reflux has been corrected surgically (20) (Fig. 10). These observations suggest that preven-

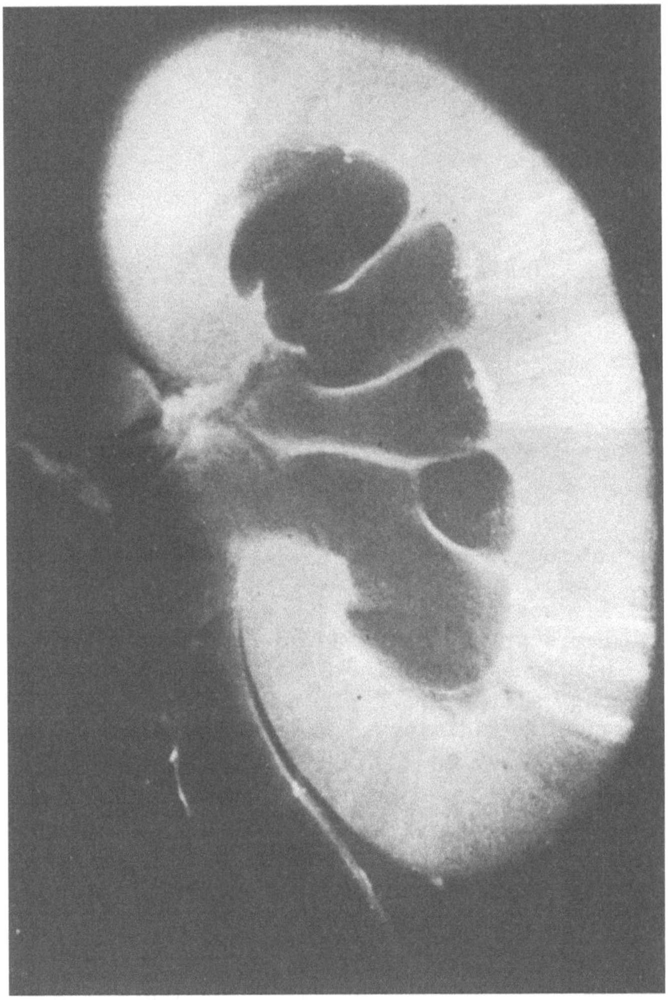

FIG. 8. Radiograph of a slice of pig's kidney subjected to severe bladder outflow obstruction reflux and intrarenal reflux for about 2 months. Immediate pre-autopsy cystogram showed scattered generalized intrarenal reflux. Note *generalized* papillary flattening and focal white streaks. These are individual ducts of Bellini which have permeated by contrast.

tion of scarring is more profitable than any form of treatment after its occurrence.

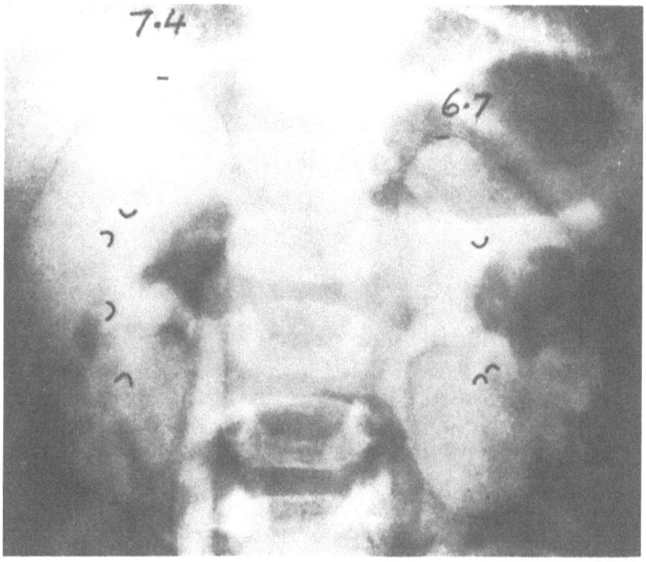

FIG. 9. Early scarring. Comparison of the 4 polar regions of this 8 month old girl, shortly after her second symptomatic urinary infection, shows obvious shrinkage of the left upper pole, even though the papilla is not yet retracted. This lesion is probably only 6 weeks, or so, old.

Patterns of Scarring

One of the most notable things about reflux nephropathy is the distribution of scarring, several varieties being commonly encountered (Fig. 11). Generalized scarring is most frequent; upper pole involvement is next, with bipolar involvement following closely. Sometimes the upper half of a kidney may be totally involved, the lower half being spared, while in total ureteric duplication the reverse is the rule. Bilateral *focal* scarring involves the two kidneys unequally, so that they are of different sizes, whereas it is not uncommon for bilateral *generalized* changes to affect them almost equally. In this context it is a fact that in a few individuals complex papillae are present throughout the kidney, and this may predispose to generalized intrarenal reflux. But it is likely that high pressure is the original main factor in these generalized changes, as exemplified by what happens when reflux complicates a high-pressure neurogenic bladder at any stage of life.

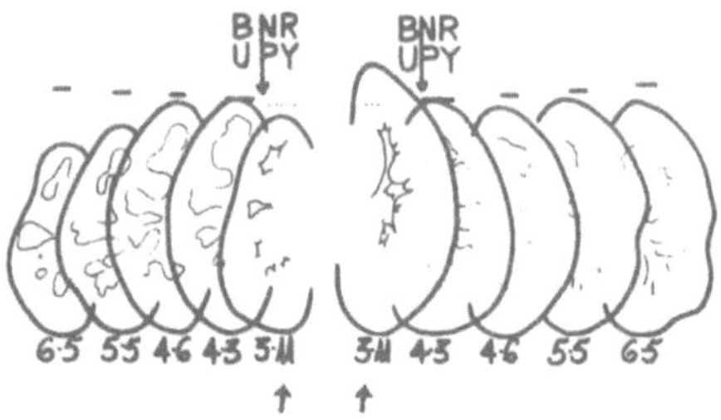

FIG. 10. Post-surgical progression of scarring. Bladder neck resection and bilateral ureteric reimplantation were performed on this girl, whose bilateral reflux was associated at the age of 4.5 months with early scarring in the upper half of the right kidney and the left upper pole. The urogram tracings show progressive decrease in size with advancing scar contraction on the right over the next 2½ years. The short line above each kidney tracing is the mean length for the child's height.

Fresh Scarring

After the age of 5, fresh scarring, i.e., scarring in a new location, is uncommon. Smellie recorded it in 10 children in her series (the members of which were on maintenance antibiotics), sometimes involving a previously normal kidney, usually coincident with a temporary gap in prophylactic treatment, and nearly always associated with reflux and one or more acute clinical episodes (73). The significance of these data is profound, as they appear to indicate that while reflux is still present, unless the urine is monitored at frequent intervals, the child remains at risk, albeit a small one, of incurring renal damage. Fresh scarring is not to be confused with the contraction of previously diseased tissue which may radiographically appear normal at the first urogram. Even if reflux is prevented such damaged tissue commonly undergoes further contraction and may continue to do so for as long as 3 years (15).

A separate problem is when reflux is produced as a result of a surgical procedure, e.g., basket removal of a ureteric stone, or fulguration near the ureteric orifice (66). If infection becomes superimposed, scarring may follow even as far as end-stage kidney disease (5).

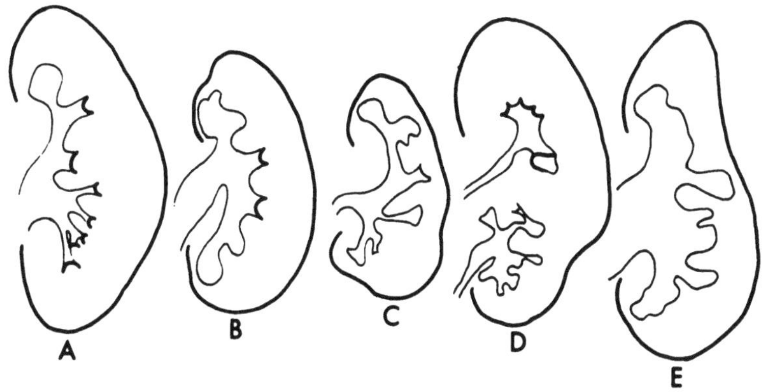

FIG. 11. Tracings of urograms: Common patterns of scarring from reflux nephropathy in man. A, advanced upper pole, early lower pole; B, bipolar, severe; C, generalized, with one spared lower pole lobe; D, severe in low portion of duplex kidney; E, generalized diffuse high-pressure effect (one of a pair of equally involved kidneys in symptomless patient with albuminuria).

HYPERTENSION

The symptoms of hypertension, headaches, dizziness, or visual disturbances, may first bring patients of all ages from 6 years onward to seek medical advice. Usually gross bilateral disease of the generalized type is present with, not infrequently, some degree of renal failure. But this is not always the case and the author has encountered four cases in which only bipolar scarring was present on one side, with hypertrophy of the opposite kidney. Nephrectomy resulted in a cure. Unfortunately these latter cases seem never to be recorded in the literature so that their prevalence is unknown. On the contrary, a number of patients with an apparently similar degree of bilateral damage may continue to eventual renal failure without any elevation of blood pressure.

Of the first 100 cases of this disease which the author documented, 49 percent had severe hypertension. Such a statistic, however, requires to be set in context. The population involved (aged 5 to 68 years) was one referred to a London teaching hospital with a well-known hypertensive clinic, and how this "cohort" relates to the general population cannot be determined. Nevertheless it coincides in degree with the two published series mentioned previously (12,23). The mean age of the hypertensive patients was 23.7 years with a range from 7 to 68 years. There is little doubt that hypertension is one of the severe complications of reflux nephropathy and that its occurrence relates largely to the degree of renal damage.

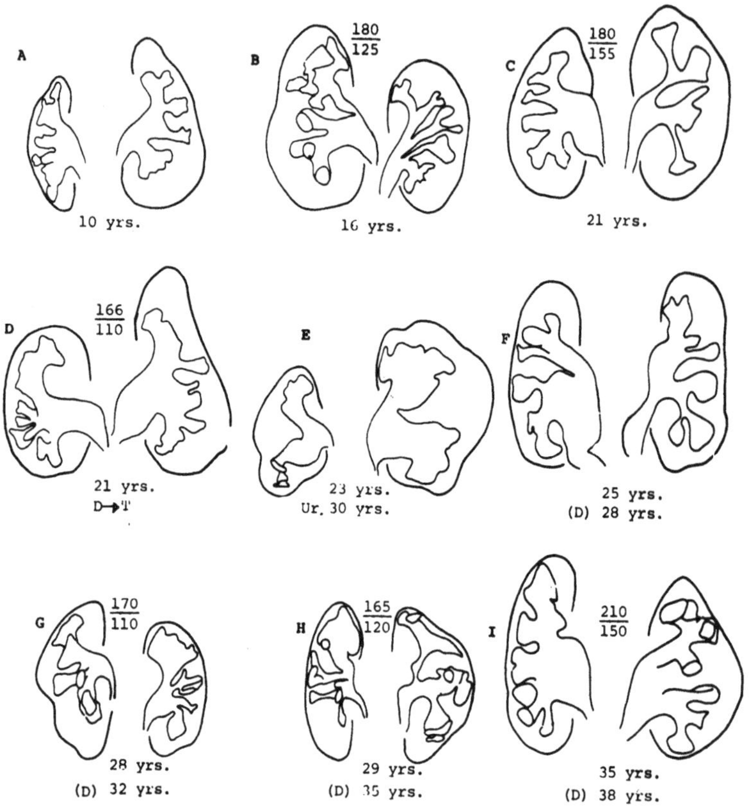

FIG. 12. Tracings of urograms of severe bilateral reflux nephropathy. D → T = dialysis and transplantation. UR, uremia. D, deceased. Blood pressures indicated. Cares B,C,D, and F were discovered on routine medical examination with albuminuria or hypertension.

RENAL FAILURE

This, too, is an aspect of this disease about which it is almost impossible yet to obtain hard data, because, as mentioned before, the criteria for its diagnosis are presently so ill-defined and are not yet on any official listing. As judged from the figures listed in the proceedings of the European Dialysis and Transplantation Association (60), reflux nephropathy probably accounts for some 30 percent of children under 16 with advanced renal failure, and 15 to 20 percent of adults below age 50 years. Its significance lies in the fact that it is the younger age groups which are mainly affected since if the kidneys are destined to fail from this disease they will mostly do so before the age of 40 years. Its financial burden, i.e., the treatment of failed kidneys, is therefore considerable.

RENAL FUNCTION AND SCARRING

From histology very little functioning tissue remains in the scars once they are even moderately contracted and yet it is a remarkable feature of many patients, even when advanced disease is present, that a) an excellent concentration of contrast medium is achieved on excretion urography (which may be the result of the water-absorbing capacity of ischemic tissue) and b) how well their general health is preserved in the presence of even severe bilateral disease. Away from the scars the laws of renal hypertrophy demand that uninvolved tissue should enlarge above the normal, and this sometimes even occurs on the side of the scarred kidney. If it remains a normal (as opposed to an increased) size it is probably involved in an ischemic process. Helin (25) has demonstrated a decrease in function (both glomerular and tubular) in prolonged sterile reflux in pigs, but only comparatively recently has the functional progress in children with reflux been studied. Aperia (6) has shown that the reduction in glomerular filtration rate relates to the area of the kidneys as measured by planimetry on radiographs. In other words, the smaller the kidneys, the worse the prognosis. This prognosis is fortified a) if the kidney fails to grow, b) if it continues to get smaller. By the same token if a kidney associated with reflux, without infection and even though scarred, has dropped into a lower growth percentile, it is at some type of risk (as yet not identified). Cure of either the infection or reflux may result in renewed growth of the kidney and recovery of an average size (85,10).

VESICOURETERIC REFLUX

This is a phenomenon about which very much has been written on an empirical basis without due control observations, which admittedly are very difficult, or ethically impossible, to perform in the child. It has been graded into 3, 4 or 5 grades of severity, but the factors governing these categories have never been satisfactorily explained. It is known that bacterial endotoxins will cause ureteric dilatation (77) and therefore tend to increase the grading severity, but what determines whether reflux is grade 2 or grade 3 has not been determined. Age may be one factor, as the upper urinary tract in the very young child is much more readily distensible than the mature ureter. The duration of reflux may be another. But both in the experimental animal and in man there is considerable evidence that pressure is perhaps the most important of all. This is a complex subject which cannot be detailed here, but the fact that it is usually the more severe grades that are associated with kidney damage, particularly the more generalized form, is in itself highly suggestive. That such reflux is sometimes designated "low pressure" because it occurs readily during bladder filling - often up wide-open ureteric orifices - may be entirely fallacious. It may, on the contrary, be the result of prolonged high-pressure reflux, and is usually associated with severe renal damage (46).

Most people personally conducting repeated cystograms are aware of the variability of reflux grading in the same individual from time to time. It may even be absent at one examination between two others in which grade 4 is demonstrated. Moreover, the techniques used for its demonstration vary widely between centers, and may even be left to technicians to perform. Inevitably the examination is conducted after infection has been treated, and the true state of affairs operating when infection is present must thereby be at least modified, if not significantly altered. An equivalent is carrying out radiography of the chest 4 weeks after a pneumonia has been treated. Often the results of surgery are assessed by the decrease in the amount of dilatation of the upper urinary tracts. This is certainly valuable, but it is the status of the kidney, after all, which is the final arbiter.

Is reflux ever congenital? It most certainly can be in cases of posterior urethral valves, as it is sometimes demonstrable in gross form at the age of 1 to 2 weeks of life, with gaping ureteric orifices which can scarcely have developed in such a short period. Indeed its presence in utero appears to be the logical explanation of the "dysplastic" kidney changes found above grossly dilated tortuous ureters, at or shortly after birth, in similar cases. Acton and Drew have also found hyalinized glomeruli in a 6 week old baby with reflux and infection (1). Whether these could develop in 6 weeks seems improbable.

Is reflux ever the result of infection? It certainly can be in tuberculosis, and it appeared to follow the onset of chemically induced cystitis in one child, so that bacterial cystitis might be expected to render the ureteric orifice incompetent and so induce reflux. It is a point on which obviously it is difficult to obtain hard data. The issue is now further complicated by the possibility that infection may give rise to bladder dyssynergia from sphincter spasm in the very young and so introduce the factor of raised pressures and the increased likelihood of reflux (44,3,78,31). On the contrary even severe reflux may cease in some children with repeated infections (8), which is an important observation. It does not appear that evidence is conclusive either one way or another.

It seems possible that the present progressive evolution of pressure-and-flow studies of the lower urinary tract will provide a much more solid basis for evaluating the factors involved in the persistence and grade, if not the actual production, of reflux.

SUMMARY

Reflux nephropathy is probably the most common kidney disease in children. It is usually diagnosed when scarring is already present. Its prevention calls for a nationwide institution by parents to look for any disorder of the infant's stream, frequent diaper wetting, and foul smelling urine. Simple home bacteriologic screening is a practical possibility. Certainly any child with fever, whatever the symptoms, should have a urine culture performed as a routine, before treatment with antibiotics. The treatment of its complications is a major sum to any national health-care budget.

Many aspects of its pathophysiology are as yet incompletely understood although enormous strides have been made in recent years. The arguments of surgery (ureteral reimplantation) versus prolonged antimicrobial prophylaxis are not yet fully defined because of a lack of factual detail regarding prolonged follow-up and the stage at which surgery may be effective.

The underlying renal damage probably relates to the pressure at which reflux reaches the kidney as well as whether infection is present or not. It also relates to the papillary morphology of any particular kidney. In some families, up to 40% of individuals may be affected, although factors governing its inheritance are not yet clear.

Interest in, and concern about, this disease are growing all over the civilized world. Its eradication should be a major medical objective.

REFERENCES

1. Acton, C.M. and Drew, J.H.: Vesico-ureteric reflux in the neonatal Period. _In_ Hodson, C.J. and Kincaid-Smith, P. (eds.): Reflux Nephropathy. New York: Masson Publishing, U.S.A., Inc., 1979, chap. 7.

2. Allan, T.: Urodynamic patterns in children with dysfunctional voiding problems. J. Urol. 117: 247-249, 1978.

3. Allen, T.D.: Vesicoureteral reflux as a manifestation of dysfunctional Voiding. _In_ Hodson, C.J. and Kincaid-Smith, P. (eds.): Reflux Nephropathy. New York: Masson Publishing, U.S.A., Inc., 1979, chap. 18.

4. Amar, A.D.: Calicotubular backflow with vesico-ureteral reflux. JAMA 213: 293-294, 1970.

5. Amar, A.D., Singer, B. and Lewis, R.: Vesico-ureteral reflux in adults. A twelve year study of 122 patients. Urol. 3: 184-189, 1974.

6. Aperia, A., Broberger, O., and Ekengren, K.: Correlation between kidney parenchymal area and renal function in vesicoureteral reflux of different degrees. Ann. de Radiol. 12: 141-144, 1977.

7. Arant, B.S., Jr., Sotelo, Avilia C. and Bernstein, J.: Segmental "Hypoplasia" of the Kidney (Ask-Upmark). J. Pediatr. 95: 931-939, 1979.

8. Ask-Upmark, E.: Uber juvenile maligne Nephrosklerose und ihr Verhaltnis zu Störungen in der Nierenentwicklung. Acta Pathol. Microbiol. Scand. 6: 383-442, 1929.

9. Bailey, R.R.: The relationship of vesico-ureteric reflux to urinary tract infection and chronic pyelonephritis - reflux nephropathy. Clin. Nephrol. 1(3): 132-141, 1973.

10. Bauer, S.B., Willscher, M.K, et al.: Long-term Results of Antireflux Surgery in Children. In Hodson, C.J. and Kincaid-Smith, P. (eds.): Reflux Nephropathy. New York: Masson Publishing, U.S.A., Inc., 1979, chap. 29.

11. Benz, G., Willich, E. and Scharer, K.: Segmental renal hypoplasia in childhood. Pediatr. Radiol. 5: 86-92, 1976.

12. Breckenridge, A., Preger, L., Dollery, C.T. et al.: Hypertension in the young. Quart. J. Med. 36: 144, October 1967.

13. Dein, R.W., Walker, D. and Hackett, R.L.: The Ask-Upmark kidney. A case report. Arch. Pathol. 96: 10-13, 1973.

14. Dent, C.W. and Hodson, C.J.: Radiological changes associated with certain metabolic bone diseases. Br. J. Radiol. 27: 605-618, 1976.

15. Drew, J.H. and Acton, C.M.: Radiological findings in newborn infants with urinary infection. Arch. Dis. Child. 51: 628, 1976.

16. Dworskin, J.Y.: Sibling uropathology. J. Urol. 115: 726-727, 1976.

17. Fairley, K.F., Becker, G.F., Butler, H.M. et al.: Diagnosis in the difficult case. Kidney Int. 8(Suppl. 4): S12-S19, 1975.

18. Fasth, A., Hanson, L.A. et al.: Autoantibodies to Tamm-Horsfall Protein associated with urinary tract infection in girls. J. Pediatr. 95: 54-60, 1979.

19. Fikri, E., Hanrahan, J.B. and Strept, L.A.: Renovascular hypertension in a child: Ask-Upmark Kidney. J. Urol. 110: 728-731, 1973.

20. Filly, R., Friedland, G.N., Govan, D.E. et al.: Urinary tract infections in children. Part II. Roentgenologic aspects. West J. Med. 121: 366-373, 1974.

21. Frey, R.N., Patel, H.R. and Parsons, V.: Familial renal tract abnormalities and cortical scarring. Nephron 12: 188-196, 1974.

22. Funston, M.: Post-mortem studies of intrarenal reflux in children's kidneys. Abstract No. S.0094. Book of Abstracts. 6th Int. Congress of Radiol., 1977.

23. Gill, D.G., Mendes da Costa, B., Cameron, J.S. et al.: Analysis of 100 children with severe and persistent hypertension. Arch. Dis. Child. 51: 951-957, 1976.

24. Habib, R., Courtecuisse, V., Ehrensperger, J. et al.: Hypoplasie segmentaire du rein avec hypertension arterielle chez l'enfant. Ann. de Pediatr. 12: 262-279, 1965.

25. Helin, I.: Clinical and experimental studies on vesico-ureteric reflux: Thesis. Lund, 1975.

26. Heptinstall, R.H.: The enigma of chronic pyelonephritis. J. Infect. Dis. 120: 104-107, 1969.

27. Hodson, C.J., Craven, J.D., Lewis, D.G. et al.: Experimental obstructive nephropathy in the pig. Br. J. Urol., Suppl. 6, 1969.

28. Hodson, C.J., Davies, Z. and Prescod, A.: Renal parenchymal radiographic measurement in infants and children. Pediatr. Radiol. 3: 16-19, 1975.

29. Hodson, C.J. and Edwards, D.: Chronic pyelonephritis and vesico-ureter reflux. Clin. Radiol. 11: 219-231, 1960.

30. Hodson, C.J., Maling, T.M.J., McManamon, P.J. et al.: The pathogenesis of reflux nephropathy. Br. J. Radiol., Suppl. 13, 1975.

31. Hoyer, J.R.: Autoimmune tubulo-interstitial nephritis induced in rats by immunization with Tamm-Horsfall Urinary Glycoprotein. Kidney Int. 10: 544, 1976.

32. Hoyer, J.R. and Seiler, M.W.: Pathophysiology of Tamm-Horsfall Protein. Kidney Int. 16: 279-289, 1979.

33. Hunt, J.S. and McGiven, A.R.: Stimulation of human peripheral blood lymphocytes by Tamm-Horsfall Urinary Protein. Immunol. 35: 391-395, 1978.

34. Hutch, J.A., Hinman, F., Jr., and Miller, E.R.: Reflux as a cause of hydronephrosis and chronic pyelonephritis. J. Urol. 88: 169-175, 1962.

35. Hutch, J.A. and Smith, D.R.: Sterile reflux. Urol. Int. 24: 460-465, 1969.

36. Javapour, N., Doppman, J.L., Scardino, P.T. et al.: Segmental renal vein assay and segmental nephrectomy for correction of renal hypertension. J. Urol. 115: 580-582, 1976.

37. Johnston, J.H. and Mix, L.W.: The Ask-Upmark kidney: a form of ascending pyelonephritis? Br. J. Urol. 48: 393-398, 1976.

38. Kaufman, J. and Fay, R.: Renal hypertension in children. In Johnston, J.H. and Goodwin, W.E.(eds.): Reviews in Paediatric Urology. Amsterdam, Excerpta Medica 207: 240, 1974.

39. Kimmelstiel, P. and Wilson, C.: Inflammatory lesions in the glomeruli in pyelonephritis in relation to hypertension and renal insufficiency. Am. J. Pathol. 12: 99-105, 1936.

40. Kincaid-Smith, P.: Glomerular lesions in atrophic pyelonephritis and reflux nephropathy. Kidney Int. 8(Suppl. 4): S81-S83, 1975.

41. Kincaid-Smith, P.: Vascular obstruction in chronic pyelonephritis kidneys and its relation to hypertension. Lancet 1: 1263-1269, 1955.

42. Kincaid-Smith, P. and Hodson, C.J.: In preparation.

43. Klauber, G.T.: Personal communication.

44. Koff, S.A., Lapides, J. and Piazza, D.H.: The uninhibited bladder in children: A cause for urinary obstruction, infection, and reflux. In Hodson, C.J. and Kincaid-Smith, P. (eds.): Reflux Nephropathy. New York: Masson Publishing, U.S.A., Inc., 1979, chap. 17.

45. Kunin, C.M.: Epidemiology and natural history of urinary tract infection in school age children. Pediatr. Clin. N. Am. 8: 509-528, 1971.

46. Lattimer, J.K., Apperson, J.W., Gleason, D.M. et al.: The pressure at which reflux occurs, an important indication of prognosis and treatment. J. Urol. 89: 395-404, 1963.

47. Lewy, P.R. and Belman, A.B.: Familiar occurrence of non-obstructive, noninfectious, vesicoureteral reflux with renal scarring. J. Pediatr. 86: 851-856, 1974.

48. Ljungquist, A. and Lagergren, C.: The Ask-Upmark kidney. A congenital renal anomaly studied by micro-angiography and histology. Acta Pathol. Microbiol. Scand. 56: 277-283, 1962.

49. Longcope, W.T. and Winkenwerder, W.L.: Clinical features of the contracted kidney due to pyelonephritis. Bull. Johns Hopkins Hosp. 53: 255-287, 1933.

50. Losse, H., Intorp, H.W., Lison, H.E. et al.: Evidence of an autoimmune mechanism in pyelonephritis. Kidney Int. 8(Suppl. 4): S44-S49, 1975.

51. Lyon, R.P., Marshall, S. and Tanagho, E.A.: The ureteric orifice: Its configuration and competence. J. Urol. 102: 504-509, 1969.

52. Lyon, R.P., Marshall, S. and Tanagho, E.A.: Theory of maturation: A critique. J. Urol. 103: 795-800, 1970.

53. McLachlan, M.S.F., Meller, S.T., Jones, E.R.V. et al.: Urinary tract infection in school girls with covert bacteriuria. Arch. Dis. Child. 150: 253-258, 1975.

54. Mathew, T.H., Mathews, D.C., Hobbs, J.B. et al.: Glomerular lesions after renal transplantation. Am. J. Med. 59: 177-190, 1975.

55. Mayrer, A.R., Kashgarian, M. et al.: Tubulointersitial nephritis and Tamm-Horsfall Antibody in rabbits challenged with homologous urine. (In press).

56. Mayrer, A.R., Ruddle, N. et al.: Tubulointerstitial nephritis and cell mediated immunity to Tamm-Horsfall Protein in rabbits challenged with homologous urine. (In press).

57. Meadow, S.R., White, R.H.R. and Johnston, N.M.: Prevalence of symptomless urinary tract disease in Birmingham schoolchildren. Br. Med. J. 3: 81, 1969.

58. Miller, H.C. and Caspari, E.W.: Ureteral reflux as a genetic trait. JAMA 220: 842-846, 1972.

59. Perale, R., Passerin, G. and Rizzoni, G.: Correlations between radiological and endoscopic findings in reflux nephropathy. Am. Radiol. 21: 241-247, 1978.

60. Proceedings of the European Dialysis and Transplant Association, 1976.

61. Randolph, M.F., Morris, K.E. and Gould, E.G.: The first urinary tract infection in the female infant. Prevalence, recurrence, and prognosis: a 10-year study in private practice. J. Pediatr. 86: 342-348, 1975.

62. Ransley, P.G. and Risdon, R.A.: Renal papillary morphology and intrarenal reflux in the young pig. Urol. Res. 3: 105-109, 1975.

63. Ransley, P.G. and Risdon, R.A.: Renal papillary morphology in infants and young children. Urol. Res. 3: 110-113, 1975.

64. Rolleston, G.L., Maling, T.M.J. and Hodson, J.: Intrarenal reflux and the scarred kidney. Arch. Dis. Child. 49: 531-539, 1974.

65. Rolleston, G.L., Shannon, F.T. and Utley, W.L.F.: Relationship of infantile vesicouretic reflux and renal damage. Br. Med. J. 21: 460-463, 1970.

66. Roper, B.A. and Smith, J.C.: Vesico-ureteric reflux following operations on the ureteric orifice. Br. J. Urol. 37: 531-534, 1965.

67. Rosenfield, J.F., Cohen, L., Garity, L. et al.: Unilateral renal hypoplasia with hypertension. (Ask-Upmark Kidney). Br. Med. J. 2: 217-218, 1973.

68. Savage, D.C.L., Wilson, M.I., McHardy, M. et al.: Covert bacteriuria in childhood. A clinical and epidemiological study. Arch. Dis. Child. 43: 8-20, 1973.

69. Scott, J.E.S. and Stansfeld, J.M.: Ureteric reflux and scarring in children. Arch. Dis. Child. 43: 468-470, 1968.

70. Selkon, J. et al.: Asymptomatic bacteriuria in school children in Newcastle-upon-Tyne. Newcastle Asymptomatic Bacteriuria Research Group. Arch. Dis. Child. 50: 2, 1975.

71. Shah, K.J., Robins, D.G. and White, R.H.R.: Renal scarring and vesico-ureteric reflux. Arch. Dis. Child. 53: 210-218, 1978.

72. Siegler, R.N.: Malignant hypertension in children with chronic pyelonephritis. Laboratory and radiologic indications for partial or total nephrectomy. Urol. 7: 474-477, 1976.

73. Smellie, M., Edwards, D., Hunter, N. et al.: Vesico-ureteric reflux and renal scarring. Kidney Int. 8(Suppl. 4): S65-S72, 1975.

74. Staemmler, M. and Dopheide, W.: Virch. Arch. Path. Ant. Physiol. 277: 713-756, 1930.

75. Tamminen, T.E. and Kapiro, E.A.: The relation of the shape of renal papillae and of collecting duct openings to intrarenal reflux. Br. J. Urol. 49: 345-353, 1977.

76. Tanagho, E.A., Miller, E.R., Lyon, R.P. et al.: Spastic external sphincter and urinary tract infection in girls. Br. J. Urol. 43: 69-82, 1971.

77. Teague, N. and Boyarsky, S.: Further effects of coliform bacteria on ureteral peristalsis. J. Urol. 99: 720-726, 1968.

78. Van Gool, J.D.: Bladder infection and pressure. In Hodson, C.J. and Kincaid-Smith, P. (eds.): Relux Nephropathy. New York: Masson Publishing, U.S.A., Inc., 1979, chap. 19.

79. Vermillion, C.D. and Heale, W.F.: Position and configuration of the ureteral orifice and its relationship to renal scarring in adults. J. Urol., 1973.

80. Wagner, E.L.: Handbuch der Krankheiten des Harnapparates. I. Der Morbus Bright. In von Ziemssen, H.W.: Handbuch der speziellen Pathologie und Therapie. 9: 309-315 (Vogel, Leipzig, 1882).

81. Weiss, S. and Parker, F., Jr.: Pyelonephritis: Its relation to vascular lesions and to arterial hypertension. Medicine 18: 221-315, 1939.

82. Williams, D.I.: Urology in Childhood. New York: Springer, 1974, p. 135.

83. Williams, D.I.: Paediatric Urology. London: Butterworths, 1968, pp. 181-182.

84. Winberg, J., Andersen, H.J., Bergstrom, T. et al.: Epidemiology of symptomatic infection in childhood. Acta Paediatr. Scand. Suppl. 252, 1974.

85. Winberg, J., Claesson, I. et al.: Renal growth after acute pyelonephritis in childhood: An epidemiological approach. In Hodson, C.J. and Kincaid-Smith, P. (eds.): Reflux Nephropathy. New York: Masson Publishing, U.S.A., Inc., 1979, chap. 20.

86. Zel, F. and Retik, A.B.: Familial vesico-ureteral reflux. Urology 2: 249-252, 1973.

87. Zimmerman, S.W., Uehling, D.T. and Burkholder, P.M.: Vesico-ureteral reflux nephropathy. Evidence for immunologically mediated nephropathy. Urology 11: 534-538, 1973.

HIGHLIGHTS

ROLE OF REFLUX IN RENAL DAMAGE

Robert H. Heptinstall, M.D.

Department of Pathology
John Hopkins University
School of Medicine
Baltimore, Maryland, 21205 USA

Reflux of urine up the ureters provides a way in which infection can be conveyed to the kidney from an infected bladder. Once infected urine reaches the pelvi-calyceal system it may invade the parenchyma by one of several routes. In the first place it may invade the parenchyma by reflux up the ducts of Bellini, the so-called intrarenal reflux or calicotubular reflux. In the rat the kidney may be invaded in the fornicial region close to the insertion of the calyceal wall and it is likely that this also occurs in the newborn. Invasion via the veins - pyelovenous route - is also considered possible but is not so well documented as the other routes. Once infection has been established in the kidney remarkable degrees of tubular destruction take place and the acute inflammatory focus heals with considerable scar formation.

It has also been claimed that reflux of sterile urine up the ureter can lead to renal damage and scar formation, but this contention is controversial.

HIGHLIGHTS

SEGMENTAL HYPOPLASIA WITH HYPERTENSION (ASK-UPMARK KIDNEY)

Renée Habib, M.D. and Michel Broyer, M.D.

Institut National de la Santé et de la Recherche Médicale
Hôpital Necker Enfants-Malades, Paris, France

We report 27 patients who presented with segmental hypoplasia (SH) and hypertension. Twenty were girls and hypertension was rarely discovered before 8 years of age. Corticopapillary scarring was unilateral in 7 cases and bilateral in the remaining 20. Nephrectomy performed in 11 cases led to normalization of blood pressure (BP) in only 4. Death occurred in 2, BP was well controlled in 2 and poorly controlled in 3. The remaining 16 children were treated with hypotensive drugs. At latest followup, 8 had progressed to terminal failure and 6 had a well controlled BP with stable renal function. In one patient there was a decreased GFR while BP was well controlled and in the remaining one, renal function was stable while BP was poorly controlled.

The radiological findings which suggest the presence of SH are: the association of notching of the kidney outline with occasional amputation of the superior pole, together with thinning of the renal cortex in these notched areas as well as pyelocalyceal abnormalities, the most common of which are blunting and clubbing of a hypotonic calyx. The size of the scarred kidneys, calculated according to Hodson's formula, is usually decreased. However, a normal sized kidney, having even limited pyelocalyceal abnormalities must be considered as affected. In fact, the disease is exceptionally unilateral. It most often predominates on one side and the best criteria for normality of the contralateral kidney, besides the absence of pyelocalyceal abnormalities, is a kidney of increased size with functional compensatory hypertrophy quantifiable by the test of fixation of mercury.

Even though these findings are suggestive of SH, they are not pathognomonic of the disease. They merely indicate the presence of segmental scars, the precise nature of which can only be determined by histopathologic examination. Three main patterns, each implying a different pathogenic process, may show similar macroscopic changes. The first one is a developmental anomaly of some renicules as evidenced by the presence of dysplastic structures in the papilla and an ill-developed overlying cortex. The second one, characterized by an extensive inflammatory process, is chronic pyelonephritis. Both conditions, which may be associated, are mainly observed in patients with recurrent urinary tract infections and obstructive or nonobstructive malformation of the urinary tract. The third one is SH. The scars of SH are characterized by a thyroid-like transformation of tubules and tortuous and obstructed vessels in the cortex and by a "desertic" papilla. This pathologic entity is often but not always associated with hypertension.

The nature of the scars of SH is still a controversial matter. In the absence of dysplastic structures it is not possible to conclude that they are due to a developmental anomaly. However, the peculiar structure of the papillae of the scarred segments indicates that they might be congenitally abnormal. In the absence of an inflammatory process it seems unlikely that the scar is related to an ascending bacterial infection of the kidney. Therefore, the term "chronic pyelonephritis" often used to designate such scars seems inappropriate. There is increasing evidence that intrarenal reflux may play a role in the development of the specific scars of SH, but more clinical, pathological and experimental data are necessary in order to confirm their relationship. Coarsely scarred kidneys do not represent a single entity and although often associated with reflux, the scars may not always be directly related to it.

From a practical point of view, nephrectomy should be performed only if the contralateral kidney is normal, i.e. in compensatory hypertrophy. Progression to renal failure in patients affected with this disease is not related to newly formed scars but rather to the progressive glomerular involvement in the "spared" zones.

HIGHLIGHTS

GLOMERULAR INVOLVEMENT SECONDARY TO VESICO-URETERAL REFLUX (VUR)

Gustavo Gordillo-Paniagua, M.D.

Div. Pediatr. Nephrol., Hosp. Infantil Mexico, Mexico

City, Mexico

Two girls, 15 and 13 years old respectively, with long-standing VUR ended in chronic renal failure. The first case was diagnosed to have bilateral grade III VUR at the age of 5 years. Reimplantation of the ureters was done twice with unsuccessful results. Mild reduction of GFR, inability to concentrate the urine, normal blood pressure and proteinuria below 0.5 g/liter were stable until the age of 9 years when the patient suddenly deteriorated. Severe hypertension developed and proteinuria increased tenfold. She started on dialysis and after bilateral nephrectomy, she was transplanted with a related donor kidney. She is doing well 5 years after transplantation. Her excised kidneys showed severe tubulointerstitial nephritis as well as "crescentic" glomerulonephritis. Ig antibodies and complement in granular pattern were detected in the tubular walls and in the glomerular capillaries. These findings explain the abrupt development of a rapidly progressive glomerulonephritis superimposed on a reflux nephropathy resulting after long-standing VUR.

The second case, presented as chronic renal failure and then she was known to have VUR. She was put on hemodialysis and nephrectomized. She died of post-surgical complications. Her excised kidneys showed interstitial fibrosis edema and mononuclear cell infiltration. Most glomeruli were sclerotic and "crescents" were seen in some of them. Immunofluorescence showed antibodies, complement, and RTE antigen in both tubules and glomeruli. TBM antigen was positive only in the tubules. These facts suggested that tubular damage resulting from long-standing sterile VUR released renal tubular epithelial antigen and antibodies that were trapped in the glomeruli causing glomerular injury. Very few reports on this subject are in the literature and are much more experimental. Clinical bases are needed for better understanding of the mechanism of glomerular involvement secondary to VUR. The hypothesis derived from this study provides a possible explanation for the progression of the renal lesion to chronic renal failure.

TREATMENT OF BACTERIAL URINARY TRACT INFECTION IN CHILDHOOD

Helen M. Gorman, M.B., B.Ch., Gaston E. Zilleruelo, M.D.
Rafael Galindez, M.D. and José Strauss, M.D.

Div. Pediatr. Nephrol., Dept. Pediatr., Univ. Miami Sch. Med., Miami, Fla. 33152 USA

The accurate identification and appropriate therapy of urinary tract infection (UTI) in childhood have been subjected to continuous scrutiny over the past two decades. Appreciation of the variability of clinical presentation, refinement of diagnostic methods and better understanding of conditions which predispose to renal parenchymal scarring have facilitated patient management.

Clinical manifestations of UTI are often indeterminate, particularly in the first two years of life. Infants may present with irritability, feeding difficulties, colic, vomiting, diarrhea, poor weight gain or jaundice (1); unexplained fever, recurrent abdominal or back pain and secondary enuresis are common symptoms in older children (2). Jaundice has been reported as a presenting feature (3,4). Classical symptoms of cystitis such as dysuria, frequency and urgency may be present; macroscopic hematuria may occur. However, symptoms may be totally absent in any age group.

The clinical presentation is not a reliable indicator of site or severity of infection, or of the possibility of permanent renal damage. Therefore, final decisions about therapy must be made after the pathogenic organism has been isolated, and not be based only on symptomatology. Initial therapeutic approaches vary, and may be categorized in a descending order of urgency, as follows:

1. <u>Possible sepsis</u>. All neonates and any children suspected of having sepsis must be admitted for treatment. After urine and blood cultures have been obtained, parenteral therapy with broad-spectrum antibiotic coverage, ampicillin plus gentamycin (5) or tobramycin, should be given. Subsequently, culture results may indicate a single, appropriate antibiotic; treatment should be altered accordingly.

2. Gastrointestinal symptoms. Children of any age whose infection is associated with vomiting, diarrhea or severe abdominal pain also warrant parenteral therapy as soon as urine cultures have been obtained. Initial choice of antibiotic should be ampicillin or a cephalosporin since the most common pathogens of the urinary tract are usually sensitive to these.

3. Other symptoms. Individuals with distressing symptoms such as fever, flank pain, urgency and dysuria may be given antibacterial treatment before culture results are available. If symptoms are mild, treatment should await results of urine culture. Oral therapy is appropriate. Agents which may be used are sulfisoxazole, ampicillin, amoxicillin, cotrimoxazole, nitrofurantoin or cephalexin (6). Sulfisoxazole is by far the least expensive, and usually is well-tolerated.

4. No symptoms. Treatment of children with asymptomatic bacteriuria should await confirmation of infection by repeat urine culture if collection was by voiding. Oral therapy is indicated.

Supportive treatment should be offered to all symptomatic children. A generous fluid intake is important since promotion of diuresis will tend to ameliorate dysuria and may expedite removal of bacteria multiplying in the urine. Acidification or alkalinization of urine is not necessary; in practical terms, efficacy of the antibacterial agents noted above is independent of urine pH.

In all children without prior history of urinary tract infection and in those with known or suspected compromise of renal function, serum creatinine and urea nitrogen should be determined at the beginning of treatment. Patients with abnormal levels of creatinine, urea nitrogen or glomerular filtration rate may require modification of the dosage of antibiotic administered. This will be described in a later section. Antibiotic therapy is generally given for ten to fourteen days after which time the urine is again cultured (7). Cultures should be repeated sooner if lack of response to treatment is suspected. Although shorter courses have been proposed and may be sufficient to eradicate infections which are confined to the lower urinary tract (8,9,10), they are as yet not recommended for children. Currently, non-invasive methods of localizing the site of infection are not sufficiently specific to guide duration of therapy (11,12,13,14).

Within one to two weeks following conclusion of successful treatment of a first-documented infection in any child, intravenous pyelogram and voiding cystourethrogram should be performed. When infection has not responded to appropriate medical treatment or if an unusual organism has been found, these two studies should be carried out without delay for discovery of structural anomalies which may require immediate surgical intervention. It has been found that lack of response often is caused by obstruction of the urinary tract.

The term "first-documented" infection is used because one cannot be certain that significant bacteriuria, either intermittent or persistent, did not exist before a child's condition was first diagnosed. The anatomy and functional capacity of the urinary tract should be characterized following elimination of the first-documented infection. This applies to both sexes and any age, although the likelihood of finding a significant abnormality is considerably greater in boys (15,16,17).

An approach to management of children after treatment of the first-documented infection is diagramed in Figure 1. In children with normal urinary tracts, infection may be defined as uncomplicated, and in those with anomalies of structure and/or function, complicated. Anomalies may be further categorized as minor or major. Minor anomalies are those not associated with reduced parenchymal mass or urinary stasis and may include certain cases of horseshoe kidney, renal ectopia, bladder diverticulum, and incomplete duplication. Major anomalies include parenchymal scarring, hypoplastic, dysplastic and cystic kidney, vesicoureteral reflux, and any other condition leading to urinary stasis whether functional or anatomic.

UNCOMPLICATED INFECTION OR COMPLICATED INFECTION WITH MINOR ANOMALIES

For at least three years following elimination of the last documented infection, urine cultures should be obtained every four to six weeks for six months, and thereafter at intervals of diminishing frequency (18). Recurrences are common and may be asymptomatic (7,19,20). The longer the interval between infections, the less likelihood there is of recurrence (21). Any reinfection should be treated as the "first" infection and the followup period extended accordingly.

Two years after the first study, radiologic evaluation may be repeated to determine whether or not renal scarring has occurred. This re-evaluation should be performed earlier if recurrences of infection are frequent and in all children with minor anomalies. A child in whom scarring has developed should then be managed according to the scheme described for those with major anomalies.

In recent years controversy has arisen about treatment of recurring asymptomatic infection in girls over five years of age who have normal urinary tracts. Evidence has accumulated to support

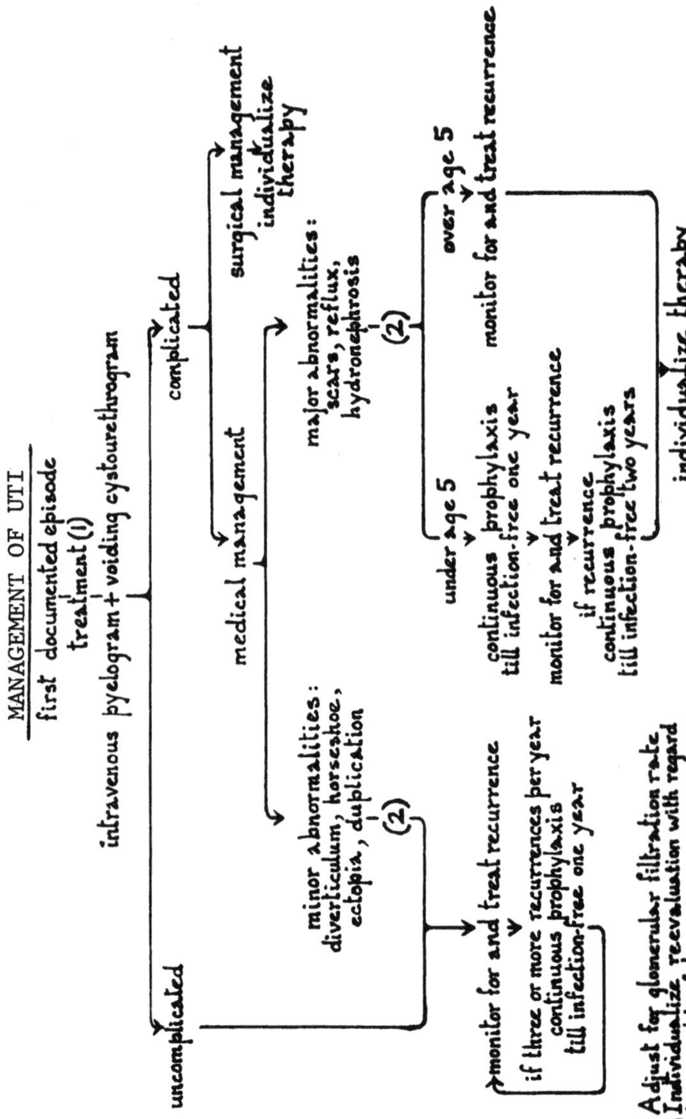
MANAGEMENT OF UTI
first documented episode
treatment (1)
intravenous pyelogram + voiding cystourethrogram
uncomplicated
complicated
medical management
surgical management
individualize therapy
minor abnormalities:
diverticulum, horseshoe,
ectopia, duplication
(2)
major abnormalities:
scars, reflux,
hydronephrosis
(2)
monitor for and treat recurrence
if three or more recurrences per year
continuous prophylaxis
till infection-free one year
under age 5
continuous prophylaxis
till infection-free one year
monitor for and treat recurrence
if recurrence
continuous prophylaxis
till infection-free two years
over age 5
monitor for and treat recurrence
individualize therapy
(1) Adjust for glomerular filtration rate
(2) Individualize reevaluation with regard to possible future surgery

FIGURE 1

the contention that such children are not at risk of renal damage (22,23,24). A child whose asymptomatic bacteriuria has been eliminated with antibiotic therapy may subsequently become more prone to develop symptomatic infection (25). Until this problem has been resolved, it is recommended that documented bacteriuria in any child be eradicated.

Children who suffer from three or more episodes of infection per year may benefit from prophylactic therapy. Agents most suitable for this are nitrofurantoin and cotrimoxazole, either of which may be administered in a single daily dose at bedtime. Effective dosage is one fifth to one half the recommended therapeutic amount (26). Methenamine compounded with mandelic acid, hippuric acid or sodium monohydrogen phosphate to lower urine pH is sometimes used; however, it is effective only when urine pH is less than 6.0. To achieve satisfactory acidification of the urine, additional medication with ascorbic acid or methionine may be required. The duration of prophylaxis must be planned on an individual basis considering age, frequency of infection and associated morbidity. Predisposing factors such as constipation and poor hygiene should be identified and eliminated if possible. The goal is to achieve at least a year of freedom from infection, following which prophylaxis may be discontinued. Urine cultures should be obtained at regular intervals for up to three years following cessation of therapy. After treatment of any reinfection within that period of time, prophylaxis should be reinstituted.

COMPLICATED INFECTION WITH MAJOR ANOMALIES

Children in this group are at great risk of progressive functional impairment, particularly if they are less than five years old (22,27). With the exception of those who present with severe obstruction of the urinary tract which requires immediate surgical intervention, management of these children is initially conservative. When a lesser degree of obstruction or any grade of reflux exists, the patient must be followed closely in conjunction with a pediatric urologist to evaluate the need for future surgery and devise a program of long-term followup.

A single recurrence of upper urinary tract infection in children less than five years of age who have major anomalies may lead to extension of old or development of new renal scars (23,26,27). After cure of their first documented infection, all such children should be placed on continuous prophylactic therapy until they have remained free from infection for one year. Then, prophylaxis may be stopped and each child monitored with monthly urine cultures to detect recurrence. Following treatment of a recurrent infection, prophylaxis should be reinstituted until the patient is infection-free for a period of two years. In this high-risk age group, the first period of prophylaxis is short because many children with major anomalies do not suffer from recurrent infection. They should not be subjected to unnecessary treatment but regular, close surveillance is imperative since it is likely that absence of infection will decrease scar formation.

The risk of complication from recurrences which are promptly detected and adequately treated diminishes with age. Children over five years old should be monitored as closely as those in the younger age group, but prophylaxis is not needed unless infection is a recurring problem.

The frequency of periodic anatomical and functional re-evaluation of kidneys and lower urinary tract must be individualized for children with major anomalies. The nature and severity of the abnormalities together with response to medical and surgical treatment must be considered. In follow-up studies, often radionuclide techniques can be used instead of x-rays, thus reducing exposure to radiation. Determination of blood electrolytes, acid-base balance, urea nitrogen and creatinine, urine concentrating ability and creatinine clearance provide essential information.

Modification of antibiotic dosage when treating UTI in children with reduced renal function must take into account the level of glomerular filtration rate and the agent's mode of excretion. Antibiotics which are removed from the body mainly by hepatic degradation do not accumulate when given in usual doses in renal failure, but their concentration in urine may fall below levels required to inhibit the infecting organism because of diminished glomerular filtration rate and urine concentrating ability. Antibiotics which are excreted mainly by the kidneys will tend to accumulate in the body as renal function deteriorates unless appropriate dose changes are introduced, and their concentration in urine also may be reduced to ineffective levels.

Studies of the half-life of most currently used antibiotics at all stages of renal function have led to the formation of guidelines for adjustment of therapy when needed (28). This adjustment may be made by 1) prolongation of the interval between normal doses, or 2) reduction of dosage given at normal intervals (29). Disadvantages of the first method are that the peak of plasma concentration after each dose is higher than normal and the trough before the next is lower. For agents which are known to be toxic at plasma levels close to the therapeutic range (such as gentamycin), this method may be dangerous. Also, the efficacy of treatment may be compromised if periods of subtherapeutic blood and urine levels are prolonged. The second method, based on reduction of the normal dose in proportion to the elimination rate of the drug, leads to more narrowly fluctuating blood and urine levels and seems to be a more logical approach. Nomograms (30) and tables (28) are available for practical application.

Further modification of therapy guided by blood and urine antibiotic concentrations measured at specified times following administration of the agent is recommended for optimal accuracy (29).

In making treatment choices, it must be remembered that nitrofurantoin is ineffective when renal function is reduced by 50% or more (31). Methenamine-organic acid compounds are contraindicated in renal failure, because hydrogen ion excretion is reduced and mandelic acid can cause crystalluria (28,32); metabolic acidosis may develop. Gentamycin may be effective until there is loss of about 90% of function (33,34). Ampicillin, cephalexin (35) and cotrimoxazole (36) are satisfactory in advanced renal failure.

In conclusion, the goals of therapy in management of childhood UTI are alleviation of the morbidity associated with frequently recurring infection and, most importantly, early identification and correction of complicating factors which predispose to progressive renal damage. Elimination or reduction of urinary stasis by timely surgical intervention, together with prevention of infections which may contribute to damage of renal parenchyma, may be life-saving. Unfortunately, deterioration of renal function may proceed inexorably in some children who receive the best management possible. These children will continue to form a significant proportion of the population with end-stage renal disease. Obviously, a better understanding of the pathogenesis of renal damage associated with infections and with obstructive tubulointerstitial nephritis is essential.

REFERENCES

1. Maherzi, M., Guignard, J-P. and Torrado, A.: Urinary tract infection in high-risk newborn infants. Pediatrics 62: 521, 1978.

2. Savage, D.C.L.: Urinary tract infection in childhood. Scot. Med. J. 16: 263, 1971.

3. Naveh, Y. and Friedman, A.: Urinary tract infection presenting with jaundice. Pediatrics 62: 524, 1978.

4. Arthur, A.B. and Wilson, B.D.R.: Urinary infection presenting with jaundice. Br. Med. J. 1: 539, 1967.

5. Bergström, T.: Studies of urinary tract infections in infancy and childhood. XII: Eighty consecutive patients with neonatal infection. J. Pediatr. 80: 858, 1972.

6. Kunin, C.M.: Urinary tract infections in children. Hosp. Prac. 11: 91, 1976.

7. Cohen, M.: Urinary tract infections in children: females aged 2 through 14, first two infections. Pediatrics 50: 271, 1972.

8. Ronald, A.R., Boutros, P. and Mourtada, H.: Bacteriuria localization and response to single-dose therapy in women. JAMA 235: 1854, 1976.

9. Fang, L.S.T., Tolkoff-Rubin, N.E. and Rubin, R.H.: Efficacy of single-dose and conventional amoxicillin therapy in urinary-tract infection localized by the antibody-coated bacteria technique. N. Eng. J. Med. 298: 413, 1978.

10. Bailey, R.R. and Abbott, G.D.: Treatment of urinary-tract infection with a single dose of amoxicillin. Nephron 18: 316, 1977.

11. Hellerstein, S., Kennedy, E., Nussbaum, L. and Rice, K.: Localization of the site of urinary tract infections by means of antibody-coated bacteria in the urinary sediments. J. Pediatr. 92: 188, 1978.

12. Anderson, H.J.: Clinical studies on the antibody response to E. Coli O-antigens in infants and children with urinary tract infections using a passive hemagglutination technique. Acta Paediatr. Scand. (Suppl.) 180: 1, 1968.

13. Hanson, L.A., Fasth, A. and Jodal, U.: Autoantibodies to Tamm-Horsfall protein, a tool for diagnosing the level of urinary tract infection. Lancet 1: 226, 1976.

14. Carvajal, H.F., Passey, R.B., Berger, M. et al.: Urinary lactic dehydrogenase isoenzyme 5 in the differential diagnosis of kidney and bladder infections. Kidney Int. 8: 178, 1975.

15. Stansfield, J.M.: Clinical observations relating to incidence and aetiology of urinary-tract infections in children. Br. Med. J. 1: 631, 1966.

16. Randolph, M.F. and Greenfield, M.: The incidence of asymptomatic bacteriuria and pyuria in infancy. J. Pediatr. 65: 57, 1964.

17. Bergström, T.: Sex differences in childhood urinary tract infection. Arch. Dis. Child. 47: 227, 1972.

18. Margileth, A.M., Pedreira, F.A., Hirschman, G.H. et al.: Urinary tract bacterial infections. Pediatr. Clin. N. Am. 23: 721, 1976.

19. Kunin, C.M., Deutscher, R. and Paquin, A.: Urinary tract infection in school-children. An epidemiologic clinical laboratory study. Medicine 43: 9, 1964.

20. Bergström, T., Lincoln, K., Redin, B. et al.: Studies of urinary tract infections in infancy and childhood. X. Short or long term treatment in girls with first or second-time urinary tract infections. Acta Paediatr. Scand. 57: 186, 1978.

21. Kunin, C.M.: The natural history of recurrent bacteriuria in schoolgirls. N. Engl. J. Med. 282: 1443, 1970.

22. Savage, D.C.L., Wilson, M.I., McHardy, M. et al.: Covert bacteriuria of childhood. A clinical and epidemiological study. Arch. Dis. Child. 48: 8, 1973.

23. Cardiff-Oxford Bacteriuria Study Group: Sequelae of covert bacteriuria in schoolgirls. Lancet 1: 889, 1978.

24. Lindberg, U., Claesson, I., Hanson, L.A. et al.: Asymptomatic bacteriuria in schoolgirls. VIII. Clinical course during a 3-year follow-up. J. Pediatr. 92: 194, 1978.

25. Lindberg, U., Hanson, L.A., Jodal, U. et al.: Asymptomatic bacteriuria in schoolgirls. II. Differences in escherichia coli causing asymptomatic and symptomatic bacteriuria. Acta Paediatr. Scand. 64: 432, 1975.

26. Smellie, J.M. and Normand, I.C.S.: Urinary tract infection with and without anatomical malformations. In Lieberman, E. (ed.): Clinical Pediatric Nephrology. Philadelphia: J.B. Lippincott Company, 1976, p. 194.

27. Shah, K.J., Robins, D.G. and White, R.H.R.: Renal scarring and vesicoureteric reflux. Arch. Dis. Child. 53: 210, 1978.

28. Bennett, W.M., Singer, I., Golpher, T. et al.: Guidelines for drug therapy in renal failure. Ann. Intern. Med. 86: 754, 1977.

29. Bennett, W.M.: Drug therapy in patients with reduced renal function. In Monographs in Clinical Pharmacology; vol. 2, Drugs and Renal Disease. New York: Churchill Livingstone, 1978, p. 21.

30. Craig, W.A., Ramgopal, V. and Welling, P.G.: The influence of impaired renal and hepatic function on antimicrobial therapy. In von Graevenitz, A. (ed.): Handbook series in clinical laboratory science. Section E: Clinical microbiology. Cleveland: CRC Press, 1977, p. 323.

31. Sachs, J., Gear, T., Noell, P. et al.: Effect of renal function on urinary recovery of orally administered nitrofurantoin. N. Engl. J. Med. 278: 1032, 1968.

32. Harvey, S.C.: Antiseptics and disinfectants; fungicides; ectoparasiticides. In Goodman, L.S. and Gilman, A. (eds.): The pharmacological basis of therapeutics, 5th Ed., New York: MacMillan Publishing Co., Inc., 1975, p. 987.

33. Whelton, A., Carter, G.G., Bryant, H.H. et al.: Therapeutic implications of gentamycin accumulation in severely diseased kidneys. Arch. Intern. Med. 136: 172, 1976.

34. Bennett, W.M., Hartnett, M.N., Craven, R. et al.: Gentamycin concentrations in blood, urine, and renal tissue of patients with end-stage renal disease. J. Lab. Clin. Med. 90: 389, 1977.

35. Kunin, C.M. and Finkelberg, E.: Oral cephalexin and ampicillin: antimicrobial activity, recovery in urine, and persistence in the blood of uremic patients. Ann. Intern. Med. 72: 349, 1970.

36. Craig, W.A. and Kunin, C.M.: Trimethoprim-sulfamethoxazole: pharmacodynamic effects of urinary pH and impaired renal function. Studies in humans. Ann. Intern. Med. 78: 491, 1973.

PANEL DISCUSSION

Moderator: José Strauss, M.D.

Div. Pediatr. Nephrol., Dept. Pediatr., Univ. Miami Sch. Med., Miami, Fla. 33101, USA

QUESTION: Studies of Dr. Hodson indicated that some type of functional obstruction causes segmental fibrosis. Could the Panel help clarify the roles played by reflux and by obstruction? Also, are there any differences in the vessels of the atrophic-fibrotic pole as compared with the rest of the kidney that would explain the hypertension found in these patients?

RESPONSE: Well, you've sort of hit the knot of the big controversy that's going on - that is whether high pressure, sterile, intrarenal reflux will give rise to total scarring. I've got to accentuate the high pressure because there is no doubt about it; one does not get the scars unless one gets the high pressure reflux going on. You may say this doesn't occur in a child unless there is an infection, but it may. We are not sure about this yet. I think that if one looks even at minor degrees of posterior urethral valves - not the very bad ones but the minor degrees - one may find striking changes. There are two patients I know whose kidneys have been dissected out. There was generalized damage (scarring) of the renal parenchyma with generalized caliectasis. I was unaware about this stuff when I first saw these specimens. I can't tell whether there was fibrosis or not. But the fact is that even minor degrees of posterior urethral valves have been very similar to the urethral rings implanted in pigs by Hodson and collaborators. Now, there were three cases written up of infants with uremic ascites. I investigated the first one that was written up; it had bad posterior urethral valves. I don't know how many of you have done voiding cystourethrograms but when you first put a catheter into the bladder, the bladder blows up in a circular manner. You can almost always tell whether or not the bladder is hypertrophied by the manner the bladder blows up; maybe as long as 10 minutes later, suddenly the urethra opens and your contrast material goes down to the valves, then if you watch it carefully, you'll see the urethra contract. Note the contrast in the urethra first, then back into the bladder and the bladder contracts and the whole upper urinary tract blows up. In this particular case the contrast media went through the right kidney into a big collection of what I could call urine underneath the capsule. Now, that little boy when he died a few weeks later, the contrast material was going through the kidney in one track and we found this track and it was epithelialized. And that kidney was quite thick. I mean there was quite a lot of renal parenchyma there. The pathologist some time later still had this kidney in blocks so he looked at the blocks for Tamm-Horsfall protein and found it in the interstitium of that child's kidney under the thick capsule. Why are we so interested in Tamm-Horsfall protein? It may be strange to some people here. This protein is only formed in the ascending limb of the Loop of Henle and in the distal convoluted tubule. It is not in urine until it gets in the ascending limb of the Loop of Henle. To get urine with Tamm-Horsfall protein in it, the urine must be "mature" - after it's been down through the proximal convoluted tubule and the descending limb of the Loop of Henle. Now, if that urine is getting back into the kidneys, this means the reflux of mature urine which contains Tamm-Horsfall protein. This protein then is like the fingerprints or footprints for refluxed urine.

The second question was related to vessels. The arterial changes are very interesting. I don't have time to talk about these in detail but in pigs allowed to grow for four years without doing anything to them, arterial blood pressure was measured. A method of estimating blood pressure was devised by having a little cuff put over the pig's tail; this cuff was then blown up and the pig became used to having this cuff blown up while it was having breakfast in the morning. Three of these pigs were hypertensive and the fourth became hypertensive while monitoring was going on. Those pigs were eventually killed and the kidneys were sent to a pathologist who found exactly the same vascular changes first described in 1955 on ischemic renal tissue of adult human beings with high blood pressure. Presumably, these are absolutely specific changes.

COMMENT: I just have to say something about these arterial changes. For those of you who are not old enough to remember, in 1955 or 1956 Dr. Kincaid-Smith put forward the thesis that the reason you got scars in chronic pyelonephritis was that during the stage of acute inflammation you got an acute arteritis that healed by occluding the lumen of the arteries and that caused ischemia beyond it and this produced the scars. Now this interested me at the time because a claim would depend on how frequently does one see acute arteritis in acute pyelonephritis. I had seen it I think in one artery in one of many cases which made me very suspicious of this whole idea. So that prompted a number of us to study this and experimental pyelonephritis in the rabbit was produced. A technique of post-mortem angiography was used to try and demonstrate vascular occlusion. To cut a long story short, we were completely unable to do that. So, at a later time Dr. Hill using a more refined method of microangiography where you can get down to these vessels in greater detail, was unable to demonstrate any changes such as Dr. Kincaid-Smith had claimed. So I'm afraid I'm very suspicious of this and I would like to know a little bit more about the specificity of these changes.

RESPONSE: I am afraid I can't help you on this. It's too complicated. I always remember when this famous nephrologist first looked at that hypertension material with the bipolar scarring and said, "My God, there they are again." I said, "What are?", thinking there was something very good there. The response was, "the same vascular changes that I saw in the adult human kidneys". When the second group of hypertensive pigs arrived, all the kidneys got these changes in them and they were larger. Will you accept what was called at that time partial or incomplete ischemia or infarction?

COMMENT: The term was "incomplete infarction". I would describe it as being a rather nonsensical term.

QUESTION: What could we compromise with? Could we call it areas or zones of ischemia?

COMMENT: That's simple ischemia. I'm not doubting the fact that you may get vascular changes in pigs because in human chronic pyelonephritis you do get changes. Currently available documentation shows that if you take a chronic pyelonephritic kidney and you look at the blood vessels, they are more severely affected in the scarred areas than they are in the others. Now, my interpretation is rather different. I don't think this is acute arthritis. I don't really know what it is. It may possibly be something akin to a disuse endarteritis such as in an older person's ovary or uterus when it has no further function; the blood vessels undergo intimal thickening to cut down the blood supply because it does not need it anymore.

Now, we might get back to the question that was raised previously in this Seminar - "can you get hypertension in chronic pyelonephritis, reflux nephropathy, or segmental hypoplasia- whatever you call it, in the absence of chronic renal failure where one may be working on the basis of hypervolemia?" I've always believed that you could do that and I think this could be a likely mechanism, as Dr. Habib showed. What could happen in chronic pyelonephritis or whatever you call it is that you could be getting these ischemic changes - you might use that term, stimulating the juxtamedullary apparatus to produce renin and then you will get changes at a later time if the hypertension was severe enough in the nonpyelonephritic parts of the kidney which is precisely what was found later on. I personally believe that hypertension can occur in chronic pyelonephritis without the patient having to be in chronic renal failure.

COMMENT: I have two comments regarding some of the things that were just said. The first one is about the reference to posterior urethral valves. Jay Bernstein several years ago studied the presence of dysplasia in various types of kidneys and found an incidence of 90% of dysplastic structures with posterior urethral valves. I have not that much experience but I would say that in my material I have found exactly the same percentage. That is, posterior urethral valves in 90% of the cases are associated with dysplasia. I think that is an important thing. Whatever high pressure reflux may cause to the kidney, you have to know that these kidneys are already extremely malformed.

COMMENT: I would like to answer that. It seems to me that posterior urethral valves are there presumably from the word "go". As soon as urine starts being formed - somewhere around the 14th week in intrauterine life - just over three months - by the first glomeruli which are formed, then the whole system will fill up. And from then on, what further develops will be developing in a high pressure situation against the posterior urethral valves. My suggestion is that the interpretation of the fact that there is dysplasia of the kidneys mean that, for the remaining renal tissue, development will be in an abnormal situation, that it is a secondary dysplasia.

COMMENT: I thought that from the embryology information we have, the presence of dysplastic structures was equivalent to saying that it had developed in the very early embryonic period. That is before 14 weeks. That's why I've been insisting about the dysplastic situation because my feeling is that these dysplastic structures might be a clue to some of these scars which might not be the consequence but the association with high pressure, reflux or whatever you want to have developed, once urine has been produced. It is in that precise situation - I don't know for the rest - but in that precise situation of dysplastic papillae, 90% of the higher pressure group with posterior urethral valves, have dysplastic structures. I don't believe that the scars you see in posterior urethral valves are only the consequence of high pressure because you have these dysplastic structures which show that probably they have been present earlier.

QUESTION: This worries me because why should posterior urethral valves - are you going to say that they are part of the dysplastic picture?

RESPONSE: Yes.

QUESTION: The two little folds of urethra?

RESPONSE: Yes. You have an abnormality of the whole urinary tract.

COMMENT: Oh no, you don't have it.

QUESTION: How do you know the relationship between that little tiny thing and the changes in the papillae? What do you want to be the consequence? It can be associated. That's my hypothesis.

My other comment concerns the problem of vascular changes. The vascular changes are also a problem of association. One is struck by the fact that there is association of these scars and these vessel changes. Of course when you have two things associated, you always must ask,is it associated or is one the consequence of the other? And you can take all the possibilities. I was also struck by the association of vascular changes in what I called segmental hypoplasia after having read the paper of Dr. Priscilla Kincaid-Smith of September 1955. I read it and I said,"I don't think she is talking about the same thing but she is calling it chronic pyelonephritis and I personally don't think that it is chronic pyelonephritis. It must be something else. I will leave the door open. I don't want to close it by calling it chronic pyelonephritis." Now, these vascular changes, either they can be considered as the cause or the result of the scar. Maybe it could be abnormality of the vessels because they are so striking that one could consider that the scar could be secondary to these vascular changes; I don't say that I have changed my mind because the reverse could also be true and that is that in a scar you have what you termed "disuse vessels. " I think that in this field we have to refer to what happens in other organs. We know very well that in the lung, the uterus and several other situations, you can very well see in scar tissue regression or hypertrophy of the vessel wall so that all these changes may very well be the consequence of the scar. So, again we are coming back to "what causes the scar?" If we are sure that it is not the vessel lesion and that the vessel lesions are the consequences, then "what causes the scar?"

COMMENT: I haven't finished with these posterior urethral valves because there are minor degrees of posterior urethral valves which don't occlude the lumen but they're not associated with dysplastic changes of the upper urinary tract. You see what I mean? You can get just a little coat of mucosa. I don't believe that just because they happen to be a little bit wider in some cases than in others that they are going to be associated with dysplasia of the upper urinary tract and kidney. It is a matter of degree.

QUESTION: Now tell me something. You know multicystic kidney?

COMMENT: I don't know about what a multicystic kidney is. Could you please tell me?

RESPONSE: Yes. Multicystic kidney - since I have been in pathology only for the last thirty years I understand that you wouldn't know what multicystic is. Clearly it is a kidney with lots of cysts.

COMMENT: Could you be a bit more precise?

RESPONSE: These extensive dysplastic kidneys have almost no more normal tissue in them, and may or may not be complicated by cysts. By the way, that's why I don't like very much the word "multicystic".

COMMENT: It is an archaic term, and we could do as well without it.

RESPONSE: Yes. It's extremely dysplastic kidneys, nearing aplasia, with or without cysts. In this condition, the ureter is more or less obstructed, not completely, sometimes, or it could be absent. Could you imagine that it is that obstruction which is responsible for the extensive dysplasia of that kidney? Or is it an association? It's a question I'm asking; I am not answering it. I just want to know how you can explain such complete absence of functional kidney with extensive dysplastic changes in that situation.

COMMENT: For people who perhaps are not completely familiar with dysplastic kidneys there is a body of thought that believes that the genesis of the dysplastic kidney is in some way related to a defect in the formation of the ureter or of obstruction of the ureter, because there are examples where you get segmental dysplasia of the kidney where perhaps the whole of a pole is involved, where you have two different ureters, where perhaps another pole might show changes of dysplasia. I think that if you are going to use the term "dysplasia" then you've got to demonstrate something unique about it. I think you clearly showed the cartilage and these cellular structures around tubules as being unique and I would agree with you on the cartilage and more or less agree with you on the other - although I'm not too sure about that. And the fact that these totally dysplastic kidneys - the one that you were referring to, multicystic - may occur without a ureter or with a stenotic ureter, is suggestive evidence that some time during the development of the kidney, something has happened to the development of the ureter and therefore the rest of the kidney can not develop properly. Now, what we don't have, though, is any good, experimental evidence of this. I think it would probably be extremely difficult to get unless you could get a person who is a master microsurgeon who could do some work with early fetal circulation. I think we are completely ignorant on that at the moment but there is some evidence to show that dysplasia arises in the presence of obstruction.

COMMENT: But if you go and look at these dissected specimens where they are on view, with beautifully dissected arteries, there is classical cystic dysplasia on one side and what looks like post obstructive atrophy on the other in a case of posterior urethral valves.

COMMENT: It is clearly associated. The problem is to know if there is a relationship - a causal effect between the two things. I vote for association and you are voting for casual effect. That's all the difference.

MODERATOR: I wonder whether what we are talking about now has any bearing on the results of the correction of the posterior urethral valves. It has been said that if you correct an obstructive uropathy before two years of age that the patient will have a good prognosis and that there will not be progression towards chronic renal failure. We have found, actually, that that is not true. Babies who were repaired in the first few days or weeks of extra-uterine life with obstructive uropathies, have gone on to develop chronic renal failure and end-stage renal disease.

COMMENT: I think your remark earlier in the discussion about urologists not following the renal results in reflux surgery is well taken. However, some urologists have followed a large group very closely for a number of years. Secondly, I think that most people in the room know that reflux surgery is a relatively young form of surgery. Only now are a large number of patients coming to 10 and 15 year followups and just a small handful to 20 year followups. Most of us in academic centers follow our reflux surgery or patients who reflux and are not operated on, very closely for such things as renal growth, GFR, and blood pressure. Most important, a group of us in the urology section of the American Academy of Pediatrics have a study going on, multicenter, in cooperation with HEW for reflux and the renal aspects of this study are most important.

My question is also a technical question. In the United States, most patients with segmental problems like Ask-Upmark kidney, if they are to be subjected to surgical procedures, most (North) American surgeons elect to do the procedure that was mentioned for duplex kidneys which are to be operated upon and that is a segmental nephrectomy. It's very simple to come back later and remove the kidney if the first, more conservative procedure is a failure. Is this done for Ask-Upmark kidney or related problems in other countries?

RESPONSE: Yes. We have performed twice partial nephrectomy. The first one was a big success. We were very happy and decided that from then on we would try to do that. The second was a failure and when the whole kidney was removed later on, we found that although there were no apparent abnormalities of the pyelocalyceal system in the remaining part of the kidney, when I had the kidney in my hand, I could see other scars which were not apparent on the various IVPs we had been performing. The big problem, and now I am convinced of that because now I have several end-stage kidneys, the big problem with these kidneys is that there are a lot of small scars here and there. Since I am absolutely convinced now that the renin is secreted in the scarred zones, if you leave one scarred zone, hypertension is going to continue.

Another problem is that the more we study this problem - now we have about 50 patients - the 27 patients I showed here were selected on the basis of having the histology to prove the nature of the process - but we have about 50 patients with the same disease. Exceptionally, we can be sure of the integrity of the other kidney. That's why we are performing less and less nephrectomies, whether partial or total. The situation where you have really a compensatory hypertrophy on the other side, which for us is the basis of the indication for nephrectomy, is extremely rare in our group. I don't know why but it is so. At the beginning we were more oriented towards surgery. Now, the more we go, the less we are doing surgery - not because we don't want to do it but just because it's exceptional to find a case with compensatory hypertrophy on the other side.

QUESTION: But they have done it on bilateral disease in the States - on a couple of cases. Isn't that so, sir? They've operated when the scars have been bilateral and with success.

RESPONSE: Yes, that is true. I think that the remarks you just made, and previous you have made, show why many of these cases have not been successful. By discussing segmental and partial nephrectomy, I am not saying that it is a wonderful operation - only that in those patients selected for surgery that it could be better. However, when one looks at all the results, one can only say that they are moderately successful. I think that the reason you just stated is in fact the reason why.

COMMENT: It's the ideal procedure but we have to analyze precisely in what cases are we going to do it. It's certainly the ideal procedure because we know that renin is secreted there; so we have to get rid of that bad part of the kidney. But, in practice, it's not that easy.

QUESTION: Since there is apparently such a close relationship between intrarenal reflux and renal damage, would you recommend to do the voiding cystogram by drip infusion to a certain height at least in infants? The reason I ask you this question is because some radiologists and my own house staff don't like it because it takes longer time to do it. Sometimes the children strain and don't let you do the procedure. What is your opinion about it?

RESPONSE: I am not at all convinced that the demonstration of intrarenal reflux is all that important. I'm certainly totally ignorant of what factors are involved in this demonstration and I'm also totally ignorant as to what height or pressure you may drip or do anything for that matter in infants. We were recently at a meeting where presentations included that of a child who had a cystogram and had gross generalized intrarenal reflux into one kidney all the way in. That cystogram was infected. I don't know where the infection got in, but the child got a very severe bacteremia following this and had to have the kidney out. I don't think one should go around pushing stuff into children's kidneys unless there is a very good reason for it. I don't really believe that there is. I think that this is a nice thing to see if you can find it, but even with a contrast of only 30 centimeters above the child you may find a patient whose VCU reveals contrast material up normal ureters and into both kidneys. These may be normal size kidneys. You're not going to operate on that child's ureters just because he showed intrarenal reflux. It's a very useful experimental thing, but I don't think that we should go and change the already complicated problem of VCUs to show intrarenal reflux. I really cannot see the logic of this.

COMMENT: I definitely agree with you. I don't think there is any need to show the intrarenal reflux. I know that it is common practice among radiologists to do the cystogram with low pressure by drip infusion, not by direct syringe injection. We have had some cases of adult paraplegics in whom we have done cystograms and we have shown intrarenal reflux. They have neurogenic bladders and high pressure reflux. In these cases we have done a gallium scan and we have shown a massive uptake of the gallium in the kidneys. So they have that evidence, both clinically and by radionucleide studies, of acute infection. I would suggest that in certain patients to be careful not to use excessive pressure since some of them develop septicemia and diffuse massive renal infection.

QUESTION: I seem to recollect that Tamm-Horsfall protein has been demonstrated in serum of patients who have had massive reflux. Can you comment on that? Second, you told us how the papillae of pigs are similar to human; I wonder if there is any major difference between the two?

RESPONSE: The Tamm-Horsfall business, that's a bag of worms. There was a beautiful, extremely good, sensitive radioimmune assay for this protein and for its antibody in animals but not in man.

In pigs, once started, it didn't stop for a week and it went to its maximum for three weeks while they were refluxing. It also happened to another pig that was obstructed. We were very excited because we thought, here at last is a simple way of picking up the significant refluxes. But we have been unable, in spite of lots of money and lots of time - 9-12 months - we have been unable to repeat that in man. I'm very sorry about that.

The other thing you asked, was about papillae - as far as I know they both have the same characteristics. The only thing is that in about 2/3 of the children, I think that's a fair estimate - you don't get the compound papillae. Theoretically they are not open to intrarenal reflux. Now, you could recognize a compound papillae on a good IVP. Of course you have a calyx which is not a simple cup. It may be just tending to two cups or it may be three cups. You can recognize this very easily. The thing is, my experience in North America is that here there are more compound papillae than there are in some European countries. This poses a very interesting question. I have the same walk as my father did. We inherit all sorts of things. Why shouldn't we inherit a particular type of kidney? You see, there are all sorts of interesting things we never mention. Why don't black children get reflux? Do they have a funny bladder? Do they have a very deep insertion of the ureter in the bladder or what? I think there are so many things around us that are opening up and need working on. I think that Ramsey's figures - I think she said 2/3 of children don't have compound papillae, is not true of this side of the Atlantic amongst the adults. We're doing papillary counts and coming up with about 50% who have midzone papillae with duplex and most of the have compound papillae.

QUESTION: I think that one of the important things in the topic we have been discussing is that if you follow a patient who already has an established scar, you can see the scar increase. There is a thinning of the parenchyma. Very seldom you will see newly formed scars. Of course, another thing which is apparent is that it's better not to be infected. These are the two possibilities of progressing to a more severe disease and to renal failure if you have scarred kidneys. The first is a newly formed scar, which is exceptional. The second one is infection, but it is exceptional. So my question is, it becomes apparent from all our studies that the glomeruli of the spared zones become sclerosed or altered. I would like to ask if there might be an immunological mechanism responsible for this deterioration of glomeruli which has been hypothesized recently. Among all the cases we have been studying for the last 20 years, we have found only two patients who developed a glomerular nephropathy - a real one - not this type of glomerulosclerosis. One was a girl who developed a membranoproliferative glomerulonephritis and recently we have had a case of membranous nephropathy in a child who had had an operation for some vesical problem ten years previously and who was not infected in between those ten years. It is exceptional to see membranous or membranoproliferative glomerulonephritis developing in such patients. Most of the glomerular damage which has been described looked more or less like focal sclerosis. I would like to ask if there may be some immunological mechanism.

RESPONSE: This is a very difficult question. I can simply tell you what is the evolution of this concept during the last 40 years. It was one of the original and a very challenging hypothesis which was proposed in Germany 40 years ago. Obviously this problem had been approached on an experimental basis first. Using several methods including the extensive use of a nephrotoxic nephritis, it was proposed that at a certain point the disease progresses because there is an autoimmune viscious circle responsible for the development of the autoantibodies. This problem was analyzed by Unanue and Dixon for a long time, and they came to the conclusion, which is still valid, that there is not such an autoimmune phenomenon. Then, the problem came back again because some antigen (Edginton's antigen) was discovered in the brush border of the tubules and which may be responsible for membranous nephropathy in some animals. All investigators found it true that this antigen may perhaps be involved in the development of glomerular or tubular pathology. Again, this is a very interesting hypothesis.

I will simply have to tell you that there are some requirements to be fulfilled in order to accept this hypothesis as valid. It is not enough to have immunoglobulin in the glomeruli. You have to show that this immunoglobulin, number one, contains antibody, and number two, that this antibody is specific for a certain renal antigen. Now, there is an autoimmune response to certain immune complex glomerulonephritis such as the response to antigen of the basement membrane which has been shown in a very few cases and obviously this is, after all, the histological mark of anti-GBM glomerulonephritis. That there is an autoimmune response to the antigen of the brush border, proposed by Dr. Gordillo, is an extremely interesting hypothesis but certainly these criteria have to be fulfilled so you have to show that this is antibody of the G class; you have to show that this immunoglobulin contains antibody that is specific for the brush border. These requirements are very difficult to be fulfilled. You have to have the kidney and you have to make an elution from the kidney and you have to show that the immunoglobulin is specific for this brush border antigen.

The presence of this antibody in the circulation is an extremely rare event. It has never been shown so far except on the occasion of one case of sickle cell anemia. Then it has never been shown in the U.S. or in England. There are several programs studying whether or not it is possible to detect this antigen or its antibody, by using radioimmune assay.

This is a very interesting hypothesis but they have to be demonstrated and we don't have the evidence so far. So, the cases like the one presented by Dr. Gordillo are interesting. Obviously it is following this trend of investigation that it will be possible to see if some damage is produced perhaps by an infection like pyelonephritis. Maybe at a certain point it is complicated by an autoimmune phenomenon. Several of us were very excited by the idea that we may have an immune complex glomerulonephritis which is the consequence of thyroid antibodies but I think it was ten years ago that we were talking about this hypothesis. It still is only a hypothesis. In order to be sure that it happens, you have to come up with hard evidence.

MODERATOR: Did you look for the circulating antibodies or complexes and you did not find them or did you not look for them?

RESPONSE: No. We didn't look for them.

COMMENT: The problem is that these antibodies are not present in the circulation. It is extremely difficult. If they are present, they are concentrated in the kidney because there is so much antigen which is available that they bind to the kidney. It's the old story of anti-GBM antibody which is very difficult to detect by using direct immunofluorescence. It is only by elution from the kidney that you can show this antibody. We are very happy that very seldom are we able to elute the antibody because, for that, the patient would have to die or bilateral nephrectomy is necessary.

MODERATOR: That patient that you referred to, it was of interest that when we initially looked for the complexes, they were not found. They were subsequently found in the cryoprecipitate.

COMMENT: I know. The systematic study of the cryoprecipitate may be a good method. There are now several new methods which have been developed but have not been applied. It is very difficult. For instance, the method of the $C1_q$ column which may be used for either complexes or immuno computing, or the Raji cell method. The latter is more complicated because there are components of the Raji cell lines which interfere with the evaluation of the components of the complex. So, it is really a very difficult area.

COMMENT: Before I stop speaking at this meeting I should just show you the last two slides I didn't have time for this morning because this is really very exciting. This is the first urinary diary which the mothers can do. What you do is, you lie the boy down in the crib and you put a diaper on it and you look at the diaper every half hour. If it's dry, you put it back. If it's damp you write down "damp"; if it's wet, you write down "wet". You go to the scales, weigh it, and see how much urine is being passed. The normal baby tends to empty its bladder as we said before, according to age at a fairly regular volume - of course according to his intake - at fairly regular periods. In between times, it's dry. Now let's get this first slide. This is a copy of the actual thing the mother wrote. Although she had a typewriter sheet, she copied this out herself. This is an 18-month-old baby, 12:00 damp, 12:30 damp, 1:00 damp, 1:30 dry, 2:00 dry. Damp, damp, dry. Damp, damp, soaked. Now, the soaking means the bladder emptied. What is it doing in between times? What is the damp stuff? This bladder isn't emptying when there is dampness. It's topping off. This means you've got a bladder residue and that you're very likely to have infection. In fact that child was infected. Then, the other thing that they are asked to note is the stream. This one has stop-go stream. Little spurt and stops, little spurt and stops. Stop, go, then dripping. Hesitation dripping. Others have noticed this stop-go thing in infected children. The mother, just looking at the baby, can tell whether there is something wrong with it's waterworks. This is then supported by a little plastic bag which is stuck on and has a double compartment. The top part fits back and what dribbles into that stays there so it's just when the baby streams that he streams into the lower compartment. So it's actually the midstream specimen. The child has to be watched until urine appears in the lower compartment and immediately taken out, a special swab which gives you .1 of an ml. Just dip it in the urine and give it a sharp shake. You get almost exactly .1 of an ml. You break that in half and count the number of colonies. The mother does this. This is working out almost as accurately as a lab test for a colony count.

Now we have the next slide of another baby. This is a normal which is dry, dry, dry, dry, dry, etc. That's 11:00 and that's 4:30. It's holding its water and then emptying its bladder, completely.

This one is 5-months-old, with a fever. Damp, damp, damp, damp, damp, damp, damp, damp, and flood. Damp, damp, damp, damp, damp, damp, damp, damp for five hours and then a flood. That's abnormal. She had an E. Coli infection, and this is her the next day. After 24 hours treatment, dry, dry, dry, dry, dry, dry, dry, dry, flood. She's back to normal. Now using this and two well drilled people in his office who are excellent at getting messages through to the mothers, two things have happened with Randolph. The first thing is that he has detected a disturbance in urinary function before infection. This is fascinating because it starts straight away to make one think of urethral spasm. The second thing is that his rate of positives is 3.5%. The highest rate I know of anybody in this age group is about 1.5%. He's picking out nearly twice as many undetected UTI patients by this method. It's a method that anybody can do - any mother who's got any brain tissue between her ears. I thought you'd be very interested to hear it because here is a message of odor.

IMMUNOLOGICALLY MEDIATED TUBULAR AND INTERSTITIAL NEPHRITIS

Bernice Noble, Ph.D. and Giuseppe A. Andres, M.D.

Dept. Microbiol. and Depts. Microbiol., Pathol., and Med., State Univ. N.Y. at Buffalo, Sch. Med., Buffalo N.Y. 14214, USA

Immunological mechanisms play an important part in the pathogenesis of most human glomerular disease. Damage to glomeruli may result either from the deposition of immune complexes along the glomerular basement membrane (GBM) or from the fixation of specific anti-GBM antibodies to the GBM. These two mechanisms are usually readily distinguished by direct immunofluorescence tests which reveal the pattern of distribution of immune reactants within the diseased kidney. Immune complex deposits have a characteristic discrete, granular appearance which can be detected by staining with fluorescein-labeled antibodies to immunoglobulins, complement, or the relevant antigen. In contrast, binding of anti-GBM antibody is recognized by a continuous, finely linear staining pattern. It is now well established that the tubules and interstitium of the kidney are also susceptible to injury initiated by the deposition of immune complexes or antibodies to the tubular basement membrane (TBM) (1,2, 3). Interstitial inflammation and abnormalities of the tubular epithelium and the TBM may result when immunoglobulin G (IgG), with or without complement (C), is present in granular or linear deposits in renal tubules and interstitium.

A great deal of our present appreciation of the contribution of immunologically mediated injury to tubulointerstitial pathology is based on studies with animal models. The recognition of immunological processes in the pathogenesis of human interstitial nephri-

Supported by the Department of Health, Education and Welfare, United States Public Health Service Grants AI-10334 and AM 26394.

tis has tended to follow observations made in the laboratory, although human disease can still be only partly explained by the available animal models. In this review, the animal models of experimental tubulointerstitial nephritis will be described and discussed. Evidence for similar mechanisms in human interstitial nephritis will be evaluated and compared with the findings in laboratory animals.

EXPERIMENTALLY INDUCED, IMMUNOLOGICALLY MEDIATED TUBULOINTERSTITIAL NEPHRITIS IN ANIMALS

Tubular and interstitial nephritis in animals can be elicited in animals which have been stimulated to produce antibodies to TBM or to the brush border (BB) of proximal tubular cells. Inflammatory lesions of the renal interstitium have also been observed frequently in association with interstitial immune complex deposits. In addition, delayed type hypersensitivity may cause an accumulation of mononuclear cells in the renal cortex.

Antibodies to TBM

An experimental model of tubulointerstitial nephritis attributable to autoantibodies directed against antigens of the TBM was first described by Steblay and Rudofsky (4). It has since been studied in a number of laboratories (5,6,7,8). To produce the disease, guinea pigs are immunized intradermally with an emulsion of Freund's adjuvant and TBM antigens prepared from rabbit kidneys. Within several weeks the guinea pigs develop a renal disease that is characterized clinically by proteinuria, glucosuria and azotemia. The kidneys of nephritic guinea pigs appear enlarged and pale, with petechial hemorrhages (4). In histologic preparations, diffuse cortical tubular damage is evident. Infiltration of the interstitium with mononuclear cells is a characteristic feature. Multinucleated giant cells have come to be recognized as the histologic hallmark of this experimentally induced renal disease (Fig. 1). The giant cells result from fusion of epithelioid cells derived from mononuclear phagocytes of the cellular infiltration (8). In addition to peritubular inflammation and tubular cell degeneration, wrinkling, splitting and fragmentation of the TBM are seen. In late stages of the disease tubular atrophy and interstitial sclerosis may be found. Not infrequently it becomes difficult or impossible to demonstrate TBM by light or electron microscopy. Peritubular giant cells appear to be active in the destruction of TBM for which cellular contact with the TBM appears a prerequisite. Contact of the epithelioid giant cells with the TBM is followed by lysis and phagocytosis of the TBM (8) (Fig. 2).

The sera from nephritic guinea pigs contain high titers of anti-TBM autoantibodies that can be measured in indirect immuno-

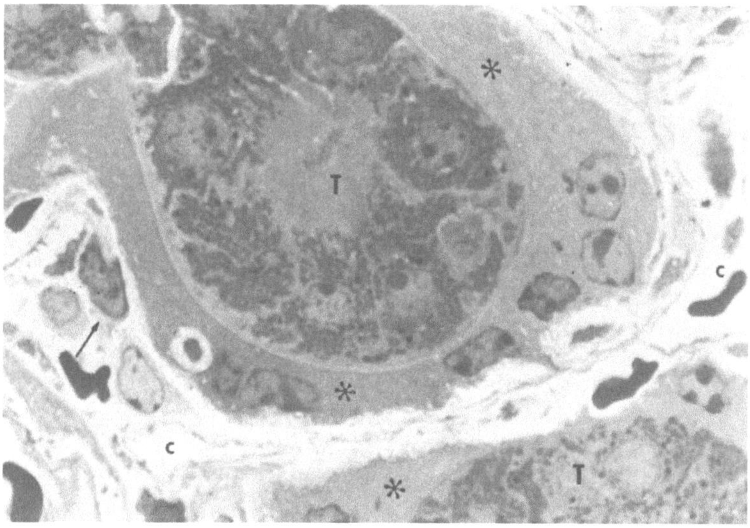

FIG. 1. Light micrograph showing a kidney section of a guinea pig 20 days after immunization with rabbit tubular basement membrane. The proximal convoluted tubules (T) are surrounded by giant cells (asterisks). The arrow indicates a macrophage; c, peritubular capillaries. (Toluidine blue, x 1000).

fluorescence tests on frozen sections of normal guinea pig kidney (4,5). By direct immunofluorescence tests, a continuous linear pattern of binding of IgG and the third component of complement (C_3) along the basement membrane of cortical tubules is demonstrable in the kidneys of the same animals (4) (Fig. 3). However, in advanced stages of nephritis, when extensive TBM destruction and loss has occurred, the linear pattern of fixation of IgG to the TBM may no longer be evident (8).

A central role of specific antibodies in the pathogenesis of this autoimmune tubulointerstitial nephritis was first suggested by the close association of TBM antibodies in sera and kidneys with the development of severe abnormalities of cortical tubular morphology (4). The passive transfer of progressive cortical tubulointerstitial disease to normal guinea pigs, using sera obtained from actively immunized nephritic animals, has confirmed the importance of anti-TBM antibodies in the induction of this interstitial nephritis (9). Passive transfer experiments have also been used to evaluate a number of factors influencing the immunopathogenesis of interstitial and tubular lesions. When guinea pigs genetically deficient in the fourth component of complement (C_4) are recipients of anti-TBM serum, a tubulointerstitial nephritis develops with all characteristic clinical, histologic and immuno-

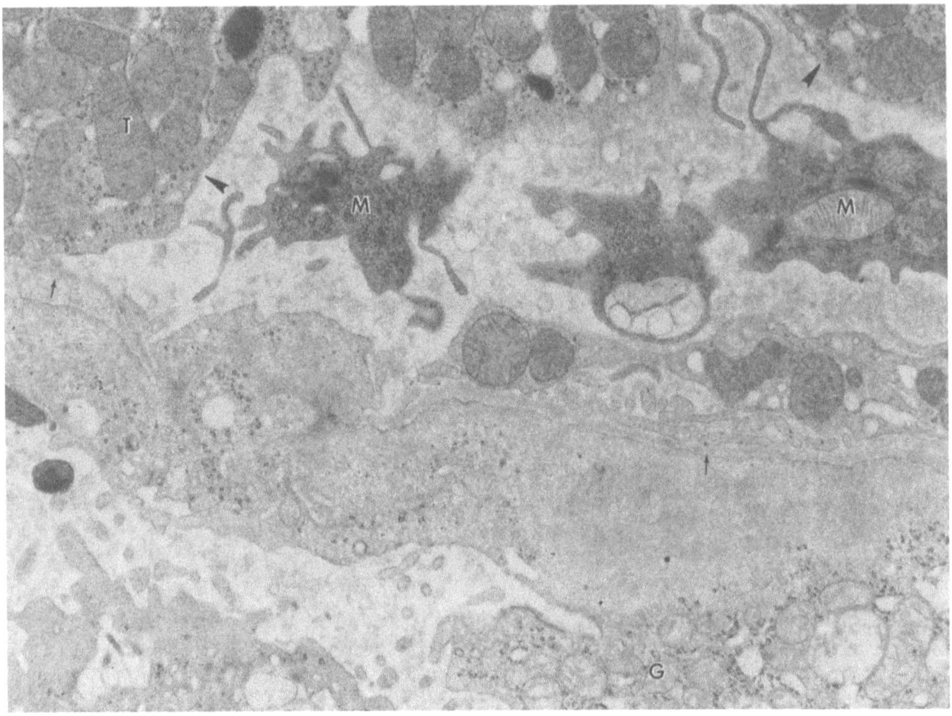

FIG. 2. Electron micrograph illustrating a kidney from a guinea pig 25 days after immunization with rabbit tubular basement membrane. A giant cell (G) adheres to the tubular basement membrane (arrows) of a proximal convoluted tubule. Parts of macrophages (M) are seen between the tubular basement membrane and the plasma membrane of epithelial cells (arrowheads) (x 15,000).

pathologic features (10). However, anti-TBM serum will not transfer disease to guinea pigs which have been depleted of complement by treatment with cobra venom factor, although IgG binds to TBM in the usual pattern (11). From these observations, it would appear that complement is required for the full development of interstitial and tubular lesions, although the alternate pathway of complement activation may be important and/or sufficient.

Expression of the disease also requires the participation of cells derived from bone marrow. Recipients, in which circulating leukocytes have been depleted by irradiation, do not develop tubulointerstitial lesions, although IgG and C_3 are seen to be deposited along the TBM (12).

The genetic basis of susceptibility to anti-TBM nephritis has been studied to the limited degree that is possible with the few

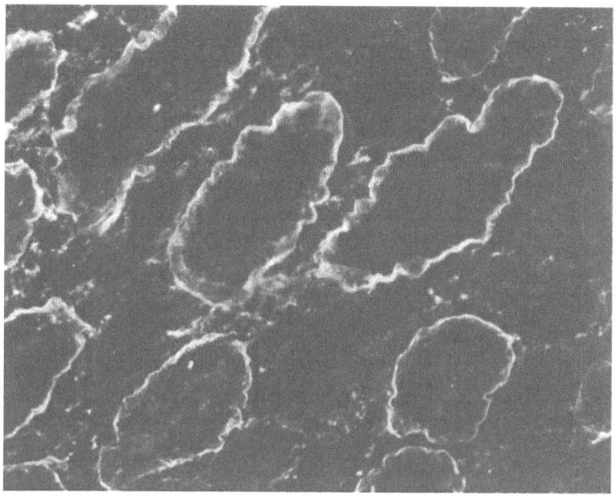

FIG. 3. Section of frozen kidney of a guinea pig with anti-TBM nephritis stained by the direct immunofluorescence technique for guinea pig IgG. Linear deposition of IgG along TBM is observed (x 300).

available strains of inbred guinea pigs. Guinea pigs of Strain 13 develop severe interstitial nephritis with conditions of immunization which fail to produce disease in Strain 2 (5). Genetic analysis has led to the conclusion that the differential susceptibility to this autoimmune renal disease is inherited as a single dominant or codominant trait linked to the major histocompatibility complex (13). Strain 2 guinea pigs also fail to develop interstitial lesions after receiving injections of anti-TBM antibodies in amounts which elicit the characteristic disease in Strain 13 animals (5). Differences in susceptibility are not absolute, however. With larger immunizing doses of TBM antigens, Strain 2 animals develop tubulointerstitial nephritis indistinguishable from that seen in Strain 13 and outbred Hartley guinea pigs, although longer time is required for the full expression of severe disease in Strain 2 (14).

The results of more recent passive transfer experiments, using highly purified subpopulations of IgG isotypes, require that some interpretations of earlier work be revised. Active immunization of guinea pigs with rabbit TBM elicits production of anti-TBM antibodies of both IgG_1 and IgG_2 isotypes. The separate transfer of either isotype induces tubulointerstitial nephritis, but also stimulates the synthesis, by the recipient, of anti-TBM autoantibodies of both immunoglobulin subclasses (15). Therefore, the demonstration of a requirement for radiosensitive cells in the passive transfer of anti-TBM nephritis may reflect an absence, in irradiated guinea pigs, of cells required for antibody synthesis. Furthermore, the resistance of Strain 2 guinea pigs to transfer of nephritis may also be attributable to a deficiency of antibody forming capacity, rather than other cellular responses. The mechanism by which transferred antibody might stimulate the synthesis of autoantibody of the same reactivity is not understood. One possibility is that the injected antibodies cause the modification or release of TBM antigens sufficient to provide an autoimmune response by the recipient. This kind of autoimmune amplification could explain the progressive nature of the disease.

Significant inhibition of tubulointerstitial nephritis can be achieved by the intraperitoneal administration of small amounts of an anti-idiotypic antiserum at the time of active immunization with TBM antigens (16). The anti-idiotypic antibodies obtained from rabbits are directed against guinea pig anti-TBM antibodies. Although the mechanism of suppression of interstitial nephritis has not been explained, similar effects in other systems have been ascribed to clonal deletion of B cells or the production of T suppressor cells. The relative amounts of idiotypic and anti-idiotypic antibody make it unlikely that a simple molecular reaction of those two antibody populations is sufficient to explain the result.

The anti-TBM antibodies produced by immunization of guinea pigs with rabbit TBM may crossreact with GBM and alveolar basement membrane (ABM) (14). Absorption experiments performed on sera and eluates of kidney and lung show that the antibodies binding to TBM and ABM are closely related or identical. Direct immunofluorescence tests confirm that IgG may be deposited in a linear pattern along the ABM in lungs of guinea pigs with anti-TBM nephritis. Fixation of IgG to ABM is associated with the accumulation of polymorphonuclear leukocytes in alveolar capillaries, thickening of alveolar septa and some proliferation of septal cells.

The histologic appearance of the interstitial infiltration is consistent with a cell mediated immune reaction. For that reason there has been considerable effort to demonstrate a role of specific cell mediated immunity in the pathogenesis of anti-TBM nephritis. The cellular infiltration in interstitial nephritis of guinea pigs with anti-TBM disease has been analyzed using hemadsorption techniques on tissue sections (6,17). Two weeks after immunization, only cells of the monocyte-macrophage series can be identified. Plasma cells, seen by light microscopy, do not react with the B lymphocyte marker. It is only three weeks after immunization that B cells are first demonstrable in the cellular infiltration (17). It is not possible to detect T cells on tissue sections prepared from kidneys taken from guinea pigs in any stage of the disease. The hemadsorption studies indicate that T lymphocytes have no important role in anti-TBM disease of guinea pigs. The failure of lymph node cells from immunized guinea pigs to transfer the disease to normal recipients of the same strain strengthens the view that specific cell mediated immunity is relatively unimportant in the pathogenesis of the disease (6).

It should be mentioned that an interstitial nephritis caused by anti-TBM antibodies has also been produced in Brown Norway and Lewis/Brown Norway rats by immunization with homogenates of rat kidney cortex or bovine TBM (18,19). Observations of immunopathology in rats are similar to those in guinea pigs. One difference is the influx of polymorphonuclear leukocytes seen in the cellular infiltration in early stages of interstitial nephritis in rats (18). Passive transfer experiments indicate that antibodies to TBM are the major factor required for development of tubulointerstitial lesions (19). Genetic differences in susceptibility are observable among inbred strains. In rats those differences have been correlated with a strain-specific nephritogenic TBM antigen that crossreacts with bovine TBM (18). Specifically sensitized cells do not appear to play an important part in the production of tubular and interstitial damage (20). The peritubular giant cells, which are associated with TBM destruction in guinea pig anti-TBM disease, are not a conspicuous feature of the histopathology of the disease in rats (19).

Anti-TBM antibodies may form following renal transplantation in rats and can be shown to be present in the allograft and in recipient sera when certain donor-recipient combinations are used (21). As binding of IgG to TBM is seen only in the transplanted kidney, it has been postulated that the antibody response is specific for an antigen present in the TBM of the donor strain and not in the recipient. It is difficult to assess the contribution of anti-TBM antibody deposition to tubular and interstitial lesions when graft rejection phenomena are superimposed.

Immune Complex Deposits

Pathologic changes in tubules and infiltration of the interstitium have been associated with the presence of immune complexes in several different laboratory models. Rabbits immunized with daily injections of a foreign serum protein, usually bovine serum albumin (BSA), develop chronic serum sickness glomerulonephritis that is characterized by the accumulation of immune complexes containing BSA, IgG and C_3 along the glomerular capillary wall (22). By immunofluorescence microscopy the immune deposits are seen to have a discrete, granular distribution; they appear as dense deposits in subepithelial and subendothelial sites of the glomerular capillary wall when studied by electron microscopy. If the daily BSA injection is increased to match individual antibody production and administered in divided daily doses to prevent fatal anaphylaxis, rabbits with a vigorous antibody response exhibit a systemic immune complex disease that is considered to be a model for systemic lupus erythematosus (SLE) in humans (23). In rabbits with systemic disease, granular immune deposits are found by immunofluorescence and electron microscopy in many organs and tissues, as well as in extraglomerular locations within the kidney (Fig. 4). Extraglomerular renal immune deposits are distributed in the walls of peritubular capillaries, in the interstitium, along Bowman's capsule and the TBM (23). The TBM deposits are not restricted to cortical tubules, but may be found in all tubular segments. Tubular cells are damaged and may become atrophic; the TBM is often thickened and split. Interstitial fibrosis and mononuclear cell accumulation are also correlated with the presence of extraglomerular renal immune deposits. It is generally believed that the complexes responsible for tubulointerstitial lesions in experimental chronic serum sickness form in circulation and deposit nonspecifically in tissues to produce pathologic changes and inflammation.

Nonglomerular kidney antigens have also been used to stimulate an autoimmune response in rabbits that causes the accumulation of immune deposits along the TBM of proximal tubules (24). In that model, a granular distribution of IgG and C_3 is associated with interstitial lesions characterized histologically by extensive interstitial fibrosis, tubular degeneration, focal mononuclear cell

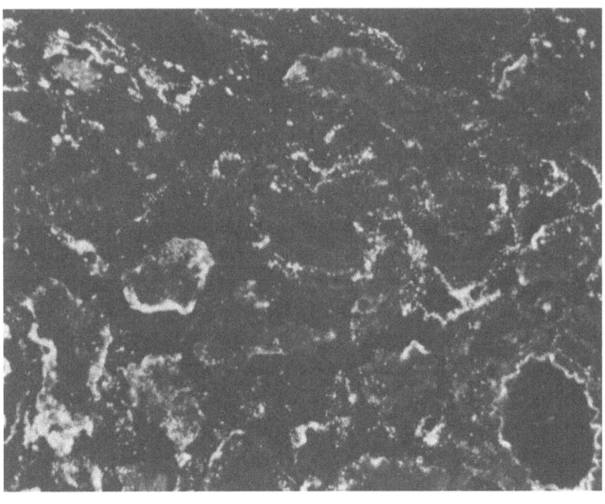

FIG. 4. Section of frozen kidney of a rabbit with chronic serum sickness produced by daily injection of BSA. The tissue has been stained in a direct immunofluorescence test for rabbit IgG. Granular to ribbon-like deposits of IgG are present along TBM. In addition, deposits can be seen in small peritubular vessels and in the interstitium (x 300).

infiltration and thickening and splitting of the TBM. Autoantibodies present in circulation and in kidney eluates stain proximal tubular epithelium (24,25). Furthermore, fluorescein-labeled kidney eluates also react with antigens present in the tubular deposits (25). Although moderate glomerular lesions may develop, this particular nephritis, characterized by the production of autoantibodies to antigens of the tubular epithelium, appears to be primarily a tubulointerstitial nephritis. It has been suggested that the immune deposits seen along the TBM do not arise as complexes preformed in circulation, but rather result from the local combination of antigen "leaking" from the tubular cells with antibody diffusing from peritubular capillaries. This autoimmune disease appears to have a complicated and, as yet incompletely described, natural history in which both antibodies to tubular epithelium and immune deposits containing the tubular antigen may be of pathogenic significance.

Similar granular deposits in the TBM of proximal tubules occur in another autoimmune renal disease, called Heymann nephritis, that can be elicited in some strains of rats (26,27). Those deposits will be described and discussed along with other aspects of Heymann nephritis in the following section of this review.

Antibodies to the Brush Border of Proximal Tubules

Damage of the tubules is found in an autoimmune disease (Heymann nephritis) produced in rats by immunization with a glomerulus-free extract of homologous kidney extract. Heymann nephritis affects both glomeruli and tubules, although most studies have focussed on the membranous nephropathy which is a striking feature of the disease (28,29,30). Several weeks after subcutaneous administration of a renal cortical extract called FxlA, granular deposits of IgG and C_3 can be detected along the GBM (31). Electron microscopy shows the glomerular immune deposits to have a subepithelial location in the capillary wall (30,32). Antibodies present in the circulation stain the brush border (BB) of cells of the proximal tubular epithelium (32). The glomerular immune deposits appear to contain BB antigen as well as the corresponding antibody and C_3 (28).

Progressive damage to the glomerular capillary wall results in an abnormal urinary protein excretion within two months of the initial immunization. At first, the kidneys of proteinuric rats with high titers of anti-BB antibody in circulation and urine are found to have IgG and C_3 fixed to the periluminal border of most proximal tubules (33,34) (Fig. 5). Alterations of the proximal tubules and the BB have been studied in tissues fixed by an *in situ* perfusion of the kidney that ensures optimal preservation of tubular architecture. The deposition of IgG, presumably specific anti-BB antibody, is correlated with extensive destruction and loss of

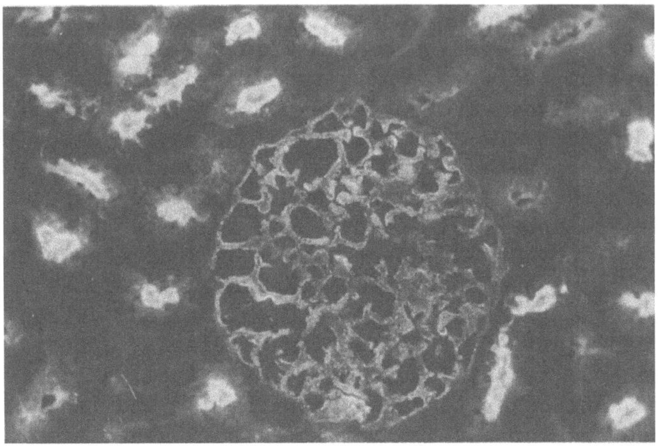

FIG. 5. Section of frozen kidney of rat in an early proteinuric stage of Heymann nephritis stained by the direct immunofluorescence technique for rat IgG. Finely granular deposits of IgG are present along the glomerular capillary wall. IgG is bound to the BB of proximal tubules (x 300).

microvilli as well as proliferation and degeneration of tubular epithelial cells (34) (Figs. 6,7,8,9). In addition to tubular damage, interstitial infiltration with mononuclear cells also occurs; mononuclear cells may be seen to cross the tubular epithelium. Cells seen within the tubular lumen may arise either from the interstitial cellular infiltration or from the damaged epithelium itself.

After 6 to 12 weeks of proteinuria, IgG and C_3 are no longer present along the luminal border of the proximal tubules, nor can the BB antigen be demonstrated by indirect immunofluorescence tests (34). By light and electron microscopy, many proximal tubules in this stage of Heymann nephritis are seen to be extensively or completely devoid of microvilli. At this time, direct immunofluorescence tests reveal instead the presence of focal granular deposits of IgG and C_3 along the TBM. By electron microscopy the immune deposits appear as dense material accumulated between the TBM and the basal plasma membrane of the epithelial cell. The TBM is tortuous and thickened, characteristic infoldings of the basal plasma membrane are gone and many epithelial cells are flattened.

In an even more advanced phase of Heymann nephritis, when proteinuria has persisted for three months or longer, anti-BB antibodies in circulation and urine are no longer detectable or are present in very low titer (34). Direct immunofluorescence tests reveal that kidneys in this stage of the disease have IgG bound along the GBM alone; BB and TBM deposits, abundant earlier, are not detectable. With anti-BB antiserum, using an indirect immunofluo-

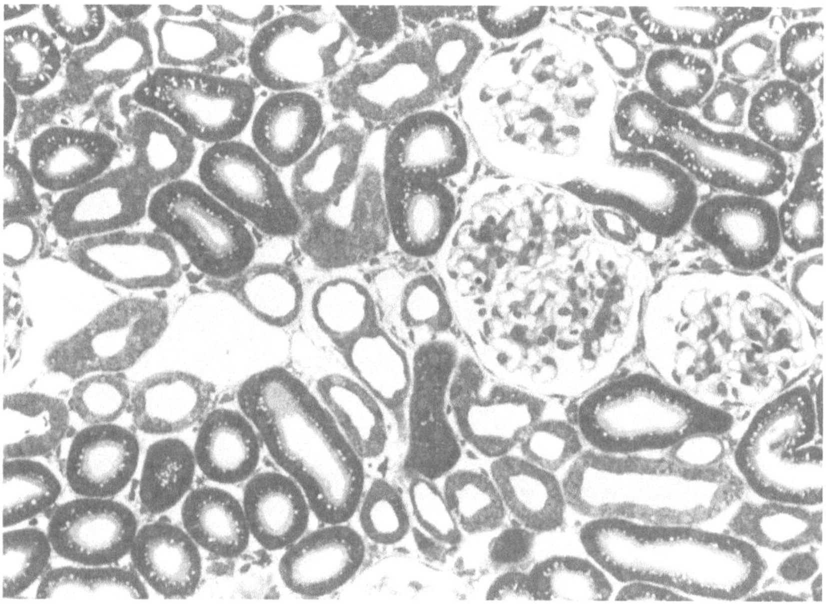

FIG. 6. Light micrograph of a normal rat kidney fixed by *in situ* perfusion (methylene blue, x 250).

rescence technique, it is possible to show that the BB antigen is present in a distribution and amount similar to that seen in the normal rat kidney. Examination by light and electron microscopy of kidneys fixed by *in situ* perfusion confirms that substantial regeneration of BB and partial disappearance of interstitial infiltration may occur in the absence of continued immunological insult by anti-BB antibody. Microvilli are present in the tubular epithelium in a near normal distribution; the cells regain a normal height; basal infoldings are restored. Newly formed TBM can be seen in close approximation to the basal surface of epithelial cells. Active cellular infiltration of the interstitium is replaced with fibrosis; intraluminal cells are reduced in number.

From the natural history of Heymann nephritis it appears that tubular and interstitial damage is the consequence of antibody mediated injury to cells of the proximal tubules. Tubulointerstitial pathology is seen only after the onset of proteinuria, when anti-BB antibody passes the glomerular filter and reaches the microvilli. An active tubulointerstitial disease persists as long as anti-BB antibody is present and able to react with antigen in the proximal tubules.

It is only possible to speculate about the nature and origin of the transient granular immune deposits found along the TBM in

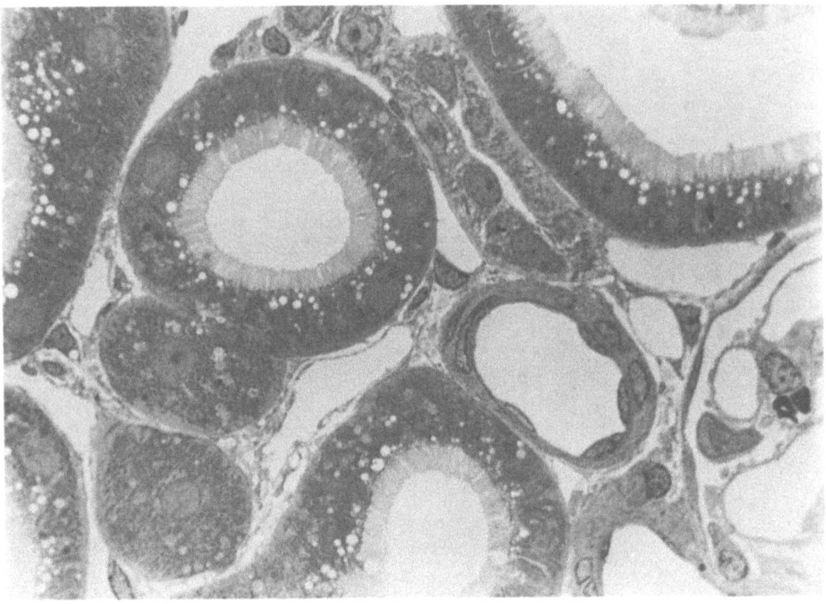

FIG. 7. Light micrograph of a normal rat kidney. The cells of the proximal tubules have a tall and uniform BB and many pinocytic apical vesicles (methylene blue, x 900).

Heymann nephritis. Granular deposits are not seen in vessel walls of the kidney or other tissues, as in chronic serum sickness. The strict limitation of the deposits to the TBM of proximal tubules also suggests that an immune reaction specific to antigens of the proximal tubular cells is responsible for their formation. For those reasons it seems unlikely that the deposits originate as complexes preformed in circulation. Substantial evidence suggests that the glomerular deposits in Heymann nephritis result from an *in situ* reaction of circulating anti-BB antibody with a fixed, crossreactive antigen which is distributed in discrete sites along the GBM (35). TBM deposits could also form by the combination of anti-BB antibodies with fixed tubular antigens or with antigens that "leak" from the cell as a consequence of the extensive degeneration that follows fixation of IgG to the BB.

Peritubular immune deposits have been described, in association with anti-BB antibody production, following renal transplantation in the rat (36). It is possible that interstitial mononuclear cell infiltration seen in the allograft is attributable, at least in part, to antibody mediated tubular damage similar to that seen in Heymann nephritis.

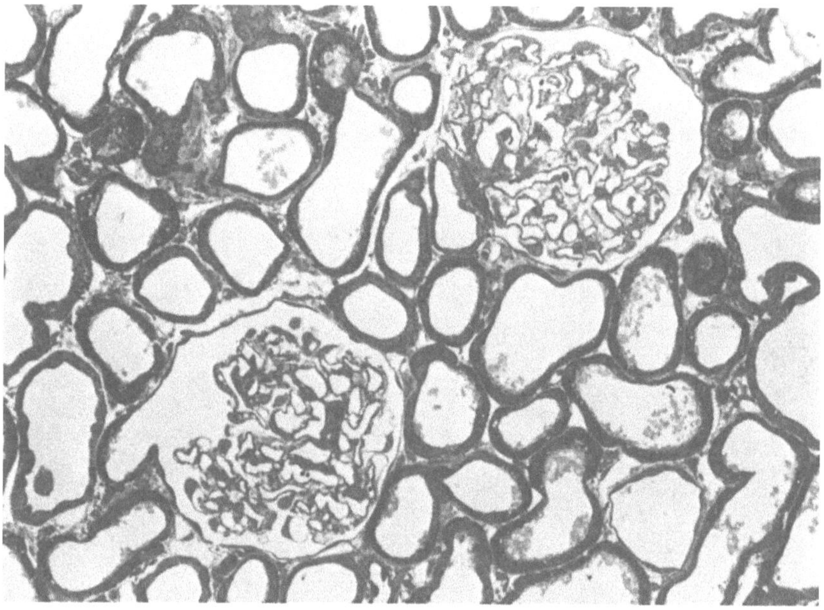

FIG. 8. Light micrograph of a kidney of a rat with Heymann nephritis at a stage in which IgG and C_3 are bound to the BB (see Fig. 5). The kidney has been perfused *in situ*. The lumina of many proximal tubules, which contain floccular debris are abnormally dilated, epithelial cells are flattened, and only a few apical vesicles are present. The BB of proximal tubules is frequently lacking (methylene blue, x 250).

Cell Mediated Interstitial Nephritis

The mononuclear cell composition of the interstitial cell infiltration found in many models of experimentally induced tubulo-interstitial nephritis is consistent with the hypothesis that cell mediated immune responses contribute to the pathogenesis. All of the available data, however, support the view that humoral mechanisms are of primary importance. It has been demonstrated that responses, analogous to delayed hypersensitivity reactions in the skin, can be elicited in the renal cortex (37). Thus, under appropriate conditions, inflammatory reactions can be produced in the renal interstitium that consist of mononuclear cells, are transferable with cells and not serum, and occur in the absence of circulating antibodies to the sensitizing antigen. It remains to be determined whether specific cell mediated immunity is a factor in the immunopathogenesis of any of the interstitial nephritides which have been produced in animals.

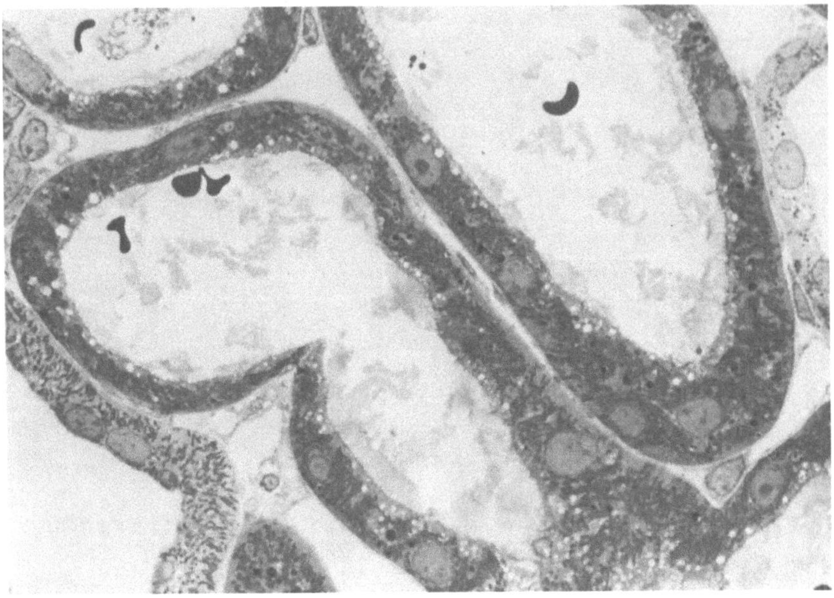

FIG. 9. Light micrograph of a kidney similar to that seen in Fig. 8 showing partial destruction of BB. Debris fills the lumen of proximal tubules. Apical vesicles are absent where BB is missing (methylene blue, x 900).

IMMUNOLOGICALLY MEDIATED TUBULOINTERSTITIAL NEPHRITIS IN MAN

Interstitial nephritis, associated with extraglomerular deposition of immunoglobulins as part of immune complexes or as anti-TBM antibody, is found infrequently in man. When observed it is often associated with immunologically mediated glomerular disease and the interstitial damage may be secondary to glomerular pathology. The information required to establish unequivocal cause and effect relationships between the immune deposits and tubulointerstitial pathology is rarely available. For that reason it is usually difficult to assess the contribution of immunological mechanisms to the development of interstitial lesions in human disease. Nevertheless, the compelling evidence from animal models and the correlations, to be described, between tubulointerstitial lesions and extraglomerular renal immune deposits in man make it appear very likely that immunological factors play a part in the pathogenesis of a variety of interstitial nephritides.

Antibodies to TBM

Antibodies to TBM in man have been detected in association with anti-GBM glomerulonephritis, in methicillin-related interstitial nephritis, after renal transplantation, and in immune complex glomerulonephritis. The observation of anti-TBM antibodies as an isolated phenomenon is very rare.

Anti-TBM antibodies are found most often in patients with anti-GBM glomerulonephritis (3,38). In those patients, serum and kidney eluates react *in vitro* with GBM and TBM, and in addition, sometimes with ABM, suggesting that antibodies may be directed against antigenic determinants common to many basement membranes. Although it is difficult to evaluate the contribution of anti-TBM antibodies to renal dysfunction in patients with a concomitant anti-GBM glomerulonephritis, the severe tubular and interstitial lesions found in anti-GBM-anti-TBM nephritis are probably partially attributable to the fixation of IgG and C_3 to the TBM. Tubulointerstitial damage is certainly more frequent and severe in patients with anti-GBM and anti-TBM antibodies than in those with anti-GBM antibodies alone (38).

Anti-TBM antibody may be seen in direct immunofluorescence tests to have a focal distribution in some patients, whereas in others the majority of renal tubules are involved (39) (Fig. 10). Antibodies in renal eluates and/or the circulation of those patients show the same patterns of reaction with TBM in indirect immunofluorescence tests. This observation suggests that anti-TBM antibodies of different specificities are responsible for the two distinct patterns of TBM staining. The tubulointerstitial lesions appear typically as peritubular and perivascular infiltrations composed of polymorphonuclear and mononuclear cells (38). Occasionally, multinucleated giant cells may be present. Cell proliferation and degeneration may be discerned in the epithelium of the tubules. The TBM can be thin and disrupted in some areas; in other places it may be thickened or duplicated. Mononuclear cells may be found between cells of the proximal tubular epithelium. The proliferation of epithelial cells seen in this human disease is not a prominent feature of anti-TBM nephritis in guinea pigs or rats, nor do the giant cells seen in human anti-GBM-anti-TBM nephritis appear to function as those described in the guinea pig model (8).

In a few patients, mostly children, anti-TBM antibodies, interstitial nephritis and severe tubular dysfunction have been observed to accompany immune complex glomerulonephritis. In one instance, formation of anti-TBM antibodies followed a severe post-streptococcal glomerulonephritis (40). Examination of sequential biopsies established that the development of tubulointerstitial disease was correlated with the appearance of anti-TBM antibodies in circulation and with their deposition along the TBM. It was

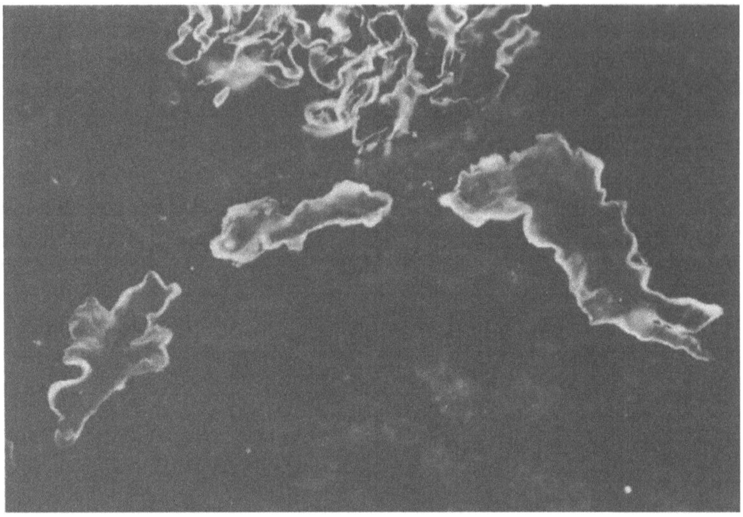

FIG. 10. Section of frozen kidney from a patient with anti-GBM anti-TBM nephritis stained for IgG. Antibody is seen to be deposited in a linear pattern along GBM and the basement membrane of a few tubules (x 300).

proposed that damage to the tubules produced by the original renal disease triggered the synthesis of autoantibodies directed against TBM antigens. In other reports, nephrotic syndrome, associated with heavy granular immune deposits along GBM and TBM was accompanied by anti-TBM antibodies in the kidney and/or in circulation, as well as with Fanconi's syndrome (3,41,42). These observations are also consistent with the hypothesis that injury to the tubules could stimulate an autoimmune anti-TBM response. One patient with linear and granular immune deposits along TBM developed pulmonary symptoms; autoantibodies reacting with ABM were found in circulation (41). This finding suggests that anti-TBM antibodies cross-reacting with ABM may also occasionally cause pulmonary lesions in man similar to those described in guinea pigs (14).

The detection of anti-TBM antibodies in a few cases of methicillin-associated interstitial nephritis has led to the suggestion that anti-TBM antibodies may play a part in the pathogenesis of drug-related nephritis (43,44). It was proposed that the dimethyl penicylloyl group, which is secreted by proximal tubules, may, when bound to the TBM as a hapten protein conjugate, stimulate an immune response that results in linear fixation of IgG along the TBM (44). Interstitial damage would be presumed to be the consequence of antibody deposition. However, as anti-TBM antibodies are not present in most cases of drug-related nephritis, including many in which penicillin analogues are implicated, anti-TBM antibodies most probably are not directly responsible for the majority of cases of interstitial nephritis associated with drug hypersensitivity (45,46,47). Taken together, the clinical manifestations of hypersensitivity, the elevated circulating IgE concentrations and the distinctive eosinophil component of the interstitial cellular infiltration seen in many cases of drug-associated interstitial nephritis provide some evidence that IgE mediated hypersensitivity may contribute to renal pathology. For this intriguing and perplexing disease an animal model would be invaluable and is lacking.

Anti-TBM antibodies in the absence of anti-GBM antibodies are sometimes found following renal transplantation (48,49,50). The rejection process may act as a nonspecific adjuvant or may cause damage to TBM resulting in the formation of anti-TBM antibodies (48). Alternatively, TBM antigens unique to the graft may be immunogenic in human recipients, as has been shown in rats (21). In any event, the pathogenetic role of anti-TBM antibodies in allograft is difficult to evaluate because the cellular immune responses important in rejection are also able to produce substantial tubulointerstitial damage.

Severe interstitial nephritis with anti-TBM antibodies in the absence of significant glomerular accumulation of IgG is rarely found (51).

Immune Complex Deposits

Granular deposition of IgG and C_3 along TBM, in the absence of anti-TBM antibodies, has been observed to be associated with histologic abnormalities of the tubules and interstitium in man. In a high percentage of patients with SLE glomerulonephritis, granular to ribbon-like extraglomerular immune deposits are also present (51). The deposits, found along TBM are associated with all tubular segments (Fig. 11). In addition, deposits may be observed in the interstitium, in the walls of peritubular capillaries and in larger vessels. Denatured DNA has been demonstrated as a constituent of the tubulointerstitial immune deposits in some cases (52). Therefore, it appears likely that the extraglomerular renal deposits in SLE arise from DNA-anti-DNA immune complexes formed in the circulation.

The pathology which accompanies deposition of immune complexes includes inflammatory cell infiltration of the interstitium, damage and degeneration of tubular cells, thickening and duplication of the TBM. Tubular dysfunction may also be the consequence of extensive tubulointerstitial accumulation of immune complexes in patients with SLE (53). These findings are anticipated from observations made of rabbits with chronic serum sickness nephritis and

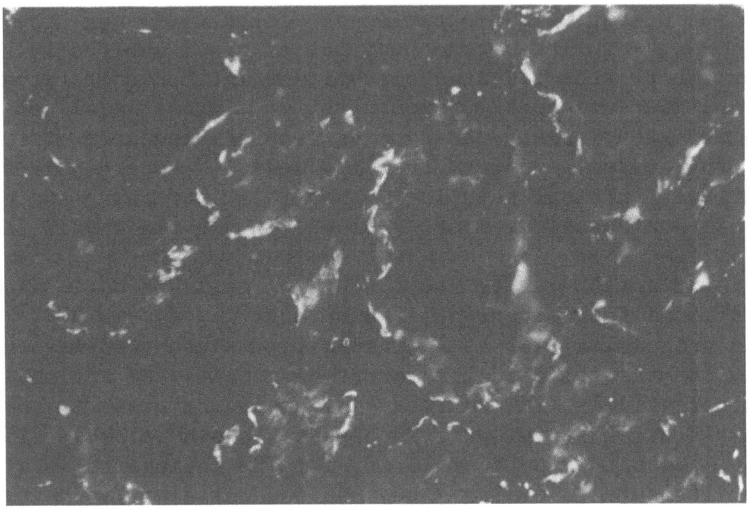

FIG. 11. Direct immunofluorescence test for IgG on a frozen section of a kidney from a patient with SLE nephritis. Immune deposits are present in a granular to ribbon-like pattern along TBM.

are a confirmation of the applicability of that animal model to the study of human disease. Granular extraglomerular renal immune deposits have been described in association with other renal diseases (54), but are so characteristic for SLE nephritis that their demonstration has some diagnostic significance.

Antibodies to Brush Border of Proximal Tubules

A role of anti-BB antibodies in human interstitial nephritis has not been demonstrated, although anti-BB antibodies have been implicated in a few cases of human glomerulonephritis (55,56). Antibodies staining the BB have also been described in allograft recipients (57). Studies of rats with Heymann nephritis suggest that antibody deposition along the periluminal border of tubular cells may be transitory, with damage difficult to discern following immersion fixation of tissue. For that reason, immune mechanisms, similar to those which produce tubulointerstitial injury in Heymann nephritis, may have been overlooked in the evaluation of human renal disease.

Cell Mediated Immunity

The histology of the interstitial inflammation seen in many cases of human interstitial nephritis suggests that mechanisms of cell mediated immunity may contribute to the development of the interstitial lesions. However, there is not yet good evidence to support that idea.

In one patient, an acute interstitial nephritis, apparently attributable to aspirin hypersensitivity, was associated with cell mediated immunity to aspirin measured in lymphocyte stimulation tests (58). This observation raises the possibility that drug hypersensitivity, manifested as a cell mediated reaction in the kidney, may produce interstitial nephritis.

The pathogenic significance of immunologic mechanisms in human tubular and interstitial nephritis is incompletely understood. The application of immunofluorescence techniques to the study of renal biopsy specimens has increased the ability to recognize immunologically mediated tubulointerstitial pathology. Animal models of tubulointerstitial renal disease have demonstrated some of the possible relationships of immunologic injury to tissue damage and renal dysfunction. Elucidation of the natural history of immunologically mediated tubulointerstitial disease in animals has aided the recognition of similar nephropathies in man. Until now, however, immunopathogenic mechanisms have been implicated in only a small fraction of human interstitial nephritides. Although immunologically mediated interstitial nephritis in man appears rare, it seems likely that an immune pathogenesis has not yet been identified in some instances in which it is important. The contribution of humoral immune factors to tissue damage, which has been greatly clarified by study of animal models, may have been overlooked in tissue specimens obtained at late stages of disease. The mechanisms by which tubular injury could lead to anti-TBM autoimmunization have not been identified, nor has a counterpart of anti-BB damage to tubules been recognized in man. In addition, animal models of tubulointerstitial disease mediated by specific cellular immunity, resembling human nephropathies, are not available. This fact may partly explain the failure to demonstrate a role of cell mediated immunity in human tubular and interstitial nephritis.

REFERENCES

1. McCluskey, R.T. and Klassen, J.: Immunologically mediated glomerular, tubular and interstitial renal disease. N. Engl. J. Med. 288: 564-569, 1973.

2. Andres, G.A. and McCluskey, R.T.: Tubular and interstitial renal disease due to immunologic mechanisms. Kidney Int. 7: 271-289, 1975.

3. Lehman, D.H., Wilson, C.B. and Dixon, F.J.: Extraglomerular immunoglobulin deposits in human nephritis. Am. J. Med. 58: 765-786, 1975.

4. Steblay, R. and Rudofsky, U.H.: Renal tubular disease and autoantibodies against tubular basement membrane induced in guinea pigs. J. Immunol. 107: 589-594, 1971.

5. Hyman, L.R., Colvin, R.B. and Steinberg, A.D.: Immunopathogenesis of autoimmune tubulointerstitial nephritis. 1. Demonstration of differential susceptibility in Strain II and Strain XIII guinea pigs. J. Immunol. 116: 327-335, 1976.

6. Van Zwieten, M.S., Bhan, A.K., McCluskey, R.T. and Collins, A.B.: Studies on the pathogenesis of experimental anti-tubular basement membrane nephritis in the guinea pig. Am. J. Path. 83: 531-541, 1976.

7. Brown, A.C., Carey, K. and Colvin, R.B.: Inhibition of autoimmune tubulointerstitial nephritis in guinea pigs by heterologous antisera containing anti-idiotype antibodies. J. Immunol. 123: 2102-2107, 1979.

8. Andres, G.A., Szymanski, C., Albini, B., Brentjens, J.R., Milgrom, M., Noble, B., Ossi, E. and Steblay, R.: Structural observations on epithelioid and giant cells in experimental autoimmune tubulointerstitial nephritis in guinea pigs. Am. J. Path. 96: 21-29, 1979.

9. Steblay, R. and Rudofsky, U.H.: Transfer of experimental autoimmune renal cortical tubular and interstitial disease in guinea pigs by serum. Science 180: 966-968, 1973.

10. Rudofsky, U.H., McMaster, P.R., Ma, W-S., Steblay, R.W. and Pollara, B.: Experimental autoimmune renal cortical tubulointerstitial disease in guinea pigs lacking the fourth component of complement (C_4). J. Immunol. 112: 1387-1393, 1974.

11. Rudofsky, U., Steblay, R.W. and Pollara, B.: Inhibition of experimental autoimmune renal tubulointerstitial disease in guinea pigs by depletion of complement with cobra venom factor. Clin. Immunol. Immunopath. 3: 396-407, 1975.

12. Rudofsky, U. and Pollara, B.: Studies on the pathogenesis of experimental autoimmune renal tubulointerstitial disease in guinea pigs. 1. Inhibition of tissue injury in leukocyte-depleted passive transfer recipients. Clin. Immunol. Immunopath. 4: 425-439, 1975.

13. Hyman, L.H., Steinberg, A.F., Colvin, R.B. and Bernard, E.: Immunopathogenesis of autoimmune tubulointerstitial nephritis. II. Role of an immune response gene linked to the major histocompatibility complex. J. Immunol. 117: 1894-1897, 1976.

14. Milgrom, M., Albini, B., Noble, B., O'Connell, D., Brentjens, J. and Andres, G.: Antibodies in guinea pigs immunized with kidney and lung basement membranes. Clin. Exp. Immunol. 38: 249-258, 1979.

15. Hall, C.H., Colvin, R.B., Carey, K. and McCluskey, R.: Passive transfer of autoimmune disease with isologous IgG_1 and IgG_2 antibodies to the tubular basement membrane in Strain XIII guinea pigs. J. Exp. Med. 146: 1246-1260, 1977.

16. Brown, C.A., Carey, K. and Colvin, R.B.: Inhibition of autoimmune tubulointerstitial nephritis in guinea pigs by heterologous antisera containing anti-idiotype antibodies. J. Immunol. 123: 2102-2107, 1979.

17. Szymanski, C., Albini, B. and Andres, G.: Subpopulations of mononuclear cells in interstitial infiltrates of nephritis. Unpublished observations.

18. Lehman, D.H., Wilson, C.B. and Dixon, F.J.: Interstitial nephritis in rats immunized with heterologous tubular basement membrane. Kidney Int. 5: 187-195, 1974.

19. Sugisaki, T., Klassen, J., Milgrom, F., Andres, G.A. and McCluskey, R.T.: Immunopathologic study of an autoimmune tubular and interstitial renal disease in Brown Norway rats. Lab. Invest. 28: 658-671, 1973.

20. Lehman, D.H. and Wilson, C.B.: Role of sensitized cells in antitubular basement membrane interstitial nephritis. Int. Arch. Allergy Appl. Immun. 51: 168-174, 1976.

21. Lehman, D.H., Lee, S., Wilson, C.B. and Dixon, F.J.: Induction of antitubular basement membrane antibodies in rats by renal transplantation. Transplantation 17: 429-431, 1974.

22. Dixon, F.J., Feldman, J. and Vazquez, J.: Experimental glomerulonephritis: the pathogenesis of a laboratory model resembling the spectrum of human glomerulonephritis. J. Exp. Med. 113: 899-919, 1961.

23. Brentjens, J.R., O'Connell, D.W., Pawlowski, I.B. and Andres, G.A.: Extraglomerular lesions associated with deposition of circulating antigen-antibody complexes in kidneys of rabbits with chronic serum sickness. Clin. Immunol. Immunopath. 3: 112-126, 1974.

24. Klassen, J., McCluskey, R.T. and Milgrom, F.: Nonglomerular renal disease produced in rabbits by immunization with homologous kidney. Am. J. Path. 63: 333-350, 1971.

25. Klassen, J., Milgrom, F. and McCluskey, R.T.: Studies of the antigens involved in an immunologic renal tubular lesion in rabbits. Am. J. Path. 88: 135-141, 1977.

26. Heymann, W., Hackel, D.B., Harwood, S., Wilson, S.G. and Hunter, J.L.: Production of nephrotic syndrome in rats by Freund's adjuvants and rat kidney suspension. Proc. Soc. Exp. Biol. Med. 100: 660-664, 1959.

27. Steinglein, B., Thoenes, G. and Gunther, E.: Genetic control of susceptibility to autologous immune complex glomerulonephritis in inbred rat strains. Clin. Exp. Immunol. 33: 88-94, 1978.

28. Edgington, T.S., Glassock, R.J. and Dixon, F.J.: Autologous immune-complex pathogenesis of experimental allergic glomerulonephritis. Science 152: 1432-1434, 1967.

29. Alousi, M.A., Post, R.S. and Heymann, W.: Experimental autoimmune nephrosis in rats. Morphogenesis of the glomerular lesion: immunohistochemical and electron microscopic studies. Am. J. Path. 54: 47-72, 1969.

30. Schneeberger, E.E. and Grupe, W.E.: The ultrastructure of the glomerular slit diaphragm in autologous immune complex nephritis. Lab. Invest. 34: 298-305, 1976.

31. Glassock, R.J., Edgington, T.S., Watson, J. and Dixon, F.J.: Autologous immune complex nephritis induced with renal tubular antigen. II. The pathogenetic mechanism. J. Exp. Med. 127: 573-587, 1968.

32. Grupe, W.E. and Kaplan, M.: Demonstration of an antibody to proximal tubular antigen in the pathogenesis of experimental autoimmune nephrosis in rats. J. Lab. Clin. Med. 74: 400-409, 1969.

33. Klassen, J., Sugisaki, T., Milgrom, F. and McCluskey, R.T.: Studies on multiple renal lesions in Heymann nephritis. Lab. Invest. 25: 577-585, 1971.

34. Mendrick, D., Noble, B., Brentjens, J. and Andres, G.: Antibody-mediated injury to proximal tubules in Heymann nephritis, submitted for publication.

35. Couser, W.G., Steinmuller, D.R., Stilmont, M.M., Salant, D.J. and Lowenstein, L.M.: Experimental glomerulonephritis in the isolated perfused rat kidney. J. Clin. Invest. 62: 1275-1287, 1978.

36. Thoenes, G., Pielsticker, K. and Schubert, G.: Transplantation-induced immune complex kidney disease in rats with unilateral manifestation in the allografted kidney. Lab. Invest. 41: 321-333, 1979.

37. Van Zweiten, M., Leber, P.D., Bhas, A.K. and McCluskey, R.T.: Experimental cell mediated interstitial nephritis induced with exogenous antigen. J. Immunol. 118: 589-593, 1977.

38. Andres, G., Brentjens, J., Kohli, R., Anthone, R., Anthone, S., Baliah, T., Montes, M., Mookerjee, B., Prezyna, A., Sepulveda, M., Venuto, M. and Elwood, C.: Histology of human tubulo-interstitial nephritis associated with antibodies to renal basement membranes. Kidney Int. 13: 480-491, 1978.

39. Wilson, C.B. and Dixon, F.J.: Renal injury from immune reactions involving antigens in or of the kidney. In Immunologic Mechanisms of Renal Disease. Editors, Wilson, C.B., Brenner, B.M. and Stein, J.H. Churchill Livingstone, New York, p. 35-66, 1979.

40. Morel-Maroger, L., Kourilsky, O., Mignon, F. and Richet, G.: Antitubular basement membrane antibodies in rapidly progressive poststreptococcal glomerulonephritis. Clin. Immunol. Immunopath. 2: 185-194, 1974.

41. Levy, M., Gagnadadoux, M-F., Beziau, A. and Habib, R.: Membranous glomerulonephritis associated with antitubular and anti-alveolar basement membrane antibodies. Clin. Nephrol. 10: 158-165, 1978.

42. Tung, K. and Black, W.: Association of renal glomerular and tubular immune complex disease and antitubular basement membrane antibody. Lab. Invest. 32: 696-700, 1975.

43. Baldwin, D.S., Levine, B.B. and McCluskey, R.T.: Renal failure and interstitial nephritis due to penicillin and methicillin. N. Engl. J. Med. 279: 1245-1252, 1968.

44. Border, W., Lehman, D., Egan, J., Sass, H., Glode, J. and Wilson, C.: Antitubular basement membrane antibodies in methicillin-associated interstitial nephritis. N. Engl. J. Med. 291: 381-384, 1974.

45. Mery, J-P. and Morel-Maroger, L.: Acute interstitial nephritis. Proc. 6th Int. Congr. Nephrol., Florence, p. 524-529 (Karger, Basel), 1976.

46. Ooi, B., Ooi, Y., Mohini, R. and Pollak, V.: Humoral mechanisms in drug-induced acute interstitial nephritis. Clin. Immunol. Immunopath. 10: 330-334, 1978.

47. Galpen, J., Shinaberger, J., Stanley, T., Blumenkrantz, M., Bayer, A., Friedman, G., Montgomerie, J., Guze, L., Coburn, J. and Glassock, R.: Acute interstitial nephritis due to methicillin. Am. J. Med. 65: 756-765, 1978.

48. Klassen, J., Kano, K., Milgrom, F., Menno, A., Anthone, S., Anthone, R., Sepulveda, M., Elwood, C. and Andres, G.: Tubular lesions produced by autoantibodies to tubular basement membrane in human renal allografts. Int. Arch. All. 45: 675-689, 1973.

49. Wilson, C., Lehman, D., McCoy, R., Gunnells, J. and Stukel, D.: Antitubular basement membrane antibodies after renal transplantation. Transplantation 18: 447-452, 1974.

50. Paul, L., Van Es, L., Stuffers-Heiman, M., Brutel de la Riviere, G. and Kalff, M.: Antibodies directed against tubular basement membranes in human renal allograft recipients. Clin. Immunol. Immunopath. 14: 231-237, 1979.

51. Bergstein, J. and Litman, N.: Interstitial nephritis with antitubular basement membrane antibody. N. Engl. J. Med. 292: 875-878, 1975.

52. Brentjens, J., Sepulveda, M., Baliah, T., Bentzel, C., Erlanger, B., Elwood, C., Montes, M., Hsu, K. and Andres, G.: Interstitial immune complex nephritis in patients with systemic lupus erythematosus. Kidney Int. 7: 342-350, 1975.

53. DeFronzo, R., Cooke, R., Goldberg, M., Cox, M., Myers, M. and Agus, Z.: Impaired renal tubular potassium secretion in systemic lupus erythematosus. Ann. Int. Med. 86: 268-271, 1977.

54. Klassen, J., Andres, G., Brennan, J. and McCluskey, R.: An immunologic renal tubular lesion in man. Clin. Immunol. Immunopath. 1: 69-83, 1972.

55. Naruse, T., Kitamura, K. Myakawa, Y. and Shibata, S.: Deposition of renal tubular antigen along the glomerular capillary walls of patients with membranous glomerulonephritis. J. Immunol. 110: 1163-1166, 1973.

56. Shwayder, M., Ozawa, T., Boedecker, E., Guggenheim, S. and McIntosh, R.M.: Nephrotic syndrome associated with Fanconi syndrome. Immunopathogenic studies of tubulointerstitial nephritis with autologous immune-complex glomerulonephritis. Ann. Intern. Med. 84: 433-437, 1976.

57. Paul, L., Stuffers-Heiman, M., Van Es, L. and de Graeff, J.: Antibodies directed against brush border antigens of proximal tubules in renal allograft recipients. Clin. Immunol. Immunopath. 14: 238-243, 1979.

58. McLeish, K., Senitzer, D. and Gohara, A.: Acute interstitial nephritis in a patient with aspirin hypersensitivity. Clin. Immunol. Immunopath. 14: 64-69, 1979.

HIGHLIGHTS

IMMUNOLOGICALLY MEDIATED TUBULOINTERSTITIAL NEPHRITIS IN CHILDREN

Renée Habib, M.D. and Micheline Levy, M.D.

Institut National de la Santé et de la Recherche Médicale
Hôpital Necker Enfants-Malades, Paris, France

Several immunologically mediated mechanisms may lead to injury of renal tubules and interstitial tissue resulting in tubulointerstitial nephritis (TIN). The distinguishing features of these mechanisms are based upon their immunofluorescent microscopic (IF) pattern. Tubular linear deposits of immunoglobulins (Ig) suggest the presence of circulating antitubular basement membrane (TBM) antibodies. Granular deposits of Ig and/or complement (C) are likely related to the presence of immune complexes (IC). In the absence of deposits, a cell-mediated reaction may be suggested. These mechanisms have been well studied in experimental models. They may also be observed in man. We report about 14 children with proven or presumed immunologically mediated TIN.

Linear deposits along TBM and circulating anti-TBM antibodies were present in two patients.

In the following six, IF showed granular deposits of Ig and/or C likely representing the interstitial location of IC (2 SLE, 1 syphilis, 1 HbsAg related membranous GN, 1 shunt nephritis, 1 post infectious proliferative GN).

The findings by IF were not significant in the remaining six patients. However, the association of renal involvement with extrarenal disorders in four of them (chronic active hepatitis and ulcerative colitis in one and *uveitis* in three) suggests that an immunologic disorder might be responsible for the TIN. In a fifth patient the diagnosis of sarcoidosis was raised because of the finding of a giant-cell granulomatous lesion in the kidney. The last patient had isolated TIN (without uveitis) but, as for the previous five patients, steroid therapy led to the disappearance of the renal symptoms.

IF allows a clear-cut distinction between the various types of TIN, each deserving a specific therapy. Patients with TIN and no significant IF findings, are usually cured by steroid therapy. Etiologically related treatments may be undertaken in IC mediated TIN (SLE, shunt nephritis, syphilis). Patients with anti-TBM antibody related TIN would most likely benefit from plasmapheresis.

HIGHLIGHTS

ACUTE NON-BACTERIAL TUBULOINTERSTITIAL NEPHRITIS (TIN)

Gustavo Gordillo-Paniagua, M.D.

Div. Pediatr. Nephrol., Hosp. Infantil Mexico, Mexico City, Mexico

Clinical material was constituted of 29 children, 51% below one year of age. There were 18 males and 11 females. Twenty-three out of the 29 patients had the antecedent of drug ingestion just prior to the onset of the renal manifestations: gentamycin, kanamycin, ampicillin, streptomycin, sulphonamides, cefalosporin, sisomycin, diphenylhydantoin, diphenylhydramine were the incriminated drugs. Four patients had salmonellosis, scarlet fever, and upper respiratory infections, respectively, at the time TIN started. There were no antecedents in two children. Most of the patients presented with hematuria and some with acute renal failure. Urinary findings were hematuria, proteinuria and glycosuria. High values of BUN and serum creatinine were found in 10 patients. Percutaneous renal biopsy was done in 9 patients: interstitial edema, fibrosis and mononuclear cell infiltration were the predominant findings. No immunofluorescence was present in the tubulointerstitial lesions.

More information from the literature on cases with TIN caused by different antibiotics pointed out that skin rash, eosinophilia, fever, edema and the nephrotic syndrome were frequent findings beside acute renal failure, hematuria, and proteinuria. TIN may be presented in association with "crescentic" glomerulonephritis, membranous nephropathy, nephrotic syndrome with focal and segmental sclerosis, lupus nephritis, graft rejection, etc. There have been cases reported with simultaneous nephrotic syndrome and Fanconi syndrome. There also have been cases of TIN associated with extrarenal diseases such as uveitis.

Pathogenesis varies from direct toxic effects to immunological processes that may be immunocomplex autoantibodies or cell-mediated.

Withdrawal of the offending agent, etiological treatment, steroids or plasmapheresis may be useful according to the etiology and the pathogenesis of any individual case.

NEWER NEPHROTOXIC AGENTS

Carlos A. Vaamonde, M.D.

Dept. Med., Univ. Miami Sch. Med., Div. Nephrol.
Veterans Admn. Med. Ctr., Miami, Fla. 33152 USA

INTRODUCTION

There are numerous substances capable of affecting the kidneys and producing renal dysfunction or disease. Nephrotoxicity has been associated with acute or chronic *poisoning*, which may be accidental or suicidal in origin ($HgCl_2$, ethylene glycol, CCl_4), while in other cases results from exposure to *industrial or environmental hazards* (lead, mercury, CCl_4, cadmium, hydrocarbons). Although these forms of nephrotoxicity are important to physicians, the most prevalent cause of nephrotoxicity now-a-days is *drug induced* (Table 1).

New drugs are continuously being introduced into our pharmacologic or diagnostic armamentarium and the number of renal (and other) problems will undoubtedly increase with time and new drugs. Although a low or nil toxicity is a goal of the pharmaceutical industry, this is seldom achieved. Thus, the physician must be aware of this situation if prevention, early detection and appropriate therapy of drug-induced nephrotoxicity are to be undertaken.

The *frequency* of drug-induced renal damage is difficult to establish. In my experience, however, it is more frequent than generally thought. Patients are usually very sick with complicated medical and surgical problems on the one hand (with possible mechanisms for renal dysfunction being concomitantly operative (dehydration, shock)), or on the other extreme only the more severe patients are called to the attention of the nephrologist. With great frequency, particularly in seriously ill patients, multiple pharmaco-

Table 1. Therapeutic and Diagnostic Nephrotoxic Agents*

Drugs	Renal Dysfunction
Antibacterials	Acute Renal Failure (ARF) Acute Interstitial Nephritis Renal Tubular Acidosis (RTA) Polyuria Hypokalemia Proteinuria
Analgesics	Chronic Interstitial Nephritis Papillary Necrosis Nephrolithiasis
Lithium	Polyuria Incomplete RTA
Fluorinated Anesthetics	Polyuria ARF
Antineoplastic Agents	ARF Chronic Renal Failure
Radiographic Contrast Media	ARF

*In this review there is no intention to make tables complete or comprehensive.

logic agents (each with capacity for renal injury) have been used simultaneously or in sequency. Thus, more often than not, it is difficult to attribute to one given drug the sole responsibility for nephrotoxicity. Indeed, in many clinical circumstances a combination of offending agents may be responsible (methoxyflurane and aminoglycosides, various combinations of antibiotics, diuretics and antibiotics, etc.).

Although acute renal failure is usually equated with drug-induced renal toxicity, it is now quite clear that there is a *spectrum of clinical syndromes associated with drug-induced nephrotoxicity* (Table 2). Nevertheless, acute renal failure remains the more commonly reported form of drug-related renal dysfunction.

Of the many diagnostic and therapeutic agents capable of inducing renal damage (Table 1) only few will be described here. The drugs which I have selected are those more frequently associated with nephrotoxicity (aminoglycoside antibiotics) and those recently recognized as causing renal damage (radiographic contrast media, antineoplastic agents, rifampin).

Table 2. Drug Induced Renal Disease Clinical Syndromes

Acute renal failure

- Acute tubular insufficiency (necrosis)
- Acute interstitial nephritis
- Acute glomerulonephritis
- Renal angiitis

Nephrotic syndrome

Obstructive uropathy

- Periureteral fibrosis
- Crystalluria

Chronic renal failure

- Chronic interstitial nephritis
- Arteriolar nephrosclerosis
- Chronic glomerulonephritis

Tubular syndromes*

- Fanconi
- Renal tubular acidosis
- Nephrogenic diabetes insipidus
- Potassium wasting
- Sodium loss
- Magnesium loss
- Hydrogen loss

*Drug-induced inappropriate ADH syndrome is not included.

The purpose of this review is not to examine the effects and clinical usage of drugs in renal failure. Excellent reviews have been recently published on this subject and the reader is referred to them for specific information (1-5). However, reference to the usage of specific drugs in uremia will be mentioned. Finally, a brief review of the fundamental rôle of the kidney in the handling of drugs will be included. Again, detailed information on this subject can be found elsewhere (1-3,5-7).

THE RENAL HANDLING OF DRUGS (Table 3)

The rate of drug eliminated by the kidney depends on the *glomerular filtration rate* (GFR), the *concentration of the drug in the*

Table 3. Renal Handling of Drugs

I. Glomerular Filtration Rate
  A. Protein-Binding

II. Tubular Reabsorption
  A. Active
  B. Passive
  C. Nonionic Back Diffusion

III. Tubular Secretion

blood and its *protein binding* (7). In addition, a number of compounds (active drugs and their inactive metabolites) appear in the urine due to *tubular secretion* processes (Table 4). Others are filtered at the glomerulus and subsequently *reabsorbed* by the proximal tubular epithelium, such as the aminoglycoside antibiotics.

The reabsorption of a number of drugs will be influenced by *nonionic back diffusion*. Drugs which are either weak acids (acetazolamide, phenobarbital, salicylic acid, sulfathiazole, nitrofurantoin, penicillin, probenecid, etc.) or weak bases (amphetamine, quinidine, chloroquine, trimethaprim, ephedrine, isoproterenol, etc.) exist in a mixture of nonionic and ionic forms, with the particular proportion depending upon the pKa of the drug and the pH of the tubular fluid or urine. In an acid environment, weak acids exist pre-

Table 4. Therapeutic Agents Secreted by Renal Tubules

Acidic	Basic
Acetazolamide	Dopamine
Ethracrynic acid	Histamine
Furosemide	
Hydrochlorothiazide	Morphine
Metolazone	Procaine
Spironolactone	
Triamterene	Quinine
Penicillins	Thiamine
Phenylbutazone	
Salicylates	
Probenecid	

dominantly in their nonionized form. Since the renal tubular epithelial membrane permits the diffusion of nonionic (but not of the ionic) molecules across it, alkalinization of the urine (which decreases the proportion of nonionic molecules) diminishes nonionic back diffusion and increases excretion of certain drugs. For example, the urinary excretion of acetylsalicylic acid (pKa 3.5), phenobarbital (pKa 7.2) and probenecid (pKa 3.3) is increased by alkalinization (pH > 7.5) of the urine.

Because of the dependence of many commonly prescribed drugs on the kidney for excretion it is obvious that the elimination of these compounds will be affected when renal function is decreased. In addition, the *protein binding* of many drugs is decreased in uremia (7) (Table 5). This, however, does not mean that their plasma concentrations and duration of action will be necessarily increased in uremic patients. Other factors (metabolism, excretion) may enhance total drug elimination, making difficult to predict with accuracy the clinical consequences of decreased protein binding in a given uremic patient.

Since renal excretion represents the major route of elimination from the body for a number of drugs, there is potential risk of toxicity for the kidney. Because of its high blood flow, elevated metabolic rate, multiple enzymatic processes and specific functions (countercurrent concentrating mechanism, tubular secretion and reabsorption) *the kidney is particularly vulnerable to drug-related damage* (Table 6).

There are two basic mechanisms whereby the kidney can be subjected to drug-induced damage: *a direct toxic effect* (unchanged drug or its metabolites) or a *hypersensitivity reaction* (Table 7).

Table 5. Decreased Protein Binding of Commonly Used Drugs in Uremia

Barbiturates Diazepam Diphenylhydantoin Morphine	Benzylpenicillin Dicloxacillin Sulfonamides
Digitoxin	Phenylbutazone Salicylate
Warfarin	Clofibrate
Diazoxide	Thyroxine
Furosemide Triamterene	

Table 6. Vulnerability of the Kidney to Nephrotoxic Agents

Large blood flow
(0.4% B. Wt. gets 25% of cardiac output)

Great metabolic activity
(high O_2 and glucose consumption)

Large endothelial surface area (by B. Wt.)
(important with agents producing hypersensitivity)

Many enzyme systems
(heavy metals chelate intracellular S-H groups on essential enzymes and block cell energetics, repair and transport processes in proximal tubule)

Countercurrent system
may raise medullary concentration (phenacetin → acetaminophen)

Mechanism for protein unbinding in uremia
(Table 5)

Transcellular transport provides local exposure
(tubular secretion (Table 4); tubular reabsorption: aminoglycosides)

AMINOGLYCOSIDE NEPHROTOXICITY

The use of many antibacterial agents can result in renal dysfunction or disease. Their clinical and morphologic expression represents a spectrum of alterations ranging from acute renal failure (ARF) and acute interstitial nephritis to renal tubular disorders (renal tubular acidosis (RTA) and various water and electrolyte derangements) (Tables 1 and 2).

Table 8 depicts *antibacterial-associated renal dysfunction* categorized by clinical syndromes. *A listing of antibacterial agents without known nephrotoxicity* as of this writing is also provided (Table 9).

The aminoglycoside antibiotics are extensively used for the treatment of gram-negative infections. The incidence of renal complications varies between 2% and 10% according to author and specific antibiotic used (8-12). It should be clarified at the very outset that, although there are variations in the incidence and severity of renal dysfunction with the various aminoglycosides, *all*

Table 7. Nephrotoxic Mechanism

I. Drug Toxicity

A. Unchanged Drug (CCl_4, aminoglycosides, lithium)

B. Metabolites

(fenacetin → acetaminophen)
(methoxyflurane → F- oxalate)
(CIS-Platinum → $PtCl_4$?)

Dose-Related

(affected by decreased renal function)

II. Drug Hypersensitivity

A. Immunologically mediated

Not dose related
Needs sensitization
(penicillins, rifampin, sulfonamides)

---

the currently available antibiotics of this type are capable of nephrotoxicity (Table 10). The comparison of gentamicin toxicity to that of newer aminoglycosides is difficult. There are not adequate comparative data and extrapolation of animal data to the human situation may be misleading. Although some authors found no individual clear superiority in terms of general clinical use (11), others single out the lesser renal- and ototoxicity of tobramycin and netilmicin (13-16). Sisomicin, used mostly in Europe and South America, appears to be definitely more oto- and nephrotoxic than gentamicin in animal studies (17). Amikacin appears not to have greater toxicity than gentamicin (11) and is usually reserved for the treatment of gentamicin-resistant bacteria. We will use as a prototypical descriptive model of nephrotoxicity, that of gentamicin.

Gentamicin renal damage is noted less often in *neonates and children* than in adults, although it may occur with prolonged therapy. Recent experiments in neonates (18) and puppies (19) have demonstrated that renal tubular damage (enzymuria, morphologic changes) may occur during gentamicin administration despite normal serum creatinine levels. It was suggested (19) that the normal redistribution of renal blood flow from deeper to superficial glomeruli that occurs after ten days of life in the dog served to

Table 8. Antibacterial-Associated Nephropathies*

I. Acute Renal Failure

A. Aminoglycosides
1. Amikacin
2. Streptomycin
3. Gentamicin
4. Sisomicin
5. Tobramycin
6. Kanamycin
7. Neomycin

B. Cephalosporins
1. Cephaloridine (†)
2. Cephalothin
3. Cephalexin
4. Cefazolin
5. Cefamandole
6. Cephapirin
7. Cephradine

C. Others
1. Colistimethate
2. Pentamidine
3. Amphotericin B
4. Rifampin
5. Sulfametazole
6. Vancomycin

II. Interstitial Nephritis

A. Ampicillin
B. Methicillin
C. Nafcillin
D. Oxacillin
E. Penicillin
F. Rifampin
G. Sulfonamides

III. Nephrogenic Diabetes Insipidus

A. Declomycin

IV. Renal Tubular Acidosis

A. Proximal

B. Distal
1. Tetracycline (outdated)
2. Amphotericin B

Table 8. Antibacterial-Associated Nephropathies* (Cont)

V. Potassium Wasting

A. Amphotericin B
B. Carbenicillin
C. Penicillin
D. Tetracycline (outdated)

VI. Metabolic Alkalosis
(renal loss of hydrogen)

A. Carbenicillin

VII. Proteinuria

A. Griseofulvin

VIII. Obstruction (Cristalluria)

A. Sulfas

---

*Partial listing.
†Should not be used since less nephrotoxic alternatives are available.

minimize gentamicin accumulation and damage to superficial nephrons and to preserve function. Furthermore, sexually immature rabbits treated with gentamicin did not develop acute tubular necrosis despite similar serum and renal tissue gentamicin levels in comparison to sexually mature animals (54% incidence) equally treated (19a).

There is a *spectrum of renal abnormalities* observed with aminoglycoside therapy (Table 11).

Table 9. Antibacterial Agents Without Known Nephrotoxicity

Amoxicillin
Clindamycin
Chloramphenicol
Cloxacillin
Doxycycline
Erythromycin
Ethambutol
Isoniazid
Lincomycin
Minocycline

Table 10. Nephrotoxic Aminoglycosides

Amikacin*
Gentamicin
Kanamycin†
Neomycin
Netilmicin
Sisomicin‡
Streptomycin
Tobramycin

Aminoglycosides antibiotics produced from species *micromonospora* have the letter "i" in their names (*), while those produced from species *streptomyces* have the letter "y" (†)(11). ‡ Used particularly in Europe and South America.

The most apparent clinical presentation is non-oliguric acute renal failure, but the oliguric variety is also found. At the University of Miami Hospitals gentamicin is probably the single most frequent cause of acute renal failure observed in adults and the majority of the cases are of non-oliguric variety. Usually, the onset of renal failure is gradual. Occasionally, the beginning of renal failure may be more insidious becoming clinically apparent only a few days after cessation of therapy. The clinical course may be prolonged, particularly in the elderly. Almost invariably this is a reversible lesion. The survival of the patient,

Table 11. Gentamicin Nephrotoxicity: Clinical Presentation*

I. Reduced GFR and urinary concentration

II. Acute renal failure

- A. Nonoliguric
- B. Oliguric

III. Enzymuria, proteinuria, aminoaciduria, glycosuria (16,20,21)

IV. Electrolyte Abnormalities

- A. Hypomagnesemia (22,23)
- B. Hypocalcemia (22)
- C. Hypokalemia (12,22)

*As a prototypical description of aminoglycoside toxicity.

however, depends on the background on which acute renal failure has developed (surgery, trauma, sepsis, severe burn, simple nephrotoxicity, etc.), and dialysis may be necessary.

There is clinical and experimental evidence of proximal renal tubular injury (Table 11). Indeed, the measurement of the urinary excretion of enzymes has been suggested as an early index of renal tubular damage (18). We have seen appearance of lysozymuria after only three days of administration of gentamicin to rats (24). Several electrolyte abnormalities have also been reported (Table 11). Of interest is the rarely reported hypomagnesemia secondary to prolonged use of gentamicin at large dosage (22,23).

Like in other forms of acute renal failure there are *known factors predisposing to nephrotoxicity*. *Age* appears to be of importance. In one study (25) the incidence of aminoglycoside nephrotoxicity was three-fold greater in patients 75 years or older compared to those younger than 30 years of age. *Pre-existing renal impairment and volume depletion* are also factors to be considered (25). Dehydration and extracellular fluid contraction increase the risk of renal damage as suggested by the animal studies by Bennett et al. (26). This may be in part related to enhanced tubular reabsorption and cortical accumulation of gentamicin (26). Finally, the administration of *aminoglycosides in combination with other potentially nephrotoxic agents* is common and has resulted in experimental and clinical toxicity. The drugs reportedly involved include the fluorinated anesthetic agent methoxyflurane (27), furosemide (28), and a variety of aminoglycosides other than gentamicin and other antibiotics, particularly cephalosporins and methicillin (29-31). The question of added toxicity with the cephalothin-gentamicin combination remains uncertain. Some authors have found that this particular combination results in a lower renal cortical concentration of gentamicin and in some protection against nephrotoxicity (32). This has been attributed to the nonreabsorbable anion effect of cephalothin, since separation of the administration of the drugs by 6 hours resulted in elimination of the protection (32). Most recently, the association of gentamicin-cephalothin with the chemotherapeutic agent Cis-platinum has been responsible for the occurrence of severe renal toxicity (see below). Thus, although the potentiating effect of these drugs remains undefined, they should be used with caution when combined with aminoglycoside antibiotics.

Pathogenesis of Aminoglycoside Nephrotoxicity

It is now clear that the kidney handles gentamicin by glomerular filtration (protein binding in plasma is minimal), and subsequent proximal tubular (bidirectional, but mostly from tubular lumen to cell) reabsorption. It is also known that the human and many animal species kidneys concentrate all aminoglycosides (with exception of streptomycin) up to 20-30 times the serum levels in the renal cortex (33,34) (Table 12). This is probably significant for toxicity since other antibiotics (Table 12) are concentrated in the renal medulla and papilla but not in the cortex, following the normal steep cortex-papillary concentrating gradient. The relationship between relative cortical drug concentration and nephrotoxicity is, however, unclear since aminoglycosides with lesser nephrotoxicity than gentamicin (tobramycin, netilmicin) achieve similar levels in the renal cortex (33).

In man and animals characteristic ultrastructural lesions in the epithelial cells of the proximal tubules have been observed after administration of aminoglycosides. These appear to be altered lysosomes which contain dark, whorled inclusions called myeloid bodies (35), interacting in some fashion with the drugs. Strongly cationic drugs (such as gentamicin) cause this type of change in many tissues by their great affinity for polyanionic phospholipid membranes. There appears to be initial binding of gentamicin to the brush border membrane of the proximal tubular cells with subsequent endocytosis and lysosomal sequestration, formation of myeloid bodies and lysozymuria. However, the exact mechanisms for gentamicin nephrotoxicity, for its intracellular transport and for the described alterations are unresolved, but it is currently accepted that the myeloid bodies are a histologic marker of aminoglycoside administration and tissue uptake rather than indicating renal toxicity (3). Changes in renal blood flow and in the glomerular capillary

Table 12. Accumulation of Antimicrobial Agents in Renal Tissues*

	Tissue-Serum Ratios	
Antimicrobial	Cortex/Serum	Papilla/Serum
Aminoglycosides		
Neomycin	36	
Gentamicin	20	6
Kanamycin	10	
Tobramycin	6	
Streptomycin	2	
Carbenicillin	2	17
Ampicillin	2	5
Cephalothin	2	5
Sulfisoxazole	2	4

*Normal hydropenic dogs. Adapted from Whelton (33).

ultrafiltration coefficient have also been implicated in experimental gentamicin renal toxicity (36,37).

The *prevention* of aminoglycoside-induced nephrotoxicity follows the same general guidelines recommended for potentially toxic drugs (Table 13). Dosage should be corrected according to the serum creatinine concentration. Table 14 shows variable interval and dose methods for the adjustment of gentamicin dosage. There is no apparent advantage of one method over the other (11), although most physicians utilize for simplicity reasons the variable interval method. It should be remembered, however, that even utilizing these methods, toxicity may appear even with adequate serum levels of the drug. When serum creatinine starts to rise, already GFR has decreased substantially. In addition, assessment of serum creatinine levels is usually done in hospitals from several to 24 hours after establishing the daily dosage; thus, the adjustment of dose runs invariably behind GFR changes.

RIFAMPIN NEPHROTOXICITY

Of the commonly used anti-tuberculous drugs only rifampin has been associated with a peculiar form of nephrotoxicity. *Ethambutol* and *isoniazid* as far as it is known are not nephrotoxic (Table 9)

Table 13. General Guidelines to Prevent Antibiotic-Induced Nephrotoxicity

1. Be aware of nephrotoxicity.
2. Avoid dehydration maintaining an expanded extraceullular fluid volume.
3. Adjust dose to continued changes in GFR (serum creatinine, endogenous creatinine clearance).
4. Check frequently aminoglycoside serum levels particularly in patients with severe infections and in patients with impaired renal function (gentamicin: peak > 10 μg/ml, through > 2 μg/ml).
5. Avoid or use with caution combination of drugs (antibiotics, methoxyflurane, furosemide, radiographic contrast media, chemotherapeutic agents).
6. Be aware of the increased risk in elderly patients.
7. Rational indication of potentially toxic antibiotic prescription.

Table 14. Aminoglycoside Dosage in Renal Failure

Gentamicin	
Standard Dose (Normal GFR)	1.0 mg/Kg/8 hours

Dosage in Renal Failure: Two Methods:

1. Unchanged Dose → Variable Interval Method
2. Unchanged Interval → Variable Dose Method

EX. Scr = 5 mg/dl
1.0 mg/Kg (8 x 5) every 40 hours
Every 8 hours $\frac{(1.0)}{5}$ = 0.2 mg/Kg

Method 1 = 1.0 mg/Kg/40 hours
Method 2 = 0.2 mg/Kg/8 hours

The dose of ethambutol, however, needs reduction in renal failure. Likewise, isoniazid dosage should be reduced in slow acetylators (2).

Rifampin renal toxicity is rare and appears exclusively with intermittent therapy (38,39). The typical course is characterized by acute onset of fever, chills, loin pain and hematuria, all appearing within 60 minutes to hours of readministration of the drug after an interval in therapy. The histopathology reveals acute interstitial nephritis (Table 8) without immunoglobulin deposits in the majority of reported cases (38,39).

The pathogenesis of this lesion appears to be an anamnestic hypersensitivity reaction with antibodies against rifampin demonstrated in the serum of patients (40). It has been suggested that the drug-antibody reaction might liberate vasoactive substances which may produce renal cortical ischemia and acute renal failure. Of interest, a recent report of gradual onset of acute renal failure associated with reinstitution of rifampin therapy described immunoglobulin deposition about the tubules (41). The authors suggested that the tubular and interstitial lesions were mediated by antibody to tubular basement membrane. Renal failure improves after cessation of therapy and with steroids.

NEPHROTOXICITY OF ANTINEOPLASTIC DRUGS

Two types of currently prescribed chemotherapeutic agents have recently been associated with the development of renal damage: Cisplatinum and nitrosoureas.

Cis-platinum (Cis-diamminedichloroplatinum II, Cis-DDP) is an inorganic platinum compound active against tumors, including testicular, ovarian, bladder, and head and neck carcinomas. The main limiting factor in the clinical use of the drug is the renal toxicity. Dose-related acute tubular necrosis has been described in a number of recent reports (42-44). Of particular importance appears to be the association of Cis-platinum with gentamicin and cephalothin (44). Four patients such treated developed severe and extensive acute renal tubular necrosis which persisted until death occurring within few days to two weeks of this combination therapy (44). Chronic decreases in GFR have been also reported in patients under treatment with Cis-DDP and followed for up to two years (45). Plasma creatinine levels may not be elevated despite the decreased GFR because of the marked wasting state of the patients (45). With repeated courses of Cis-DDP chronic renal failure may develop.

The mechanism of the Cis-DDP renal damage is unknown. It has recently been shown that renal tissue protein-bound SH groups were decreased in the rat treated with Cis-DDP (46). This effect appears specific, since other models of acute renal failure in the rat (glycerol) did not change renal SH concentration. Platinum accumulates in renal cortex (mitochondria and cytosol) and it was suggested that its toxicity may be mediated by cellular accumulation and subsequent conversion to a metabolite ($Pt-Cl_4$) which causes tissue injury by reacting with SH groups (46).

Hydration and mannitol may ameliorate Cis-DDP renal dysfunction (44,45). Cis-DDP can also induce a renal tubular defect in magnesium conservation resulting in serious clinical syndromes of magnesium deficiency (47). Nitschke et al. (48) observed the occurrence of hypocalcemia and hypomagnesemia in several children receiving Cis-DDP for advanced tumors. The hypocalcemia is probably secondary to the hypomagnesemia causing diminished PTH secretion or end-organ resistance to PTH.

Nephrotoxicity has recently been reported with the use of two *nitrosoureas:* *BCNU* (1,3 Bis {2 chloroethyl}-1-NU) and *CCNU* (methyl chloroethyl-cyclohexyl NU) (49,50). These alkylating agents are the currently favored chemotherapy for solid brain tumors. Interstitial nephritis and renal failure developed in 14 of 160 children and adults treated with at least six courses of BCNU or CCNU (49). Exposure to more than 1500 mg of methyl CCNU per m^2 of body-surface area over at least 17 months led to severe renal damage in all the six children so treated (50). Renal biopsy revealed tubular atrophy, interstitial fibrosis and glomerular sclerosis in the absence of proliferation or immunoglobulin deposition. The striking fact of this new drug-induced renal damage is that nephrotoxicity occurs without a phase of renal failure and in the absence of significant urinary abnormalities or hypertension.

RADIOGRAPHIC CONTRAST MEDIA NEPHROTOXICITY

Acute renal failure is an uncommon but increasingly recognized complication of the use of iodinated radiographic contrast media. There is a growing awareness that its true incidence may be considerably higher than previously thought, since only the more serious patients tend to be seen by the nephrologists. This indeed has been our experience at the University of Miami Medical Center. A renewed attention has been given to this problem and numerous publications have appeared recently in major medical journals (51-55).

Renal dysfunction can occur following the administration of virtually *any* intravascular contrast agent and has been reported after urography, angiography, multiple dose cholecystography (56) and, most recently, computerized tomography with intravenous radiocontrast (55,57,58). Of note, in a most recent review seven of 23 patients who developed acute renal failure post-contrast media had been studied with computerized tomography (5).

In recent years a number of *risk factors* for the development of contrast media renal dysfunction have been identified (Table 15). These are: (a) advanced age (60 years or older). Review of four recent series comprising 70 patients shows that 50 (71%) were 60 years of age or older (55). It is not known if underlying vascular disease or progressive reduction in renal mass and renal blood flow associated with aging (59,60) are in part responsible. (b) Pre-

Table 15. Risk Factors in Radiographic Contrast Media Nephrotoxicity

Advanced age (60 years or older)
Pre-existing renal insufficiency
Dehydration
Specific diseases
Diabetes mellitus
Multiple myeloma
Vascular disease
Overdose (multiple exposure)
Hyperuricemia, hyperuricosuria
Proteinuria

existing renal insufficiency appears to be of great importance (61). (c) Likewise, dehydration, although not universally accepted (62), appears to contribute, particularly in susceptible patients (63,64). Patients are usually kept hydropenic for many hours in preparation or during multiple x-ray studies.

The *diabetic patient* population has emerged as probably having the highest risk of developing contrast media renal dysfunction. This can occur whether the patients have normal renal function (65), pre-existing renal disease (53,55,57,58,62,66-68), were subjected to a major angiographic procedure or only computerized tomography with contrast (55,57). A review of 88 reported patients with diabetes and radiocontrast-induced acute renal failure indicated that 89% had pre-existing renal insufficiency (55). Multiple myeloma is generally considered a risk factor; recent experience, however, casts some doubt about this (55,69).

Although there is considerable controversy, other factors thought to increase the risk are hyperuricemia, proteinuria and high contrast dose (52,55). The latter may be in the form of multiple contrast media exposure within 24 hours.

The *pathogenesis* of contrast media-induced acute renal failure has not been established. Associated with the administration of contrast media into the renal artery there is a biphasic response, with a transient rise followed by a more prolonged phase of decreased renal blood flow. It has been assumed that the hyperosmolality of the contrast media is responsible for these renal vascular changes (70). In addition, distinct red blood cell changes occur with these agents (crenation and agglutination of RBC's, increased blood viscosity) (71), but what their relationship is to contrast-induced nephrotoxicity is unknown. Some experimental evidence suggests that contrast material may produce direct tubular toxicity. There is decreased extraction of PAH (70), enzymuria (72) and altered tubular transport of sodium in the isolated toad bladder (73). Finally, intratubular obstruction by urinary protein (myeloma, Tamm-Horsfall mucoprotein), uric acid and oxalate crystallization (uricosuric effect of some contrast media agents) have been suggested (55,74,75). The significance of these alterations to the nephrotoxicity of radiographic contrast material, however, remains undetermined.

In general, contrast media-induced renal failure has a good *prognosis*. In some high risk patients, however, mortality may be as high as 5%-10% (55). Some of these patients may develop chronic renal failure (62).

Prevention of these forms of acute renal failure follows the same guidelines for nephrotoxins in general (Table 13). Specific guidelines to prevent contrast media renal damage are outlined in Table 16. It has been suggested recently that prevention of renal

Table 16. Guidelines for the Prevention of Contrast Media Nephrotoxicity

1. Careful assessment of benefit of x-ray procedure, particularly in high risk patients (aged, renal insufficiency, diabetes).

2. Avoid dehydration. This is mandatory in high risk patients.

3. Limit total dose of radiographic agent. Avoid multiple radiographic procedures within 24-hours or in subsequent days.

4. Select other diagnostic procedures when possible (sonography, computerized tomography without contrast).

5. If hyperuricemia and hyperuricosuria use hydration.

6. In high risk patients try mannitol.

failure may be achieved in diabetic patients at risk (older patients with pre-existing renal disease) by the administration of mannitol after intravenous pyelography (76).

Physicians should be aware of the possibility of nephrotoxicity derived from the use of commonly prescribed drugs for therapeutic or diagnostic purposes. Newer drugs should be considered potentially nephrotoxic until extensive and controlled experience proves the contrary. Specific patient populations at risk should be identified and preventive measures established. Finally, the specter of nephrotoxicity should not deter the physician from the rational indication of diagnostic procedures or the prescription of life-saving drugs.

REFERENCES

1. Reidenberg, M.M.: Renal Function and Drug Action. Saunders, Philadelphia, 1971.

2. Anderson, R.J., Gambertoglio, J.G. and Schrier, R.W.: Clinical use of drugs in renal failure. Thomas, Springfield, 1976.

3. Bennett, W.M., Porter, G.A., Bagby, S.P. and McDonald, W.J.: Drugs and Renal Disease. Churchill Livingstone, New York, 1978.

4. Bennett, W.M., Singer, I., Golper, T., Feig, P., and Coggins, C.J.: Guideline for Drug Therapy in Renal Failure. Ann. Intern. Med. 86: 754, 1977.

5. Rubin, A.L., Stenzel, K.H. and Reidenberg, M.M.: Symposium on drug action and metabolism in renal failure. Am. J. Med. 62: 459-562, 1977.

6. Cafruny, E.J.: Renal tubular handling of drugs. Am. J. Med. 62: 490, 1977.

7. Reidenberg, M.M.: The binding of drugs to plasma proteins and the interpretation of measurements of plasma concentrations of drugs in patients with poor renal function. Am. J. Med. 62: 466, 1977.

8. Falco, F.G., Smith, H.M. and Arcieri, G.M.: Nephrotoxicity of aminoglycoside and gentamicin. J. Infect. Dis. 119: 406, 1969.

9. Fillastre, J-P. (ed.): Nephrotoxicity. Interaction of drugs with membranes systems Mitochondria-lysosomes. Masson Publishing USA, Inc., New York, 1978.

10. Hewitt, W.L.: Gentamicin: toxicity in perspective. Postgrad. Med. J. 50: (Suppl. 7) 55, 1974.

11. Appel, G.B. and Neu, H.C.: Gentamicin in 1978. Ann. Intern. Med. 89: 528, 1978.

12. Cronin, R.E.: Aminoglycoside nephrotoxicity: pathogenesis and prevention. Clin. Nephrol. 11: 251, 1979.

13. Gilbert, D.N., Bennett, W.M., Houghton, D.C. and Porter, G.: Comparative nephrotoxicity of gentamicin and tobramycin. Clin. Res. 25: 376A, 1977.

14. Dikman, S., Bosch, J., Chung, J. and Kahn, T.: Gentamicin and netilmicin nephrotoxicity. Antimicrob. Agents Chemother. 10: 827, 1976.

15. Ormsby, A., Plamp, C., Bennett, W., Gilbert, D., Houghton, D. and Porter, G.: Comparison of the nephrotoxic potential of gentamicin (G), tobramycin (T) and netilmicin (N) in the rat. Clin. Res. 26: 141A, 1978.

16. Luft, F.C., Bloch, R., Sloan, R.S., Yum, M.N., Costello, R. and Maxwell, D.R.: Comparative nephrotoxicity of aminoglycoside antibiotics in rats. J. Inf. Dis. 138: 541, 1978.

17. Robbins, G. and Tetterborn, D.: Toxicity of sisomicin in animals. Infection 4 (Suppl.): 349, 1976.

18. Zakauddin, S. and Adelman, R.: Urinary enzyme activity in neonates receiving gentamicin therapy. Clin. Res. 26: 142A, 1978.

19. Cowan, R.H., Jukkola, A.F. and Arant, B.S., Jr.: Pathophysiological evidence of gentamicin (G) nephrotoxicity in the neonatal puppy. Kidney Int. 14: 628, 1978.

19a. Karniski, L., Chonko, A., Stewart, R., Cuppage, F. and Hodges, G.: The effects of gentamicin (G) on renal function in the sexually mature vs. sexually immature rabbits. Kidney Int. 14: 726, 1978.

20. Plummer, D.T. and Ngaha, E.O.: Urinary enzymes as an index of kidney damage by toxic compounds <u>In</u> Nephrotoxicity. Fillastre, J-P., Masson Publishing USA, p. 175-191, 1978.

21. Cronin, R.E.: Aminoglycoside induced glycosuria in the dog. Clin. Res. 26: 461A, 1978.

22. Holmes, A.M., Hesling, C.M. and Wilson, T.M.: Drug-induced secondary hyperaldosteronism in patients with pulmonary tuberculosis. Q.J. Med. 39: 299, 1970.

23. Patel, R. and Savage, A.: Symptomatic hypomagnesemia associated with gentamicin therapy. Nephron 23: 50, 1979.

24. Teixeira, R.B., Alpert, H.C., Kelley, J and Vaamonde, C.A.: Protection from gentamicin-induced acute renal failure in the rat (unpublished observations).

25. Lane, A.Z., Wright, G.E. and Blair, D.C.: Ototoxicity and nephrotoxicity of amikacin. Am. J. Med. 62: 911, 1977.

26. Bennett, W.M., Hartnett, M.N., Gilbert, D., Houghton, D. and Porter, G.A.: Effect of sodium intake on gentamicin nephrotoxicity in the rat. Proc. Soc. Exp. Biol. Med. 151: 736, 1976.

27. Barr, G.A., Mazze, R.I., Cousins, M.J. and Kosek, J.C.: An animal model for combined methoxyflurane and gentamicin nephrotoxicity. Br. J. Anaesth. 45: 306, 1973.

28. Adelman, R.D., Conzelman, G., Spangler, W. and Ishiyaki, G.: Furosemide potentiated gentamicin nephrotoxicity: early detection by monitoring of urinary enzymes. Kidney Int. 12: 538, 1977.

29. Cabanillas, F., Burgos, R.C., Rodriguez, R.C. and Baldizon, C.: Nephrotoxicity of combined cephalothin-gentamicin regimen. Arch. Intern. Med. 135: 850, 1975.

30. Plager, J.E.: Association of renal injury with combined cephalothin gentamicin therapy among patients severely ill with malignant disease. Cancer 37: 1937, 1976.

31. Yuer, L., Becq-Giraudon, B., Pourrat, O. et Sudre, Y.: La néphrotoxicite de l'association méthicilline-gentamycine. Sem. Hôp. Paris 52: 1903, 1976.

32. Dellinger, P., Murphy, T., Barza, M., Pinn, V. and Weinstein, L.: Effect of cephalothin on renal cortical concentrations of gentamicin in rats. Antimicrob. Agents Chemother. 9: 587, 1976.

33. Whelton, A.: Intrarenal antibiotic distribution in health and disease. Kidney Int. 6: 131, 1974.

34. Luft, F.C., Patel, V., Yum, M., Patel, B. and Kleit, S.: Experimental aminoglycoside nephrotoxicity. J. Lab. Clin. Med. 86: 213, 1975.

35. Kosek, J.C., Mazze, R.I. and Cousins, M.J.: Nephrotoxicity of gentamicin. Lab. Invest. 30: 48, 1974.

36. Baylis, C., Rennke, H.R. and Brenner, B.M.: Mechanisms of the defect in glomerular ultrafiltration associated with gentamicin administration. Kidney Int. 12: 344, 1977.

37. Baylis, C.: Mechanisms involved in gentamicin-induced acute renal failure. Kidney Int. 15: 445, 1979.

38. Mattson, K., Riska, H., Forsström, J. and Kock, B.: Acute renal failure following rifampin administration. Scand. J. Resp. Dis. 55: 291, 1974.

39. Campese, V.M., Marzullo, F., Schema, F.P. and Coratelli, P.: Acute renal failure during intermittent rifampin therapy. Nephron 10: 256, 1973.

40. Kleinknecht, D., Homberg, J.D. and Decroix, G.: Acute renal failure after rifampin. Lancet 1: 1238, 1972.

41. Gabow, P.A., Lacher, J.W. and Neff, T.A.: Tubulointerstitial glomerular nephritis associated with rifampin. Report of a case. JAMA 235: 2517, 1976.

42. Hardaker, W.T., Jr., Stone, R.A. and McCoy, R.: Platinum nephrotoxicity. Cancer 34: 1030, 1974.

43. Gonzalez-Vitale, J.C., Hayes, D.M., Cvitkovic, E. and Sternberg, S.S.: The renal pathology in clinical trials of Cis-platinum (II) diamminedichloride. Cancer 39: 1362, 1977.

44. Gonzalez-Vitale, J.C., Hayes, D.M., Cvitkovic, E. and Sternberg, S.S.: Acute renal failure after Cis-Dichlorodiammineplatinum (II) and gentamicin-cephalothin therapies. Cancer Treat. Rep. 62: 693, 1978.

45. Dentino, M., Luft, F.C., Yum, M.N., Williams, S.D. and Einhorn, L.H.: Long term effect of Cis-diamminedichloride platinum (CDDP) on renal function and structure in man. Cancer 41: 1274, 1978.

46. Levi, J., Jacobs, C., McTigue, M. and Weiner, M.W.: Mechanism of Cis-diamminedichloroplatinum (Cis-Pt) nephrotoxicity. Clin. Res. 27: 422A, 1979.

47. Schilsky, R.L. and Anderson, T.: Hypomagnesemia and renal magnesium wasting in patients receiving Cisplatin. Ann. Intern. Med. 90: 929, 1979.

48. Nitschke, R., Starling, K.A., Vats, T. and Bryan, H.: Cis-diamminedichloroplatinum (NSC-119875) in childhood malignancies: a Southwest Oncology Group Study. Med. Pediatr. Oncol. 4: 127, 1978.

49. Schacht, R.C. and Baldwin, D.S.: Chronic interstitial nephritis and renal failure due to nitrosourea (NU) therapy. Kidney Int. 14: 661, 1978.

50. Harmon, W.E., Cohen, H.J., Schneeberger, E.E. and Grupe, W.E.: Chronic renal failure in children treated with methyl CCNU. N. Eng. J. Med. 300: 1200, 1979.

51. Shafi, T., Chou, S., Porush, J. and Shapiro, W.B.: Infusion intravenous pyelography and renal function effects in patients with chronic renal insufficiency. Arch. Intern. Med. 138: 1218, 1978.

52. Swartz, R.D., Rubin, J.E., Leeming, B.W. and Silva, P.: Renal failure following major angiography. Am. J. Med. 65: 31, 1978.

53. Van Zee, B.E., Hoy, W.E., Talley, T.E. and Jaenike, J.R.: Renal injury associated with intravenous pyelography in non-diabetic and diabetic patients. Ann. Intern. Med. 89: 51, 1978.

54. Heneghan, M.: Contrast-induced acute renal failure. Editorial Am. J. Roentgenol. 131: 1113, 1978.

55. Byrd, L. and Sherman, R.L.: Radiocontrast-induced acute renal failure: A clinical and pathophysiological review. Medicine 58: 270, 1979.

56. Canales, C.O., Smith, G.H., Robinson, J.C., Remmers, A.R. and Sarles, H.E.: Acute renal failure after the administration of iopanoic acid as a cholecystographic agent. N. Engl. J. Med. 281: 89, 1969.

57. Berezin, A.F.: Acute renal failure, diabetes mellitus, and scanning. Ann. Intern. Med. 86: 829, 1977.

58. Hanaway, J. and Black, J.: Renal failure following contrast injection for computerized tomography. JAMA 238: 2056, 1977.

59. Takazahura, E., Sawabu, N., Handa, A., Takada, A., Shinoda, A. and Takeuchi, J.: Intrarenal vascular changes with age and disease. Kidney Int. 2: 224, 1972.

60. Hollenberg, N.K., Adams, D.F., Solomon, H.S., Rashid, A., Abrams, H.L. and Merrill, J.P.: Senescence and the renal vasculature in normal man. Circ. Res. 34: 309, 1974.

61. Ansari, Z. and Baldwin, D.S.: Acute renal failure due to radiocontrast agents. Nephron 17: 28, 1976.

62. Harkonen, S. and Kjellstrand, K.M.: Exacerbation of diabetic renal failure following intravenous pyelography. Am. J. Med. 63: 939, 1977.

63. Dudzinski, P.J., Petrone, A.F., Peroff, M. and Callaghan, E.E.: Acute renal failure following high-dose excretory urography in dehydrated patients. J. Urol. 106: 619, 1971.

64. Kamdar, A., Weidmann, P., Makoff, D.L. and Massry, S.G.: Acute renal failure following intravenous use of radiographic contrast dyes in patients with diabetes mellitus. Diabetes 26: 643, 1977.

65. Veseley, D.L. and Mintz, D.H.: Acute renal failure in insulin-dependent diabetics. Episodes secondary to intravenous pyelography. Arch. Intern. Med. 138: 1858, 1978.

66. Pillay, V.K., Robbins, P.C., Schwartz, F.D. and Kark, R.M.: Acute renal failure following intravenous urography in patients with long-standing diabetes mellitus and azotemia. Radiology 95: 633, 1970.

67. Barshay, M.E., Kay, J.H., Goldman, R. and Coburn, V.W.: Acute renal failure in diabetic patients after infusion pyelography. Clin. Nephrol. 1: 35, 1973.

68. Diaz-Buxo, J.A., Wagoner, R.D., Hattery, R.R. and Palumbo, P.J.: Acute renal failure after excretory urography. Ann. Intern. Med. 83: 155, 1975.

69. DeFronzo, R.A., Humphrey, R.L., Wright, J.R. and Cooke, C.R.: Acute renal failure in multiple myeloma. Medicine 54: 209, 1975.

70. Norby, L.H. and DiBona, G.F.: The renal vascular effects of meglumide diatrizoate. J. Pharmacol. Exper. Ther. 193: 932, 1975.

71. Lasser, E.C.: Contrast-material red blood cell reactions. Editorial. Invest. Radiol. 8: 189, 1973.

72. Talner, L.B., Rushman, H.N. and Goel, M.N.: The effect of renal artery injection of contrast material on urinary enzyme excretion. Invest. Radiol. 7: 311, 1972.

73. Ziegler, T.W., Ladens, J.H., Fanestil, D.D. and Talner, L.B.: Inhibition of active sodium transport by radiographic contrast media. Kidney Int. 7: 68, 1975.

74. Postelthwaite, A.E. and Kelley, W.N.: Uricosuric effect of radiocontrast agents. Ann. Intern. Med. 74: 845, 1971.

75. Gelman, M.L., Rowe, J.W., Coggins, C.H. and Athanasoulis, C.: Effects of an angiographic contrast agent on renal function. Cardiovasc. Med. 4: 313, 1979.

76. Anto, H.R., Chou, S-Y., Porush, J.G. and Shapiro, W.B.: Mannitol prevention of acute renal failure (ARF) associated with infusion intravenous pyelography (IIVP). Clin. Res. 27: 407A, 1979.

CASE REPORT

RENAL FAILURE ASSOCIATED WITH HYDANTOINS ADMINISTRATION IN NUTRITIONAL RICKETS

Ricardo Gastelbondo-Amaya, M.D., Ricardo Muñoz-Arizpe, M.D., Felipe Mota-Hernández, M.D., Gustavo Gordillo-Paniagua, M.D., Dept. Nephrol., Hosp. Infantil, México City, México

The clinical presentation of bone disease and renal failure in a given patient strongly suggests a close relationship between both entities, rickets being secondary to long standing renal failure.

Herein, we report a case of rickets presenting concomitantly with renal failure secondary to tubulointerstitial nephritis, with no direct relationship between each other. Rather, it seems that the renal lesion was the result of iatrogenic administration of phenylhydantoin and that Vit D deficiency rickets was secondary to chronic malnutrition. Both conditions reversed clinically and biochemically after appropriate management.

CASE REPORT

This girl aged 11 months was admitted to the hospital with the main complaint of recurrent seizures. Past family history was unremarkable. Home and family environment was deplorable, with poor hygienic conditions. Her mother was unmarried; the patient was left alone all day long while her mother was at her job. There were no other siblings. The patient was never exposed to sunlight and no vitamin supplements were given; her milestones were all below normal range for her age. Her mother noticed increased deformities of all four limbs at six months of age. At seven months of age she developed generalized tonic-clonic convulsions with upward rolling of the eyeballs, that lasted a few minutes and disappeared spontaneously. She was seen by a private physician who prescribed oral phenylhydantoin. However, she continued having seizures intermittently during the following four months. Hydantoins were withdrawn eight days prior to admission due to the appearance of skin rash. She was admitted to the hospital during a convulsive episode, with carpopedal spasm, positive Chvostek's sign, respiratory distress, stridor and peripheral cyanosis. She was severely malnourished, weight 6.2 kg (< 3 percentile), height 62 cm (< 3 percentile), head circumference 43 cm (< 2 SD), heart rate 100 beats/min, blood pressure 80/50 mmHg. Intravenous administration of anticonvulsants (diazepam) given in the emergency room did not relieve her symptoms. Calcium gluconate was given intravenously after blood was drawn for laboratory studies, with immediate disappearance of the convulsion and accompanying symptoms. Ribs and four extremities showed marked deformities characterized by bowing and distal thickening. Seizures did not recur, but she remained limp, with poor physical activity, barely strong enough to suck her bottle.

Laboratory: serum pH 7.30, TCO_2 19 millimol/liter, Na 129 millimol/liter, K 4.6 millimol/liter, total calcium 1.55 millimol/liter (6.2 mg/dl) before and 2.05 millimol/liter (8.2 mg/dl) after calcium gluconate administration. CBC: Hgb 10.4 g/dl (6.4 millimol/liter), Hct 32%, WBC 11,800/mm^3. Serum urea 12.5 millimol/liter (75 mg/dl), serum creatinine 477 millimol/liter (5.4 mg/dl), phosphates 1.97 millimol/liter (6.1 mg/dl), alkaline phosphatase 17 B.U. Urinalysis: specific gravity 1004, pH 6, proteinuria +, no hematuria and normal sediment. No glucosuria, aminoaciduria, hyperphosphaturia or hypercalciuria were detected in a 24-hour urine sample.

Skull X-rays showed wide open anterior and posterior fontanelles with osteoporosis. Long bones x-rays showed changes compatible with rickets (Fig. 1).

Initially, she was diagnosed as having chronic renal failure of unknown etiology, based on the presence of azotemia, anemia, hypocalcemia and severe bone deformities. Percutaneous renal biopsy was performed to clarify the etiology, showing focal tubular atrophy and diffuse interstitial fibrosis. The histological lesions involved tubules and interstitium, sparing glomeruli (Fig. 2,3).

She was treated with oral dihydrotachysterol (Hytakerol), 0.125 mg q 8 days during one month and adequate sunlight exposure. Her improvement was remarkable in a short period of time, becoming more alert, active, with good appetite. Urea and serum creatinine declined progressively and the bone lesions improved clinically and radiologically. Tetany and seizures did not recur. At 22 months of age her weight was 9.2 kg and height 75 cm. Even though these measurements still were within the third percentile for age, she was catching up adequately. She was then able to run, play normally, climb stairs, etc.

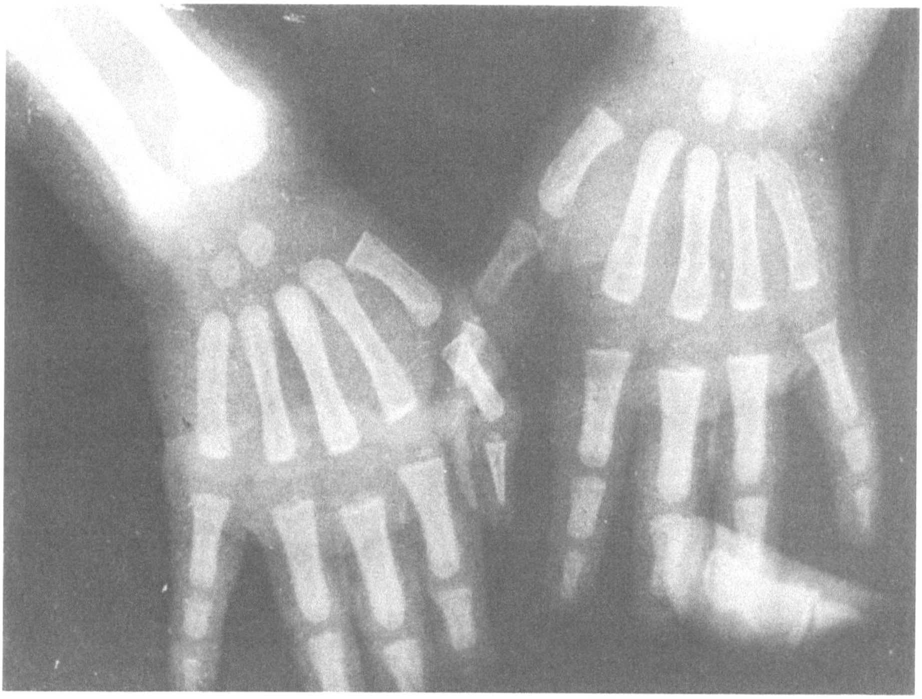

Figure 1. Bone x-rays showing bowing and distal thickening compatible with rickets.

Laboratory: serum urea 2.5 millimol/liter (15 mg/dl), serum creatinine 70.7 millimol/liter (0.8 mg/dl), total calcium 2.3 millimol/liter (9.2 mg/dl), phosphates 1.7 millimol/liter (5.2 mg/dl), alkaline phosphatase 15 B.U. Long bones x-rays showed sequelae of rickets with active healing of the lesions.

DISCUSSION

Vit D deficiency rickets is infrequently seen due to widespread use of vitamin D supplements. However, it is rather common in malnourished children with no exposure to sunlight. The response to Vit D administration is prompt, with bone remineralization and healing of the process.

Bone disease accompanying renal failure (renal osteodystrophy), though manifested as rickets in children, is a completely different

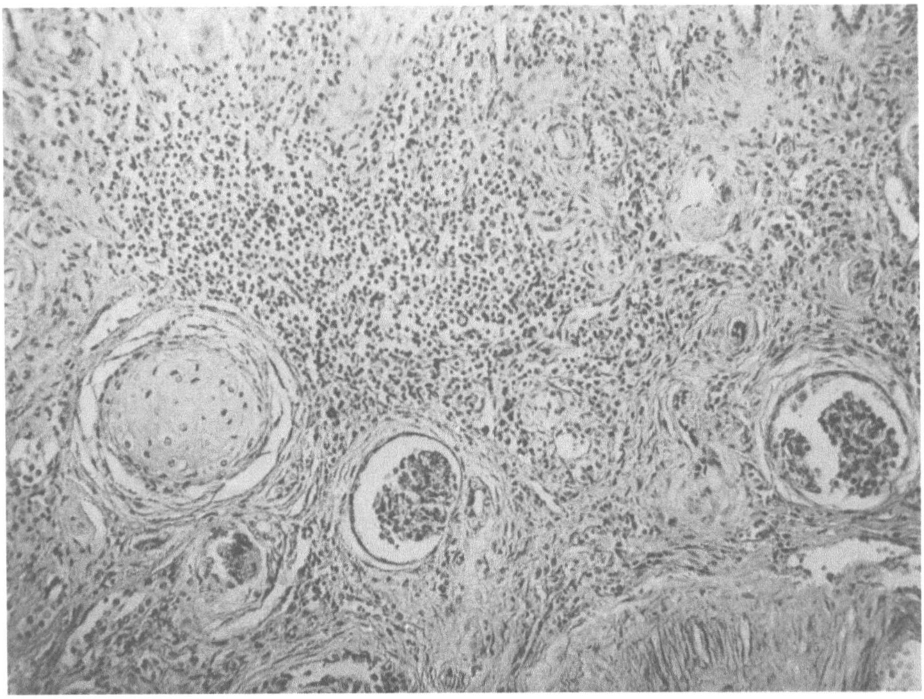

Figure 2. Renal biopsy specimen stained with H & E stain showing focal tubular atrophy, leukocyte infiltration and diffuse interstitial fibrosis (10x).

disease since the etiopathogenic mechanisms involved and the response to Vit D administration are substantially different from those observed in Vit D deficiency rickets. Hyperphosphatemia, hypocalcemia, depressed intestinal absorption of calcium, metabolic acidosis, compensatory hyperparathyroidism and lack of production of 1-25 dehydrocholecalciferol (active Vit D_3) by the kidney, are the main factors involved in the development of bone disease secondary to chronic renal failure (1,2). Bone alterations do not improve with regular or even high doses of Vit D in patients with renal osteodystrophy. However, administration of Vit D analogues (1α-hydroxy Vit D_3) have improved bone disease in these patients (3,4).

On admission to the hospital our patient was diagnosed as having renal osteodystrophy secondary to renal failure. However, tetany and convulsions were the hallmark of the clinical picture. Besides, the patient was severely malnourished and she was never exposed to sunlight, arising suspicion that she may have Vit D deficiency rickets, leading to recurrent convulsive episodes.

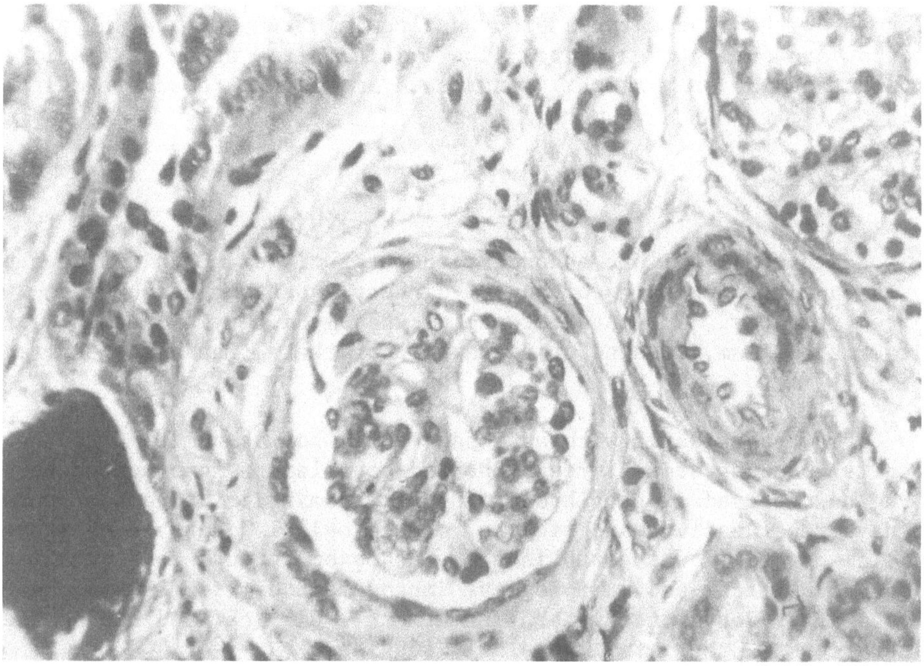

Figure 3. Renal biopsy showing normal glomeruli with H & E stain (40 x).

It seems that since the initial convulsion hydantoins were prescribed to treat what was thought to be epilepsy. Recently, the relationship of tubulointerstitial nephritis and renal failure with hydantoin administration was reported (5,6,7). Hyman considers that renal damage is due to humoral and cellular immunologically mediated mechanisms (8). Therefore, it is quite possible that the administration of the drug to this patient led to tubulointerstitial nephritis presenting as renal failure. Renal biopsy revealed tubulointerstitial nephritis, without alterations of the glomeruli.

There is also information regarding interference of Vit D metabolism with hydantoin administration (9,10). This mechanism may have been involved in worsening pre-existing rickets in this patient (2,11,12).

It was then considered that the patient had primary Vit D deficiency rickets independently of renal failure, which was also present. Renal failure was secondary to tubulointerstitial nephritis, which in turn may reasonably be thought to be the result of iatrogenic hydantoin administration. Both alterations were reversible, since urea and creatinine serum levels decreased steadily until reaching normal values. Concomitantly, there was rapid radiologic and clinical improvement of the bone lesions secondary to rickets, with disappearance of hypocalcemia after dehydrotachysterol therapy and sunlight exposure. The initial serum value of alkaline phosphatase was only slightly increased, maybe due to severe malnutrition (13).

SUMMARY

Acute renal failure secondary to interstitial nephritis caused by therapeutic ingestion of sodium diphenylhydantoin has been reported recently. The interference of sodium diphenylhydantoin with Vit D metabolism, causing or aggravating rickets, has also been reported.

This report deals with an infant girl who was admitted to the hospital because of seizures. She had convulsions four months before and received diphenylhydantoin until admission. She was found to have renal failure and rickets. Histological diagnosis of interstitial nephritis was established by means of percutaneous renal biopsy. Clinical and radiological improvement of rickets was observed after dehydrotachysterol treatment. Clinical and biochemical alterations of renal failure slowly subsided.

She had a clear-cut history of vitamin D deficiency rickets. Seizures were due to hypocalcemic tetany but were erroneously treated as "grand mal" epilepsy, with diphenylhydantoin. Interstitial nephritis complicated with acute renal failure was probably caused by diphenylhydantoin administration.

REFERENCES

1. Avioli, V.L. and Teitelbaum, L.S.: Renal osteodystrophies. In Brenner, B.M., Rector, F.C. (eds.): The Kidney. Philadelphia: W.B. Saunders, 1976, 1542.

2. Beale, G.M., Salcedo, J.R. and Ellis, D. et al.: Renal osteodystrophy. In Chan, J.C.M. (ed.): The Pediatric Clinics of North America. Pediatric Nephrology. Philadelphia: W.B. Saunders, 1976, 885.

3. Nielsen, H.E., Romer, F.K. and Melsen, F. et al.: 1-hydroxivitamin D_3 treatment of non-dialyzed patients with chronic renal failure. Effects on bone, mineral metabolism and kidney function. Clin. Nephrol. 13: 103, 1980.

4. Brickman, A.S., Sherrard, D.J., Jomsey, J. et al.: 1,25-dihydroxicholecalciferol. Effect on skeletal lesions and plasma parathyroid hormone levels in uremic osteodystrophy. Arch. Intern. Med.

5. Alfrey, C.A.: Chronic renal failure: manifestations and pathogenesis. In Schrier, R.W. (ed.): Renal and Electrolyte Disorders. Boston: Little, Brown, 1976, 319.

6. Heptinstall, R.H.: Pathology of the Kidney. 2nd Ed. Boston: Little, Brown, 1976.

7. Michel, J.R. and Mitch, W.E.: Reversible renal failure and myositis caused by phenylhydantoin hypersensitivity. JAMA 236: 2773, 1976.

8. Hyman, L.R., Ballow, M. and Knieser, M.R.: Diphenylhydantoin nephropathy. Evidence for an autoimmune pathogenesis. Kidney Int. 8: 450, 1975.

9. Popovtzer, M.M.: Disorders of calcium, phosphorus, vitamin D and parathyroid hormone activity. In Schrier, R.W. (ed.): Renal and Electrolyte Disorders. Boston: Little, Brown, 1976, 167.

10. Stamp, T.C.B., Round, J.M., Rome, D.J.F. et al.: Plasma levels and therapeutic effect of 25-hydroxicholecalciferol in epileptic patients taking anticonvulsant drugs. Br. Med. J. 4: 9, 1972.

11. Richens, A. and Rome, D.J.F.: Disturbance of calcium metabolism by anticonvulsant drugs. Br. Med. J. 4: 73, 1970.

12. Pierides, A.M., Kerr, D.N.S. and Ellis, H.A.: 1 alpha-hydroxycholecalciferol in hemodialysis renal osteodystrophy. Adverse effects of anticonvulsant therapy. Clin. Nephrol. 5: 189, 1976.

13. Barnes, L.A.: Nutritional disorders. In Vaughn, V.C. and McKay, R.J. (eds.): Nelson Textbook of Pediatrics. Philadelphia: W.B. Saunders, 1975, 183.

PANEL DISCUSSION

Moderator: José Strauss, M.D.

Div. Pediatr. Nephrol., Dept. Pediatr., Univ. Miami Sch. Med., Miami, Fla. 33152, USA

QUESTION: How often do you see patients with Goodpasture disease and tubular damage? Is it common? Do you think that these cases of Goodpasture disease that we have been seeing in the past probably are just a more severe form of all these cases you have been presenting?

RESPONSE: Your question is about how many cases of Goodpasture are being produced by an antibody to basement membrane with tubular damage mediated by antibody to tubular basement membrane?

QUESTION: In those cases, do you see in the tubuli the same thing that you see in the glomeruli? Will you see a linear formation?

RESPONSE: In our experience only about 20% of patients with anti-GBM disease have Goodpasture - a variety of pneumonitis. If we consider that about 50% of our patients with anti-GBM disease have also anti-TBM disease, probably 10% of patients with pulmonary hemorrhagic and renal diseases have anti-TBM antibodies and tubulointerstitial nephritis.

QUESTION: In tubulointerstitial nephritis, when you have linear deposits do you always have anti-TBM antibodies?

RESPONSE: No. I don't think it's constant. That's why I think that perhaps we try to simplify this pathology but probably more than one pathogenetic mechanism may be operating simultaneously, or consecutively. Perhaps one may trigger the other. Most cases of severe tubulointerstitial nephritis probably develop when we have an antibody mediated injury and then on top we have a second problem.

We are not able to dissect and make a generalization but I think it's possible that sometimes we have antibody to TBM without the interstitial nephritis. Recently there was a case in which there was antibody to alveolar basement membrane without hemorrhagic pneumonitis.

I would like to make some comments concerning an earlier presentation. I would like to say how much I have been impressed by this beautiful study of the patient who had immune complex glomerulonephritis and then developed antibody to renal basement membrane. As you know, sometimes this is associated with antibody to alveolar basement membrane. To me this means that we have an immune complex disease which perhaps produced release of basement membrane antigen and autoimmunization. How this patient responded to this injury may perhaps be the answer to a different kind of pathology. Some of them may develop anti-GBM antibody, some of them may develop anti-TBM antibodies, and some of them may develop anti-alveolar basement membrane antibody. There is one point which should be considered. If you have immune complex glomerulonephritis and then the patient develops anti-GBM antibody, we cannot make this assessment on the renal biopsy because there is already granular staining and so we cannot detect the linear staining. We have to have antibody in the serum and we have to detect the anti-GBM antibody by indirect immunofluorescence. It is obviously more easy to predict that the patient has an anti-TBM antibody as a consequence of an immune complex glomerulonephritis if you find in the same biopsy the linear deposits in the tubular basement membrane. For me, it has always been interesting the possibility that the basement membrane - and I don't mean necessarily the renal basement membrane - may have the ingredients for the production of antibody response or an immune complex response. Perhaps the same individuals may have an antibody mediated injury plus an immune complex mediated injury. This idea came to me in 1968 when Dr. Dixon gave me the blocks of his and his collaborator's experiments in which they were able to produce anti-GBM glomerunephritis in the rabbit immunized with GBM antigen isolated from the urine of normal rabbits. As you know we eliminate normally basement membrane in the urine as a consequence of the normal catabolism. So, they isolated GBM from the urine and then they immunized the rabbits and produced an anti-GBM antibody. So he told me these are the blocks, this is a linear staining, this is an anti-GBM nephritis, please have a look.

One of my students went to work with Dr. Dixon; he did this study by electronmicroscopy and he found a few subepithelial deposits. So I told him, look, this is immune complex glomerulonephritis. This is impossible. This is an anti-GBM glomerulonephritis. So then I said, perhaps some of these animals which are immunized for prolonged periods of time, at a certain point had the ingredients necessary for the formation of immune complex glomerulonephritis which is that the antigen must be present in the circulation for a prolonged period of time. This was not written in the paper that we published in the Journal of Immunology but these animals had evidence by electronmicroscopy and suggestion by immunofluorescence because the deposits are very, very fine. But I was always fascinated by this possibility. Then I was looking every time that I had a patient with anti-GBM disease for presence of immune complex in the glomeruli. Then when one finally came, it was really not so very good. And then Dr. Glassock who as you know, recently published a Goodpasture disease classic and then he had a serial biopsy and then after two-three months he had immune complex glomerulonephritis in the glomeruli presumably formed by GBM-anti GBM complexes. So we were trying to study the problem - how is it possible to produce an anti-GBM or anti-renal basement membrane disease which at a certain point may be complicated by immune complex disease? Complexes which are formed by GBM or basement membrane antigen and specific antibody complexes. This model is available and it's pertinent to the kind of discussion we are having. We were trying to stimulate production of increased amount of basement membrane. On the basis of data which are available to us from pharmacology studies in vitro and in vivo, we know that mercury produces immune complex nephritis; so, we started to study these problems. The animals, the rabbit to which you give a minimum amount of mercury, develops antibody to glomerular, tubular, and alveolar basement membranes which are detectable by radioimmunoassay, by direct immunofluorescence, by the presence of linear deposits in glomeruli and in the tubules. Then, these animals, after two or three weeks, one month, they started to develop circulating complexes detectable by the C_{1Q} method, with the Raji cell method, and you can see the shape from linear deposits to granular deposits. If you isolate the complexes or if you make an elusion from the kidney, in the early stages of disease when there are linear deposits and in the late stages of disease when there are granular deposits, you can show that these immunoglobulins have the same reactivity as the basement membrane. With the basement membrane all over the body, with the basement membrane of the vasculature, especially the reticulum of the spleen, with the basement membrane-like material which is present between smooth muscle cells of the artery. There is recent evidence that these animals have a variety of antibodies and a variety of immune complexes including fibronectine, laminin, collagen type 4. So, we have an antibody response to the collagen proteins which are present in the collagen matrix. Presumably the different clinical and pathologic aspects may be due to the prevalent response to one versus the other antigen. I was wondering if perhaps the patient mentioned earlier had not developed antibody to tubular and alveolar basement membrane because he had mainly antibody to fibronectine which was recently shown to be localizing in tubular and alveolar basement membranes. So, this is an open field and I think that antigens in the collagen matrix are important and perhaps we should keep our minds open to the possibility that immune complex glomerulonephritis is produced from the very beginning by immune complexes which contain antigens of the collagen matrix. We use the terminology of the biochemist which includes basement membranes all over the body, the ground substance of collagen and the reticulum of the spleen. Perhaps this patient could have immune complexes formed to this antigen and then at a certain point, because of immunological equilibrium changes, they could form more antibody or the antigen secretion may no longer be detectable, may no longer be present so complexes may no longer be formed and so antibody may be free for reaction since it may no longer be saturated. It may be available for reaction with the tissue antigen. So we can imagine that perhaps we had immune complexes first and linear binding later. As you can see, there are a lot of possibilities that we should consider.

COMMENT: I am very happy about your comment because this case has really been puzzling to us. The reason why there was a delay between our presentation and the real publication is because we were trying to take all the possibilities and analyze them and we couldn't find satisfactory explanations. I would like to tell you - this is not the answer but a small detail which I am sure you will be interested in - something like 20 years ago I saw a case of nephrotic syndrome with DeToni-Debre Fanconi syndrome. The histology showed that it was a typical membranous nephropathy with a huge interstitial inflammation. Of course, again it was investigated, does he have pyelonephritis or not? Of course he had not.

He progressed to terminal renal failure in something like six years. This patient for me was unique. I'm sure that he was identical to this case - the first one I presented. Because we just mentioned that in a paper we wrote on nephrotic syndrome, some people sent me their case and they said "we would like to know if you have already seen a case of membranous nephropathy with tubulo-interstitial nephritis" and they sent me the immunofluorescent slides, but there were only granular deposits. Their case had membranous and DeToni-Debre-Fanconi syndrome. The same week they sent me the slide, we had our case with membranous and linear deposits. So, I wrote back saying this was "a very well known association" except for the first case we had seen a long time ago - that we had a similar case, but that in our observation, there were antitubular basement membrane antibodies and that there were linear deposits. They wrote back saying that they were unable to find anti-TBM antibodies. So the situation was like that. Two months later they wrote back saying that then they had found anti-TBM antibodies. So the immunofluorescence at the beginning, except for the DeToni-Debre-Fanconi syndrome, was that of the association of granular deposits in the glomeruli and in the tubules. But there was a Fanconi syndrome and because of that, they looked for anti-TBM and they found it. In the other case there was first, granular deposits, and then anti-TBM antibodies although they couldn't find linear deposition along the tubules. This is the difference in the two cases. I'm sure that the strict limit of granular on one side and linear on the other side which has been so interesting since Dixon presented his first data, I think that probably it will have to be completely revised. Between these two things, we might find an explanation for many of the clinical and experimental situations.

QUESTION: I'd like to ask about the comment regarding immune complex nephritis associated with Myastemia Gravis. I remember two years ago we had a patient with Myastemia Gravis and he developed immune complex disease following thymectomy. L.E. cells test was negative and the ANA factor was of lower titer. I believe that case also had tubulointerstitial changes but we thought that they were due to SLE. Since lupus has been described following thymectomy, we took for granted that it was SLE. We didn't look for the anti-TBM antibody. I was wondering; since patients tend to have auto-immune disease and nephritis, and, in our patient, since the nephritis developed after the thymectomy, what is the pathogenetic mechanism involved?

ANSWER: In lupus there probably is a broad hyperreactivity to a variety of stimuli so I am not surprised that the patient may have an association with some pathology like Myastemia Gravis which is produced by antibodies to acetylcholine receptors. I am not aware of the simultaneous development of antibodies to acetylcholine receptors and for lupus, but it is possible. We have several other combinations. What is interesting and pertinent in the work we just heard described before, is that the very first description of antibody to tubular basement membrane was a description many, many years ago in four patients with Sjögren syndrome. They described very nicely the presence of linear deposits of IgG and complement to tubular basement membrane but they were interested in Sjögren syndrome and they did not make any comment about the renal pathology; they mentioned that the patient had a defect in concentration capacity, the tubular acidosis, etc. Probably, there is some link in this pathology; this link may be a new response to certain collagen components. We certainly don't know. However, there is another interesting case which is different from a certain point of view but similar to the one just mentioned. A recent report of a patient with Goodpasture syndrome, a lady who developed antibodies to sarcolemma and she developed a severe myopathy. She went to see a physician at the hospital because she had severe myopathy. She was admitted to the hospital and by muscle biopsy showed linear deposits of IgG and complement in the muscles and then when she was in the hospital after a few weeks she developed a classic Goodpasture disease with antibodies to GBM. So again, it shows there is a similarity in the antigenic stimulation. The sarcolemma may contain antigens which are shared by GBM and TBM.

COMMENT: Some people still diagnose chronic pyelonephritis for anything that comes along. We should undermine this very prevalent concept that arose during the 30's, the 40's and 50's that pyelonephritis was a very, very common condition. One of us, many years ago saw a specimen of a patient with interstitial nephritis and uveitis. The specimen was shown to a health service pathologist who diagnosed it as chronic pyelonephritis. This was a very prevalent idea at the time, that whenever in the kidney you saw the combination of tubular loss with very few glomerular changes or possibly only sporadic segmental changes, plus interstitial fibrosis, interstitial inflammatory cells, this was automatically chronic pyelonephritis. We must destroy this belief and show that this is a nonspecific picture that may have many different backgrounds to it.

QUESTION: I have been very interested in a lot of what has been said here. I just have one question on sort of a practical point. It has been known for many years that there are various conditions, particularly diabetes, where you may get a false, linear fluorescence in the glomeruli when you do not have antiglomerular basement membrane disease. Mention was made of this but it wasn't very clear whether the same thing obtains for tubular fluorescence. Can you assume that when you see linear fluorescence in tubules that you are automatically dealing with anti-TBM disease or is it the same state of affairs as with the glomeruli - that this is nonspecific and then you have to demonstrate by other means the presence of anti-TBM.

ANSWER: This is a good point. I think I already stressed this point in the experimental part of my presentation. Certainly whatever we know about glomeruli, it's got to be true about tubules. I think nobody should make a diagnosis of anti-TBM disease simply on the basis of linear stain. We have stressed this concept for many years concerning the linear deposits in glomeruli. I think one has to show that the linear deposits contain immunoglobulin and contain antibody and be able to show that this antibody has specificity for tubular basement membrane. This obviously requires demonstration of presence of antibody in the circulation or presence of antibody in the renal eluate. We radio-labeled the antibody and we did a passive transfer injecting the antibody in a mononephrectomized monkey and showed that the antibodies were highly concentrated in the kidney of the monkey and that they were able to produce the linear deposits in the kidney of the monkey and able to develop the nephritis. I agree completely that you can see linear deposits in non-immunologically mediated conditions. We have seen kidney that has been perfused because of transplantation, malignant hypertension, in several cases of sclerosing glomerulonephritis of unexplained etiology, familial nephropathy, and so on.

QUESTION: I'll have my last question. I mentioned in my general overview presentation that, to my knowledge, there is only one case in existence of interstitial nephritis due to anti-tubular basement membrane antibody in the absence of any glomerular disease. Are there in fact anymore? Also, I will extend that to immune complex disease. Are there any cases where, if you exclude generalized diseases like systemic lupus, that you may get an isolated case of immune complexes in the tubules with nothing going on in the glomeruli?

RESPONSE: I mentioned that in the series of 26 patients that we published with anti-renal basement membrane disease, we have one with pure anti-TBM antibody disease. This is a patient with severe interstitial nephritis who died; so in about 2000 renal biopsies, we had only one case with anti-TBM disease.

The only difference from the case which you mentioned is the fact that there was a minimal amount of anti-GBM antibody but negligible. There was no real glomerular pathology. The second question concerning the immune complexes in the disease, I think that now there are more frequent reports of tubulointerstitial nephritis in lupus without associated glomerular pathology.

Now, excluding systemic disease like SLE, I have some thoughts. Our group had six cases of tubulointerstitial nephritis mediated by immune complexes. Retrospectively, I am not sure that two of the cases were not lupus. So, some of these cases were described as tubulointerstitial nephritis mediated by immune complexes the etiology of which we considered unknown but retrospectively, I am not so sure.

QUESTION: If I remember right, one of the six cases was a case of lipoid nephrosis or minimal change type, whatever you would like to call it. I think case number 6 could possibly fall into this category where it was no known disease; it was purely tubular. Is that correct?

RESPONSE: It is correct but I doubt about it retrospectively. I have never seen again a case like this.

COMMENT: He might be right about the case I was referring to.

COMMENT: Really, I don't know. As I told you, I spent a month during the summer. I asked my associate to turn out their cases of interstitial nephritis so that I could look at them. That was the only one with uveitis that he showed me. There might be others. And then they showed me another one that had an iridocyclitis and I think they had one with an iritis, too. I was always very interested in the association with eye lesions.

QUESTION: The second thing that I would like to ask you is, why do you feel accused of diagnosing chronic pyelonephritis everywhere?

RESPONSE: Well, you kept saying that this is what I would call...

COMMENT: I didn't say that. I never said that. I think that on the contrary, I've always insisted on the fact that you had helped tremendously the decrease of the incidence of chronic pyelonephritis in the field of nephrology. So, I don't think anybody has ever said that. I only accuse you of calling chronic pyelonephritis what I call segmental hypoplasia. That's all.

COMMENT: One of these days we are going to convert you!

QUESTION: In the slides that you showed of shunt nephritis, the immunofluorescence was IgM. Do you make anything particular out of this?

RESPONSE: Yes. We have studied eight cases now of shunt nephritis. The predominating immunoglobulin has been IgM in the eight cases. I don't make anything of it; it's just that I don't know why. Maybe my colleague has an explanation for everything, but it seems that in shunt nephritis IgM is the predominant immunoglobulin.

COMMENT: In shunt nephritis as well as in acute bacterial endocarditis, you have the highest levels of rheumatoid factor and of IgM. In this condition you can show that these are rheumatoid factor immune complex like aggregates. Finally, if you take a section of the kidney and soak the section in high concentration of aggregated IgG which presumably is the antigen, then you are able to solubilize these aggregates. Accordingly, the proposal is that perhaps one of the methods for treatment of immune complex glomerulonephritis is to shift the patient to antigen excess, something that the WHO is considering. Some of these studies and proposals include cases of children with malaria immune complex glomerulonephritis. Obviously, this has never been done. You cannot inject a large amount of antigen in man. I think this is an interesting event - the fact that you have rheumatoid factor like substances in the glomeruli. Perhaps this is a condition in which you can try to manipulate the human system.

MODERATOR: May I expand the question a little? What determines the reversibility of the changes in shunt nephritis or in any of the other conditions that were described today? We had a case which Rawle McIntosh helped us diagnose; he thought that the case would completely recover. It has been two or three years since the shunt was removed and the patient changed from a ventriculoatrial shunt to ventriculo-peritoneal shunt. This patient continues with some urinary abnormalities though markedly improved. Is there any way to determine the reversibility of these situations? Somebody made a comment during the morning that the presence or absence of immunofluorescence may help along these lines. Would you care to comment.

COMMENT: Our methods are either immunohistologic when we try to see by immunofluorescence what we have in the tissue, or methods for isolation of these immune complex like substances or immune complexes in the circulation. Rheumatoid factor or real antigen-antibody complex, is an example. These methods are just being developed. There are methods which are being successfully applied only recently for identification, quantification and possibly for removal of immune complexes from the circulation of patients with parasitic diseases and very high level of complexes. For instance, patients with leishmaniosis have a very high level of complexes, in the range of 40% of $C1_q$ binding activity. In these patients, if you pass the serum through a $C1_q$ column, you can remove these complexes. Obviously you also have to eradicate the infection, the most important goal of the treatment of these patients. Perhaps in the future it will be possible to remove the complexes from the circulation. It's already possible in animals where you can use $C1_q$ or immunoconglutinin columns.

COMMENT: I think personally that the two most fascinating diseases we know are shunt nephritis and syphilis because first of all, they are the two we can get rid of; second, they beautifully demonstrate that the important thing in glomerular disease is not to treat patients with any of these dirty drugs we are using, but to try to identify the antigen and therefore, get rid of the immune complexes. Shunt nephritis, you can cure a patient extremely easily by suppressing the cause, and syphilis, the same thing. So that every time somebody asks me something about treatment, I always answer with the example of shunt and syphilis because that proves that we are not on the right wave length when we talk about "is it better to give cyclophosphamide or chlorambucil or this or that?" What we should do is try to be in the same position with all the other immune complex diseases in the situation we are with shunt and syphilis.

MODERATOR: Yes. But you do not in all cases of shunt nephritis get complete recovery. Like this example. Rawle McIntosh had some case or cases in which the same thing had happened but he believed that it was the duration of the insult that determined outcome. In syphilis we know that we treat the infection and the renal problem goes away.

RESPONSE: No. I'll tell you. The secret of shunt nephritis is that like any other type of glomerular disease, you can have very mild glomerular involvement and extremely severe glomerular involvement. What is interesting in having eight cases to look at is that we cover almost all the renal pathology except membranous nephropathy which is something I don't understand, but that is how it is. You have anything from a very, very mild mesangial hypercellularity (almost nothing) to extremely severe crescentic glomerulonephritis. So, if you cannot get rid of a nephropathy, it's not because it lasted too long. It's just because the severity of the glomerular damage has been such that even if you get rid of the immune complexes, sclerosis of the glomeruli by itself will lead to terminal renal failure. The damage is already done when you remove the antigen. That's why the results in shunt nephritis are so variable. It's just based on the fact that you can have any type of glomerular involvement with shunt nephritis-except membranous.

COMMENT: Have there been any studies in myeloma patients regarding tubular basement membrane deposits? I am intrigued by the fact that the tubular damage in myeloma has always been attributed to a toxic effect of the myeloma protein - whether there is an IgM antibody staining in the tubular membrane because of the reported relationship of the renal tubular acidosis in some of these patients (distal and proximal) and also of the interstitial involvement. Likewise, in amyloid patients, where you may get reversibility of the nephrotic syndrome in some of these patients with treatment of the inciting disease.

RESPONSE: As you know, several people have worked on the hypothesis that in myeloma a light chain protein may produce this renal damage by toxic effect. Certainly the incidence of myeloma has greatly decreased now that we have started to have better control of the imbalance of calcium and phosphorus in these patients. There was evidence that the calcium and phosphorus imbalance was responsible for a great part of the tubular interstitial damage. We don't see now, with the modern treatment of myeloma, the same frequency of tubular interstitial pathology that we used to see before. I can categorically deny that in myeloma or in amyloidosis you have these antibodies to tubular basement membrane. However, your question gives me the chance to make a remark that may be pertinent to the discussion that we had before. As you know, secondary amyloidosis is due to tissue polymerization of SAA protein. SAA protein is a protein which is present in connective tissue. As a consequence of the toxic injury or stimulus usually produced by endotoxin, gram negative bacteria, or chronic infection, this protein is released from the connective tissue into the circulation in large amounts and then, for reasons we do not well understand, polymerized in tissue.

So, we have a condition in secondary amyloidosis in which the amyloid is formed by polymerization of a protein of the connective tissue. In the last years two or three papers have been published about membranous glomerulonephritis in association with amyloid and two of these papers show that the membranous glomerulopathy was reversible either by treatment of the infection or by amputation of a leg which had osteomyelitis. Is it possible that some of these proteins are released and then may form immune complexes in the circulation which produce membranous nephropathy? Maybe this is the pathogenesis of membranous nephropathy associated with amyloidosis. There are more and more reports that, by using $C1_q$ or Raji cells, there are circulating immune complexes in amyloidosis. This is a very challenging area of research for the future. Some of my colleagues in the Panel have seen patients with amloidosis and membranous nephropathy. This is one of the conditions in which membranous nephropathy seems to be reversible. What do you think?

RESPONSE: I haven't seen that but I have seen a form of amyloid in the glomeruli that could be mistaken by a not very good pathologist for membranous glomerulonephritis. This is the type that an old friend of mine described. I think he called it "spikey amyloid", where you get structures very similar to deposits on the outside of the basement membrane but they are in fact amyloid. I am not suggesting that the finding is necessarily that of a "not good" pathologist; I'm simply saying that one of these cases of "spikey amyloid" I was shown had been diagnosed as a membranous nephropathy.

COMMENT: I was going to refer to the same thing. I have been personally involved in two cases which were diagnosed as being membranous and then when we looked at the electronmicroscopy they were typical cases of amyloidosis. But, I don't think that is what is being referred to; what you are referring to is the actual association of the two things.

COMMENT: I know we have been talking about this too long already, so I am going to change the subject with a question. Very infrequently we still see cases of methoxyfluorine induced hydrogen output after renal failure in my country. This is a very particular situation. We usually see oliguric acute renal failure from other etiologies. So, it is a very interesting situation. Is there any explanation regarding the renal pathophysiological mechanisms involved in sodium and water excretion or retention in this phenomenon?

RESPONSE: I assure you people that I don't know this gentleman. He was in some areas of research in my lab years ago but I didn't talk about this because in this country methoxyfluorine is very little used now. Since its nephrotoxicity was discovered, it's only used for analgesia in obstetrics, not as an anesthetic agent; at low dose it produced no toxicity. Methoxyfluorine is a fluorinated anesthetic agent which was very good from the point of view of an anesthetic agent because it was stable, non-explosive, and had a lot of qualities. It was for ten years approved by FDA and then it was discovered that it had a certain degree of nephrotoxicity. Actually, looking back, there was a paper that pointed this out but nobody paid attention. As far as I can tell, in man, rat and dog, there is no evidence that salt would be involved. We looked carefully at the possibility of the decreased transfer of sodium by the kidney of the dog and man. Other people looked at the rat and there is no evidence of that. The molecule of this agent is being broken down in the liver and in the kidney by special enzymes called fluorinases which break the molecule in several steps. They release fluoride, organic and inorganic, which appears in the blood and the urine and also oxalic acid, lots of it. As far as I know, the animal and human experience with oxalic acid is oliguric or almost anuric acute renal failure. Most of the cases (there were over a hundred reported years ago) were high output as you described, and I think what happens is fluoride most likely produces nephrotoxicity and a nephrogenic type of diabetes insipidus. I say that because if you take a dog and put it to concentrate the urine maximally, it will concentrate the urine up to 2,000-2,500 mOsm/kg. If you start an infusion of fluoride, you will rapidly (depending on the plasma concentration you achieve, between 15 and 40 minutes) induce a urinary concentrating difficulty. It's not associated with increase of sodium or urea excretion - just purely water excretion. We did some other studies of how fluoride affects ADH action or increases medullary blood flow. Here at the University of Miami ten patients who received anesthesia with methoxyfluorine were compared to ten patients who received anesthesia with halothane. There was absolutely no change of renal function with halothane. In all the 10 patients with methoxyfluorine, there was a decrease in concentrating ability. The study included evaluation right after surgery, two days after surgery (which has the peak plasma level), and then five to ten days after surgery. If you ask me why they had acute renal failure, I wouldn't know and I wouldn't be surprised if it was a volume phenomenon. The initial patients were identified clinically because they were extremely polyuric patients, passing 2,3,4 liters of urine following surgery when they were not receiving that amount of fluid. Almost everyone, until the problem was discovered and corrected, was dehydrated.

MODERATOR: We are running out of time. I would like to close with a final question. As you know, we have a study of nephrotic patients regarding food manipulation. We have looked for changes of IgE in the serum. The late Rawle McIntosh looked for IgE in the biopsy material and we have not been able to document any changes along those lines. What do you make of the cases in the literature where there is evidence of hypersensitivity in various other areas, skin, respiratory tract, GI tract, etc.?

RESPONSE: Well, I have no answer to that. Certainly there is evidence of accumulation of eosinophils in the interstitium and the coincidence of extrarenal pathology produced by an intermediate IgE type hypersensitivity but we cannot draw any conclusions. We have no proof that the renal pathology is produced by IgE mediated hypersensitivity because we don't have a suitable technique. By immunofluorescence you can show whatever you want. The controls are not good enough; I think everybody agrees that so far it has not been possible to show presence of IgE immunoglobulin in minimal glomerular disease. If we could do so, we would be able to prove that the British clinicians that put forth the concept of asthma and nephrosis were right. Sometimes IgE immunoglobulin is not present in lupus but there are many types of immunoglobulin and we don't know what may be the significance. Certainly, we have no evidence that they may be responsible for renal pathology.

MODERATOR: Thank you very much. Thanks to the panelists for their fine contributions.

WORKSHOP:

CLINICOPATHOLOGIC CORRELATIONS

Moderator: José Strauss, M.D.

Div. Pediatr. Nephrol., Dept. Pediatr., Univ.
Miami Sch. Med., Miami, Fla. 33152 USA

MODERATOR: The first case will be presented by Dr. Helen Gorman.

DR. GORMAN: This case is a 14-year-old white boy with history of primary enuresis; polyuria and polydipsia together with constipation became evident at about age 6 ys. In August 1973 IVP and cystoscopy were normal. In November 1973 urine concentrated only to 328 mOsm/kg after water deprivation and aqueous vasopressin, with a rise of serum osmolality from 296 to 305. Serum creatinine was 1.1 to 1.5 and BUN 17 to 26 mg/dl. Creatinine clearance was 62.5 ml/min, corrected for surface area (1.73 m^2). Renal biopsy showed 50% sclerotic glomeruli, foci of marked tubular atrophy and interstitial fibrosis and infiltrates of chronic inflammatory cells. Right hydronephrosis and hydroureter were present at that time by IVP. VCU showed no reflux. In February 1974 renal arteriogram showed multiple minute radiolucent defects located predominantly in the inner cortex and medulla, each 1 mm in diameter or less, in the right kidney. Both kidneys were mildly enlarged. He was treated with NaCl and KCl supplementation because of a salt-losing tendency and persistent hypokalemia. In the past 4 years he has been asymptomatic except for 2 or 3 episodes of UTI, treated with sulfonamide. His growth has been impaired. At age 4½ he was above the 90th percentile; age 9, 75th; now at age 14 he is between the 25th and the 50th percentile. At the present time, his blood pressure is 130/90 mm Hg, and physical examination is normal, except for pallor. Fundi are normal. U/A: trace of protein, sediment within normal limits. Serum creatinine 4.5, BUN 54 mg/dl. Hb, 8.9 g/dl. He is being treated with vitamin D, Amphojel and supplementary potassium. There is no family history of renal disease.

DR. PARDO: On low magnification (Fig. 1) there were a few atrophic tubules but the most impressive change was the interstitial infiltrate with lymphocytes and plasma cells. There are a few atrophic tubules. In Figure 2 there are some totally obsolete glomeruli and the remainder of the glomeruli were normal morphologically. Figure 3 is a high magnification. There are a few eosinophils here and there and the infiltrate shows lymphocytes, plasma cells and a few polymorphonuclears. Mainly there are normal cells and a few eosinophils.

When I saw this biopsy, I didn't know the clinical history. This is an outside case. What I found was extensive inflammatory infiltrate with round cells and a few eosinophils; also, some abnormal glomeruli and some normal glomeruli, an interstitial fibrosis and focal tubular atrophy.

COMMENT: In this case it wouldn't be necessary to look at the slides to make the diagnosis. The clinical diagnosis is absolutely evident. It's a typical case of nephronophthisis for me and of course the finding of these tubulointerstitial lesions only confirms the clinical possibility that it is nephronophthisis. I must insist about the fact that no one, no one can make the diagnosis of nephronophthisis from the histology alone. This is much too unspecific to allow anyone to make the diagnosis without knowing the clinical history. So, it's the combination of the clinical presentation and of these histological findings that helps, especially in a case where you have only a biopsy. One of the good clues to the diagnosis, according to my good friend here, is the presence of cysts in the medulla. This is the reason why the disease was called Medullary Cystic Disease in this country. At the same time, Fanconi was describing nephronophthisis in Europe.

The second thing which I think is very important but here it was difficult to see because we had no PAS stain, is that I have more than an impression that there are very special tubular basement membranes in nephronophthisis. Reviewing again, I'm always quoting that but I learned a tremendous amount of things--reviewing all the end stage kidneys removed at time of transplantation--I was very surprised that these extensive tubular basement membrane changes which are seen in nephronophthisis couldn't be found in more than three or four cases of terminal renal failure of other origin and even then, they were only very focal. So, now, after having looked at about eighty cases of nephronophthisis, I think that this, even if we haven't seen cysts in the medulla, these tubular changes are so extraordinary that they can be taken as good evidence for the disease. But I insist, I think that without the clinical history, nobody should dare make the diagnosis.

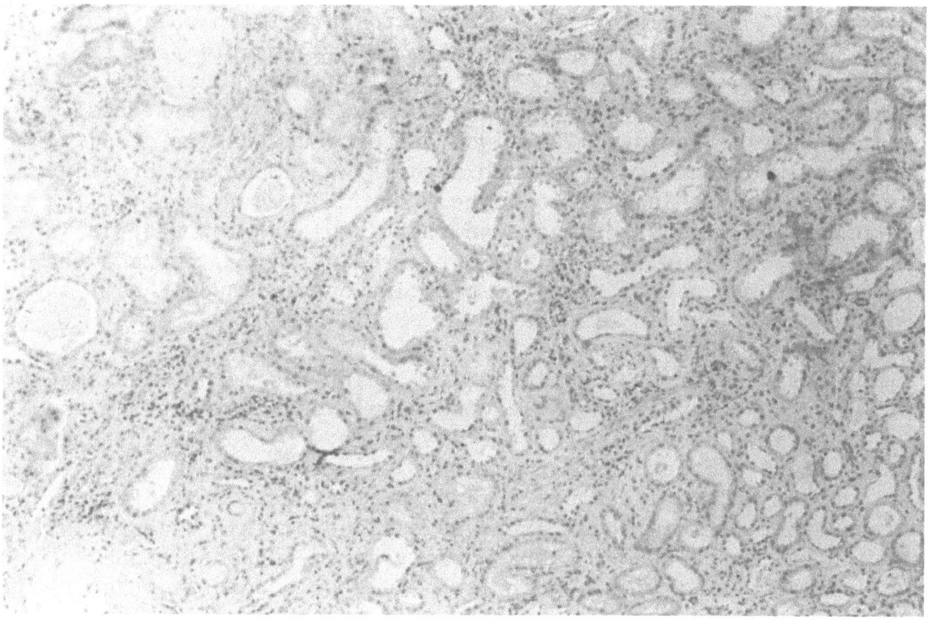

FIGURE 1

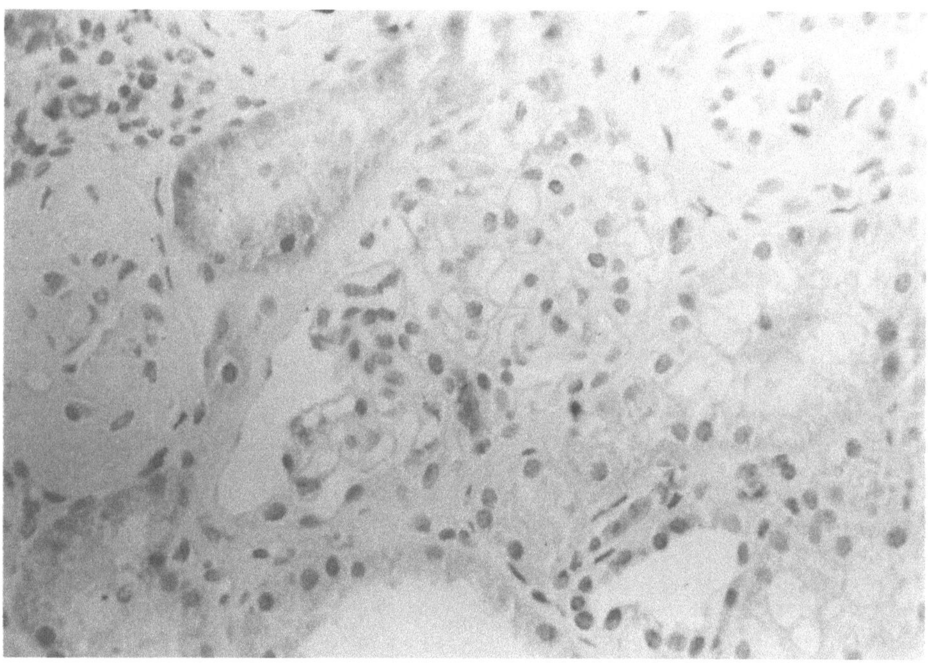

FIGURE 2

COMMENT: I must say I am inclined to agree with what has just been said. I think that this case is diagnosable from the clinical history without having to do anything else. Enuresis is a very frequent feature with people who have what we call Uremic Medullary Cystic Disease. There you get a concentration defect which goes into renal failure with a normal sediment and proteinuria. There aren't many things it could be. I would put my money particularly in view of having seen the histology--not that it is all that helpful--but it's ruling out certain things, perhaps the negative features rather than the positive ones. I would call this Uremic Medullary Cystic Disease.

The business of the cystic part, I think has been overexaggerated in the past. We have seen these with hardly any cysts at all and I don't think it's necessary for the diagnosis. My colleague here is probably right in that it is not a terribly good term to use for this. This term has caused in people's minds a great deal of confusion with the other forms of medullary cystic kidney. This is especially true with the so-called--I think wrongly named--"sponge kidney" which is a condition with a much less sinister prognosis which tends to come on in later years. Now, the only thing that I really don't know about are these tubular changes, these basement membrane changes which were mentioned just now. Perhaps you might let me into the secret of that.

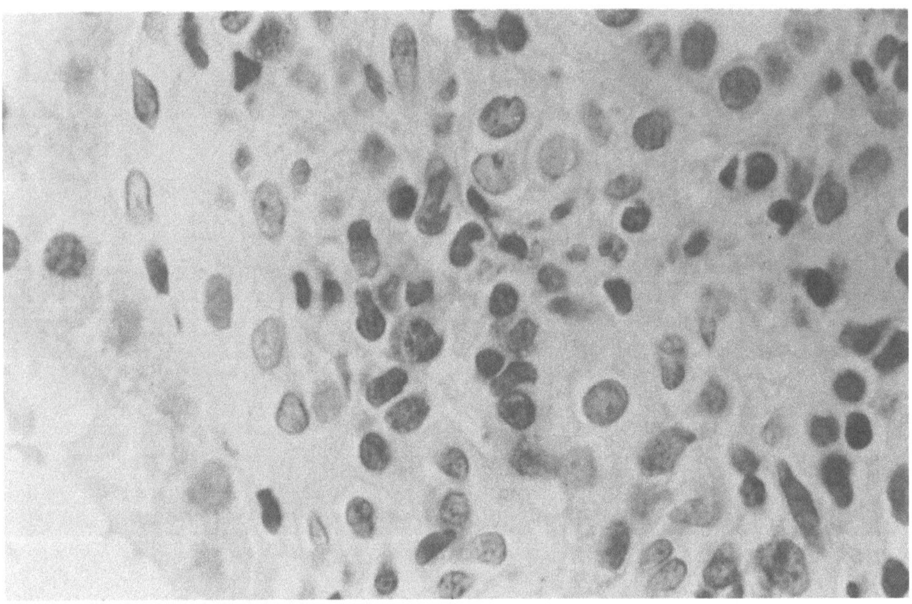

FIGURE 3

COMMENT: It's a laminated basement membrane with extremely queer wrinkled rings and you have at least 3-4-5-different... like concentric layers, but extremely disorganized. It's too bad that I haven't got the slide of that to show you. It is really something; I think special. I can tell you I insisted about that in my first paper on nephronophthisis and ever since I have noticed that feature in all the cases I have seen.

MODERATOR: In the description that you make of the basement membrane, how would you differentiate that appearance from the glomerular basement membrane described in the Alport Syndrome? Is there any comparison?

RESPONSE: It has absolutely nothing to do because in Alport Syndrome, first of all you can hardly see it by light microscopy. The second thing is that it is in the basement membrane. These rings around the tubular basement membrane are like transformation and then accumulation of...it's like new basement membrane. You see what I mean? I don't think you can compare one with the other.

QUESTION: I was curious about the hydronephrosis and hydroureter. Is there any relationship to this patient's underlying disease? Or perhaps this is related to the constant diuresis this patient has?

RESPONSE: I have no opinion but it might be related, I guess.

MODERATOR: In practical terms, we know that polyuria can be present with various types of glomerular involvement and tubular involvement. Some people say with infection. By history, how would you differentiate a patient like this from the others? From the point of view of polyuria and enuresis, how would you approach the workup or the clinical impression of a patient like this?

RESPONSE: In a school age boy or girl with polyuria and nothing else in the history, we would suspect first nephronophthisis. Then, the second feature that is quite common is the pallor, anemia, which is out of proportion to the renal function deterioration. I don't exactly know what this is due to but it's a very common finding. So, when we find this we have to learn exactly what has been going on. We do the IVP's and so on. We do the renal concentrating test and we discover the inability to concentrate which was found here. I think that by exclusion of all the other things, we have to suspect that it is nephronophthisis.

COMMENT: And salt-losing nephritis, too. It's a very good laboratory finding in this disease.

QUESTION: I would like to ask, what do you think about the work of a group extensively involved with the problem of Medullary Cystic Disease using isolated nephrons? They have special techniques by which they can study the resistance of the tubules to distension. Their findings suggest that in Medullary Cystic Disease there is an abnormality of tubular basement membrane and the intraluminal pressure is normal in this condition, whereas in the normal condition it is possible to produce the cystic formation only by increasing the intraluminal pressure. Their conclusion is that in this disease there is an abnormality of the tubular basement membrane which they don't think has a nephrologic counterpart. They think that it probably is a condition in which a normal intratubular pressure produces cystic dilatation because the tubular basement membrane is abnormally distensible. It's a type of investigation which falls on one group of physiologists because it requires a very sophisticated technique of isolation of tubules and study of the tubular distension.

RESPONSE: I didn't know of this work. I think it is a very interesting thing. There is one fact which I think is important and that is that most of the classifications of cysts will include nephronophthisis with only one variety of cysts. Personally, I don't think that it belongs to any type of cyst. I think that these cysts are secondary. The best proof of that is that we have several patients with early biopsies where there are no cysts although the biopsies were taken surgically and they consisted of medulla. Then, we have autopsy cases where there are some cysts in the same patient and then something interesting appears from hemodialysis patients: the cysts tend to increase and the more the kidneys stay, the more there are cysts. For instance, we have a patient from whom we had to remove one of the kidneys at time of transplantation. The transplant didn't work very well and had to be removed. The child was put on hemodialysis again and there was another kidney transplantation performed. Then, they removed the second original kidney. The comparison showed that there were much more cysts in the remaining kidney than in the first kidney removed. There were two years in between and there was almost no more renal parenchyma in the second kidney. I think that these cysts may very well increase with time; so it's not a cystic disease. Something is happening which allows cyst formation. It could well be that the answer is that maybe there is some abnormality in the tubular basement membrane which allows cystic dilatation. I don't know but I am very interested.

QUESTION: I really didn't quite understand exactly what you said. You mean that they have measured intratubular pressure from isolated tubules in man?

RESPONSE: Yes, they have a technique by which, using kidneys obtained at nephrectomy, they can isolate the single tubule and measure the intraluminal pressure. It's probably the only group in the United States working in this area but it is recognized as the leading authority.

QUESTION: As a general morphologist, being a shadow man and dealing with kidney size, it surprises me that you can get a normal IVP of kidneys which are in failure. There's something wrong. I thought that these kidneys were never normal. I thought that the medullary cystic disease kidney was usually smaller than normal.

COMMENT: End stage. This again brings up what I keep saying. The accurate measurement of the kidney is the most important part of the intravenous pyelography or excretion urography. I don't believe that was a normal pyelogram. I think that if you measured this it would be well below 2½ centimeters. What's more, occasionally you actually see contrast medium going out into these cysts. I've got a couple of these patients with IVP's in which there is lots of contrast out in these cysts.

COMMENT: In this I think that there was something.

COMMENT: That's an arteriogram. That's interesting. Two milimeter spaces in an arteriogram. Very high quality arteriogram.

QUESTION: Is this the only child in the family or are there other family members?

RESPONSE: There are other family members. I really can't remember exactly. There are about four, I think. Most are older than he is, up to about 25, all normal.

QUESTION: Have they been investigated?

RESPONSE: I am not quite sure, you see, this child came to us very recently-bringing all this data with him. None of this investigation was done here; it was all done somewhere else. I am not aware of any of the details about family workups-except they have been tissue typed and he has one good donor. That's all I know.

COMMENT: Maybe this should be investigated more thoroughly because a concentration defect could be found in other members of the family. You see, in this disease it's not always evident in young age. There are some adults now who are known to have the disease, too. It can appear later. So, it would be worthwhile to have documentation on the rest of the family.

MODERATOR: In that regard, I remember discussing with you a family that we had reported a number of years ago with so-called nephrogenic diabetes insipidus. You thought at the time that it may have been a family with nephronophthisis. Could you clue us in about the workup of such a family-how the inheritance of nephrogenic diabetes insipidus, being so questionable and with different reports-for some, females do have the disease; for others, they don't, or have less penetrance, etc. In the family we reported, the mother of the propositus and his maternal aunt did not think they were sick. Their family history had been described by themselves as being normal. Actually, they used to go to sleep with a pitcher of water on the night table because they had to drink all night long. They really had severe polyuria which they didn't realize was abnormal.

COMMENT: There are only two things I can say. First, with diabetes insipidus the kidney is always morphologically normal. Renal biopsy at least solves this problem. The second thing is, there are extremely few cases of dominant inheritance in this disease. That's all I can tell you. There are so few that we are wondering if these cases with dominant inheritance are the same thing as nephronophthisis.

MODERATOR: Regarding the anemia, do you have any thoughts? The question may be interpreted more broadly if you like. What is the mechanism of the anemia in this disease or in renal disease in general? Right now we have a patient who had a very mild, presumably post-infectious glomerulonephritis who has had severe anemia which has not been identified in any fashion after thorough workup. Probably the patient will end up receiving cortico-steroids as the usual solution for problems which we don't understand. Do you have any idea as to whether there is any immunological mechanism involved?

RESPONSE: No. We know very little about the origin of anemia in this type of renal disease. The obvious hypothesis is that it is due to marrow depression secondary to uremia when uremia is advancing. The only disease in which there is some hint that an immunological mechanism may be cooperating in the genesis of anemia is anti-GBM disease. Some people, especially in England, have reported that complement is involved in the destruction of the erythrocytes. But, it is work which probably requires confirmation.

MODERATOR: The degree of anemia is not in proportion to the renal failure or you may even have anemia in the absence of renal failure. Am I correct?

RESPONSE: That is correct.

MODERATOR: This is the situation we are facing with this new patient. We have looked into the possibility that there may be a problem with the erythropoietin production. We found in this patient erythropoietin increased but not to the level we would have expected with a marked anemia. At the same time, the bone marrow looked normal but obviously insufficient to maintain a good level of hemoglobin in the blood or of red cell production. Is there anything like erythropoietin acceptability or performance? Rejection? Do we know anything about receptors?

RESPONSE: Not to my knowledge. Some people have proposed that some patients may have antibodies to erythropoietin...

QUESTION: Do you have any ultrastructural studies of the basement membrane of these patients?

RESPONSE: Very few. Very few.

QUESTION: Did you find anything?

RESPONSE: No.

MODERATOR: Dr. Gaston Zilleruelo will present the next case.

DR. ZILLERUELO: This patient was a male Latin boy from San Salvador referred to us in March 1977 at 2½ years of age with a history of a familial nephropathy with progressive renal disease and associated with certain peculiar physical findings, liver compromise and congenital heart disease. He had a history of two episodes of UTI in the newborn period with mild anemia and jaundice. At that time liver was palpable 3 cm below RCM. Also mild proteinuria was found in the urinalysis. Patient had an IVP and VCU that only showed a normal size kidney with slight distortion of the right upper calyceal system. He persisted with mild proteinuria up to 1+; moderate polyuria and polydipsia were noted. In December 1975 (1 yr 4 mos) a gr II/VI holosystolic murmur was found and cardiac evaluation was consistent with a VSD. Also appeared evident some abnormal physical findings such as enlarged forehead (frontal bossing), high palate, short and broad fingers. Liver was 5 cm below RCM, hard, nontender. Spleen tip was palpable. Serum creatinine was 1.3 mg/dl and a decreased creatinine clearance (16.3 ml/min/m^2) was found. Proteinuria was 13 mg/ml/hr; there was a decreased urine concentrating ability (U max 550 mOsm/l). In January 1976, repeated IVP and VCU were WNL. Otherwise, patient was doing well, with a normal development for age, including normal psychomotor and intelligence. However, in February 1977 he had to be admitted to a local hospital because of vomiting and abdominal pain. BP was found to be elevated (170/120 mm Hg) for the first time and liver was 8 cm BCM; BUN was 19, s. creatinine 1.4 mg/dl and urinalysis showed increased proteinuria to 2+. A kidney biopsy was done which showed severe tubulointerstitial fibrosis with microcysts formation, tubular atrophy and glomerular fibrosis. Patient was treated with parenteral and oral reserpine with good results and referred to us for evaluation of his renal disease.

Past history: recurrent bronchitis. UTI and jaundice in the newborn period. Psychomotor: sat at 7 mos., walked at 11 mos. Normal speech for age. Family history: a sister died at 2½ years of age (October 1974) after a short course of severe anemia (non-hemolytic type), hypertension and renal failure. She also presented with enlarged liver and cardiac murmur (interpreted as secondary to congestive heart failure). No post mortem examination was done. Mother was found to have slight hypertension (February 1977), renal failure (s. creatinine 2.4 mg/dl) and same abnormal fingers. However, urinalysis and IVP were WNL.

Physical examination in March 1977 showed a well-developed, well-nourished male in no acute distress. Alert, active, intelligent. Frontal bossing, epicanthal fold of right eye, anteverted nostrils. High palate. Lungs clear. HR 90/min, reg., gr III/VI holosystolic murmur irradiated to axilla and back. Abdomen: soft, nontender liver was palpable 6 cm below RCM, spleen tip was palpable. Extremities with short hands and broad fingers and with overriding of second toes. BP was 100/60 mm Hg, supine. Patient was admitted to UM/JMH Medical Center where a complete re-evaluation was done. Lab results showed: Hb 10.9 g/dl, Hct 30%, BUN 25 mg/dl, creatinine 0.8 mg/dl, uric acid 7.7 mg/dl, serum electrolytes WNL, total protein 6.8 g/dl, albumin 4.2 g/dl, total bilirubin 0.4 mg/dl, PT-PTT normal. Urinalysis was negative for protein and blood. Creatinine clearance was 36 ml/min/1.73 m^2. Selective renal vein renins were normal and a renal arteriogram also was normal. Chromosomal study was found to be normal. Patient returned to San Salvador on same treatment for his hypertension. However, a progressive renal function deterioration and progressive severe hypertension were observed during the following months. He was placed on antihypertensive drugs (Apresoline, Inderal, Ismelin, Lasix) without good results. He had several admissions for treatment of hypertensive crises. In November 1977 BUN was 20 mg/dl and serum creatinine 1.8 mg/dl. In February 1978 BUN was 38 mg/dl and serum creatinine 2.8 mg/dl. In April BUN was 58 mg/dl and serum creatinine 5.5 mg/dl. He had a progressive tormentous course until his death a few weeks later. Post mortem examination was done from which we have available histopathological slides from liver and kidney.

MODERATOR: Dr. Victoriano Pardo will present the histological sections.

DR. PARDO: There are sections from the kidney and the liver. I took photomicrographs without any knowledge of the clinical history. They showed patchy fibrosis with inflammatory infiltrate; no wedge-shaped scarred areas. The glomeruli appeared normal. The most prominent finding was an inflammatory infiltrate with fibrosis and tubular atrophy with concentric thickening of the basement membrane and obsolete glomeruli. Most of the glomeruli showed very advanced peri-glomerular fibrosis. No intrinsic lesions of the glomerular tufts were observed.

The liver (autopsy material) shows a marked septation of the parenchyma. There were no fibrous bridges between the portal spaces and the central vein. So, I think there was not a true cirrhosis. There is hyperplasia of the bile ducts which do not appear dilated (Fig. 4).

QUESTION: I am interested to know if there were findings of microcystic changes either on the initial biopsy or at autopsy.

RESPONSE: I didn't see the gross pathology. I don't have data on the gross appearance of the kidney. I didn't see any cystic spaces there, either in the biopsy or the autopsy material. I didn't see any dilated tubules.

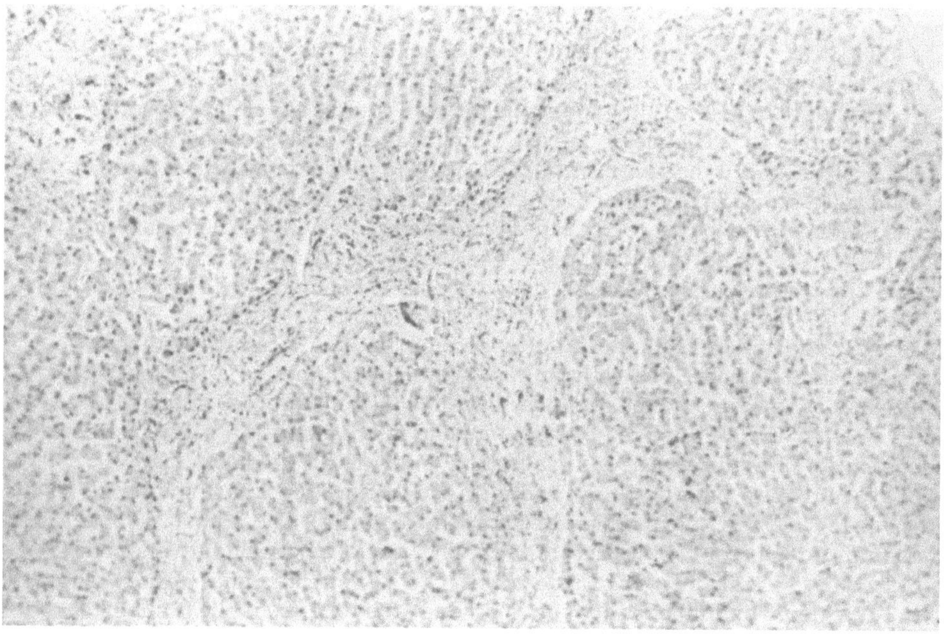

FIGURE 4

DR. ZILLERUELO: There was no finding of cysts in the macroscopic examination of the autopsy material.

QUESTION: At microscopy, were there some areas that could be called cystic? You didn't find any dilatation of the tubuli?

MODERATOR: The answer is no. No cystic formations were found.

COMMENT: I think the liver is extremely interesting here. It's true that in congenital hepatic fibrosis, which is part of the polycystic kidneys, you can have these big strands of fibrosis; but it is absolutely necessary that you have dilated bile ducts. If not, it is not congenital hepatic fibrosis. That is, the type described in polycystic disease. So, I think that this diagnosis has to be completely eliminated. It does not stand. Let's talk about the kidney first. It has chronic tubulointerstitial nephritis. So, maybe it could be diagnosed as being nephronophthisis, again. But first there was hypertension and for me that is against the diagnosis of nephronophthisis.

COMMENT: There are only a few but we have seen some that are hypertensive, particularly when there are advanced lesions. The liver enlargement is not against that; it's just all related to the hypertension and it's a congested liver.

COMMENT: But hypertension has been a major problem in this child. I'm very interested to know that you have seen some cases of nephronophthisis with hypertension. I must say that in our experience it is extremely rare. Very rare. The second thing is that this child has very special findings such as enlarged forehead, high palate, short and broad fingers, and a lot of other things. Then, we have that liver problem. I don't know how to classify this. The only thing I can tell you is that, in the recent literature, there have been several reports which have been published. One is called the Boichis Syndrome. It's our friend in Israel who described that. He showed me the slides several years ago and I made the diagnosis of nephronophthisis on the kidney but then he showed me the liver which had this fibrosis just like that. I must say that we don't think we have ever seen fibrosis of the liver in our patients but also, we have few complete autopsy cases. So, I don't know exactly the incidence or the possibility of this fibrosis in the liver. The other publication is about two patients who had liver cholestatic jaundice and had exactly the same kind of fibrosis in the liver but the kidney looked just like nephronophthisis, too. These are the two published associations of kidney disease with liver fibrosis. But in Israel, we had the meeting of the European Society of Pediatric Nephrology and among the free communications and poster sessions there were at least three papers presented which showed something which looked like nephronophthisis in the kidney with liver fibrosis. In one case presented by someone from Iran, there were several things including abnormalities of the palate, short fingers. So, my feeling at the moment is that there are several syndromes, call it Boichis Syndrome or several other people's syndromes. I'm afraid to include all these types of abnormalities in nephronophthisis. Already we were wondering if retinitis pigmentosa should be included. I wonder if we have to separate all those things and keep the name "nephronophthisis" just for the kidney disease or if we have to add all these compound syndromes which associate other types of involvement.

COMMENT: We spent the whole morning on this problem of semantic associations, and now we are again on this problem. My colleague here is a specialist in saying what is the primary, most important thing and what is the secondary thing. I would say that nephronophthisis is the primary finding and all other findings are secondary associations, some in the liver, others in the eyes, and so on. I cannot see why we don't restrict the name "nephronophthisis" to the renal findings, knowing that it can be associated with many other things.

QUESTION: Could you have hepatic fibrosis with polycystic disease of the kidney without portal hypertension?

RESPONSE: Of course, all the cases of polycystic kidneys, recessive type, have that liver involvement and not all have portal hypertension. I think that my colleague does not agree.

COMMENT: It is not that I disagree with you. In matters like this, I have to defer to you because you see so many more pediatric cases than we do, but the very few cases of congenital hepatic fibrosis, if you like to use that term, associated with polycystic kidney, the few that I've seen have invariably had portal hypertension. I was going to ask whether the spleen, for example, was enlarged in this particular patient. I really wasn't impressed with the amount of fibrosis.

COMMENT: The reason I asked is because in a book it is mentioned that that is the main reason for the portal hypertension in this kidney disease.

COMMENT: It mentions that the portal hypertension is the main cause of death. Of course, if you don't die of your kidney, you die of your liver. Ninety percent of the cases of polycystic, infantile type, die at birth. So, it's finished. You get rid of the majority of cases immediately. Some of them live longer because they have less holes and more kidney. Then the liver starts being involved. I think it's a matter of how long you live. If you live with polycystic kidneys you might, as a matter of fact, die of your liver. But, in the infantile type--I would rather call it recessive type--it's a constant feature to have liver involvement with what is called congenital hepatic fibrosis. But not all have portal hypertension, at least at the beginning. It may be that they can develop it later.

COMMENT: I find this an extremely confusing case. The liver part, I don't know whether we have overplayed the liver hand; I think we probably have. It's very difficult to give an opinion when you just see one or two kodachromes. I certainly wasn't very impressed with what I saw in the liver. The few cases I've seen of the association of congenital hepatic fibrosis and cystic kidneys, I would exclude that. As has been said here, there are many features that are very consistent with the diagnosis of nephronophthisis or medullary cystic disease. The presence of hypertension has been very rightly pointed out here. I don't think I've seen hypertension in spite of what you are saying.

I can't get over the fact that there are certain other abnormalities in this patient; the short and broad fingers, high palate, and they seem to be present in relatives, too. I think this may be something new. I'm not really familiar with it.

COMMENT: Regarding what one of you was saying, "why don't you accept the features as secondary and keep the nephronophthisis business?", as I emphasized in the preceeding case, I think that we don't have enough histological clues to the diagnosis of nephronophthisis to be sure that there is not another disease which can give exactly the same type of chronic diffused tubulointerstitial nephritis and which might be something completely different. I am always open to the development of what is going to be found as the cause of nephronophthisis. Suppose it's a deficient enzyme. It might very well be something like that. Maybe it will be some other deficient enzyme which is responsible for these other diseases associated with something else. We must be very careful not to put in the same bag all the things because we have no other diagnosis to propose. That's why, personally, I would rather have nephronophthisis when there is only the kidney involvement alone. Then, the same type of kidney involvement may be found in association with eye abnormalities, liver abnormalities, face or anything and they may be the same disease but they may be something else. I think that we should not confuse everything because what we are doing now is trying to do good nephrology so that people who are working in other fields can find the solution to our problems. Maybe in ten years' time we will laugh to have been able to confuse these things. As I remember Professor Debre the day he realized that the case he had been describing, DeToni-Debre-Fanconi Syndrome, some were cystinosis and others were something else. There is DeToni-Debre-Fanconi Syndrome, but we well know now that it covers a tremendous amount of different things. It's not a disease; it's a syndrome. Maybe that's the type of mind we should have when we are dealing with such non-specific things. When you find cystinosis, cystine crystals in the kidney, you know that it's cystinosis. That's a specific feature. But chronic tubulointerstitial nephritis, what is it? We've been talking of that since yesterday morning. We are going to talk about that tomorrow and you are going to see that it covers so many different things that I don't think we can consider that as a specific feature.

QUESTION: Yes. In the first case that was discussed, you were very emphatic that the concentric layers around the tubules in nephronophthisis were a very distinctive feature. Yet, when they were shown in this case, you seemed to show some reluctance in accepting this as nephronophthisis. Is it not tied up for you, completely and absolutely?

RESPONSE: I don't want to answer because I haven't looked at the whole kidney. I haven't looked at PAS stain. I'm not sure that what we saw, these big rings there, cover what I consider as being, though not specific, extremely good evidence for. I don't know with the English, but "good evidence for" does not mean "specific". It's different.

COMMENT: What other conditions have you seen it in?...I'm sorry. I let you off the hook. You are absolutely right in being put on the spot in trying to make a diagnosis on just kodachromes, possibly not of the magnification you would like to see it, nor with the stain. I withdraw that.

QUESTION: Did you say that if you do not see bile duct dilatation you are not going to call it hepatic fibrosis and/or polycystic kidney? I recollect a patient of mine two years of age with liver enlargement, a slight rise in bilirubin and no liver compromise by SGOT or SGPT. We biopsied the liver and the pathologist claimed that it either had to be galactosemia, fructose intolerance, or cystinosis. We worked him up for that and it was all negative. There was very minimal fibrosis. I went ahead and did an IVP because whenever I find something in the liver, especially if there is mild fibrosis, I evaluate the kidneys. To my surprise we found tubular ectasia. I took this case to a famous pathologist. I first sent him just the liver biopsy and he gave me the same diagnosis: acinar formation, mild fibrosis. When I told him the IVP findings, he said "this would have to be infantile polycystic disease". I just wondered, since the liver biopsy was so striking-it was just acinar formation, no ductal proliferation, no dilatation, just minimal fibrosis.

QUESTION: But you had no specimen of the kidney? You just had seen the IVP?

RESPONSE: Correct. We didn't do a kidney biopsy.

COMMENT: It is a common association, tubular ectasia and hepatic fibrosis.

COMMENT: Except that what was striking was the acinar formation in the biopsy. Yes, I am aware that there is tubular ectasia and hepatic fibrosis. What I was surprised to see on the liver biopsy was acinar formation. That's why I consulted various pathologists who said that without the IVP they would have made the same diagnosis. But the IVP, since there was tubular ectasia, no matter whether the liver showed acinar formation or not, one of them was going to put it into the category of infantile polycystic kidney disease.

COMMENT: We have another very similar case. In fact, the other way around. The first sibling died of liver disease. I can't recall exactly but post-mortem showed the liver fibrosis and also the kidney changes. So, initially we thought that it was infantile polycystic kidney disease. Then later on, about ten years later, we saw him again when he came down with renal disease. Now, the changes are compatible with juvenile nephronophthisis; the patient also has retinitis pigmentosa. So, then we were puzzled as to whether or not this was juvenile nephronophthisis. Maybe this happens in some of the cases; it's very difficult to differentiate various entities.

QUESTION: In the liver there was congenital hepatic fibrosis?

RESPONSE: Right. The child died.

QUESTION: With dilatation of bile ducts or not?

RESPONSE: No. I won't say that.

COMMENT: That's the big problem. We shouldn't give people's names to diseases of nephronophthisis with congenital hepatic fibrosis. I don't like the English word either. I'll tell you the one I have invented. I think it is much better. "Fibro-adenomatosis of biliary ducts". I think that is much better because you see, that avoids the confusion. If you call it congenital hepatic fibrosis, then all types of hepatic fibrosis are included in that. The characteristic feature of polycystic kidney, infantile type, is the dilatation of bile ducts which is surrounded by fibrosis. In the name "congenital hepatic fibrosis", you don't hear that. You see, again the problems of nomenclature.

COMMENT: Actually the first case initially was diagnosed as polycystic disease. Later on, the sibling, ten, fifteen years later, had a similar disease but with retinitis pigmentosa and the histological study revealed the picture of nephronophthisis.

QUESTION: I would like to ask about a recent article-monograph on polycystic disease of the kidney in which the authors describe perinatal, neonatal, infantile and juvenile types. They start with mild hepatic fibrosis in the early part. In juveniles it is really predominant in that it's also dilatation of the biliary tree. They say that the juvenile kind might be picked up on routine examination just with hepatosplenomegaly. We did have a patient like this who was picked up by routine examination and who was referred for workup of hepatosplenomegaly and had portal hypertension, the venous pressure was high and because at the time of the radiological study the kidneys were big, at the time of liver biopsy we did go in and do a kidney biopsy too. It did show polycystic disease and liver-you could hold it up to the slide and see that there was fibrosis. Would you make some comments on that article?

RESPONSE: I can. I think that it's not a very good idea separating by age different things. In fact, for me the problem of infantile polycystic disease is the proportion of holes in the kidneys. Period. You may have different types in the same family; I have seen a family where there were three types. One died at birth and had very enlarged kidneys, full of holes. Another one started having hypertension when he was two years of age, and the third one, when he was seven years of age developed portal hypertension and the kidney disease was found. The same thing in the same family. So, it's just my feeling that the big difference among these three children was that one was born with a lot of holes and the other one had small holes predominating in the medulla and the liver was the first one to have symptomatology. So, that's why, even though I think that paper is an excellent paper, beautiful paper, I am not sure that this kind of classification according to age is reasonable. That's my opinion.

COMMENT: I would like to ask for comments on analgesic nephropathy and the nephropathy seen with rheumatoid arthritis. We had a 10 year old white girl who was diagnosed as having pulmonary TB, treated with anti-tuberculosis drugs during two years. Subsequently, she had onset of new problems at seven years of age with joint pains, recurring fever and weight loss. LE preparation was negative. IVP revealed 2 kidneys of 13 cm each in length and an irregular contour. Bone deformities in both hands were noticed one year prior to admission. She received prednisone and salicylic acid during two years and eight months. Then she developed a tubulointerstitial nephropathy (confirmed by biopsy) due to salicylate ingestion.

QUESTION: That was the proposed diagnosis? That is, that she took so many aspirins?

ANSWER: Yes.

COMMENT: But, you don't know what analgesic, how it started. This could be papillary necrosis but I would expect small kidneys in that case. But this is a young girl and analgesic nephropathy has been described more in adults and maybe contraction takes some years, too. So, it is possible that at the beginning it's an interstitial nephritis with an enlargement of kidneys and then they shrink.

COMMENT: No. The time factor in analgesic nephropathy does not follow the time factor in any other form of kidney disease. We were talking about this yesterday. Analgesic nephropathy appears to start in the middle of the papilla and then, if that's so, the papillary necrosis, an obstruction there, follows. So, you will get a fan of intrarenal obstructive nephropathy whether it's infected or anything else, it's like tying off these tubules. So you get essentially a scar and that doesn't take long to happen. If you tie this off you will start getting this in six weeks. What we saw was a much more extensive type of analgesic nephropathy, the type where the whole papilla is gone and this is sort of extending out into the medulla. Now, if you've got that kind of lesion and you've got multiple papillae involved, usually you get a history of colic, because they are passing debri and they are aware of it. This may happen, as you say, in people the age of 45 or 50. The youngest one, I think, that they've had in Australia, down in Melbourne, was a boy 21. So, then you've got this kidney which measures 13 centimeters and usually the kidneys at this age are about 11½ to 12 centimeters, and they have this slightly irregular contour. This may be analgesic nephropathy complicating some other kidney disease. I really can't tell; I'm sorry, I really can't think any more definitely than that without more information.

COMMENT: There is another possibility, to interpret the interstitial findings as being drug-induced interstitial nephritis. But, then, maybe we wouldn't have this modification of the IVP. I don't know. I have a question. The other diagnosis raised is that of lupus or of rheumatoid arthritis. The findings of immunofluorescence consisted exclusively of IgM and fibrin in the mesangial areas of the glomeruli, and nothing around the tubules. Is that correct? Would you accept that as being diagnostic for lupus?

RESPONSE: Certainly these findings are not very characteristic. Usually in lupus, in the minimal variety of glomerular pathology, there are several classes of immunoglobulins in the mesangium. So, these very mild changes would be more consistent with the diagnosis of mesangial pathology, that you can see in some patients with rheumatoid arthritis and positive rheumatoid factor, a condition where you have IgM in the kidney because the rheumatoid factor is followed.

by IgA antigen reacting with an IgM antibody. But considering the possibility that this tubulointerstitial nephritis may be due to the same pathogenetic mechanism which produces glomerular pathology, I would be really rather reluctant to accept this interpretation. In the tubulointerstitial nephritis of lupus, it's usually present due to local deposition of antigen-antibody complexes in the severe diffuse proliferative glomerulonephritis. In this condition, it's present perhaps in 50% of patients with glomerulonephritis. But again, in this condition you have a very definite deposit of immunoglobulin and complement in tubular basement membrane rather than in the interstitium. So, I would say that if this is a lupus serologically, there is some suggestion although the titer of the antibody is not very high, but there are no positive LE cells. If this is a lupus you certainly will have to find another explanation for the tubulointerstitial pathology. I'm very sympathetic with the other hypothesis that perhaps it's a drug induced reaction-perhaps aspirin or some other drug.

QUESTION: Have you seen this change in rheumatoid arthritis?

RESPONSE: Well, that's a very difficult question to answer. It's difficult to say what you have in the kidney of rheumatoid arthritis because it is a condition in which you have circulating immune-complex-like substances, but you don't frequently see glomerular pathology. You don't have frequent positive urinary findings. So, really, I don't know what there is in the kidney of rheumatoid arthritis. I am not aware of tubulointerstitial nephritis in rheumatoid arthritis.

COMMENT: You get tubulointerstitial nephritis in rheumatoid arthritis but it is usually a result of the therapy.

RESPONSE: Oh yes, I agree.

COMMENT: I think that those are about the only circumstances under which you would see it. As you know, for years and years people talked about a mild form, a proliferative form of glomerulonephritis in rheumatoid arthritis. I have never seen it but what is also interesting in rheumatoid arthritis is the membranous nephritis, membranous nephropathy (whatever you like to call it) as a result of gold therapy. I had occasion to review a paper some time ago from a series of patients with rheumatoid arthritis who had developed a membranous glomerulonephritis without any gold having been taken. I have just very vague recollection of reviewing this and I don't think it's appeared yet but I was very surprised when I read this. For those who are not familiar it has been described on several occasions that people with rheumatoid arthritis being treated with gold injections may develop proteinuria and on biopsy will be found to have what is called membranous nephropathy in which you have an electron dense deposit on the epithelial side of the basement membrane. This has been produced experimentaly too, and I think a very interesting idea was put forward to explain it-the gold was possibly damaging tubular epithelial cells which was putting tubular antigen in contact with antibody producing cells and you were getting something analogous to the Heyman-Edgington autologous immune complex. It was never really proved completely but there were these two or three cases in this paper of the membranous picture without gold having been used.

COMMENT: Another paper like this one has been published recently in Finland. They frequently have membranous nephropathy patients with rheumatoid arthritis. Again, in this series there were two patients who developed membranous nephropathy without gold treatment. In some of these patients the kidney eluate was tested for antibody specificity and there was no evidence that the tubular antigen was involved. There is another paper on this subject which is very controversial but it has been published. It is concerned with an extractable antigen which is present in the liver, kidney, and several other organs. These patients seem to have periodically a high level of this antigen in the circulation and periodically a high level of antibody, a situation similar to the one described in lupus before we knew that lupus was produced by an antigen-antibody complex. So the interpretation was that perhaps the cellular cytoplasmic antigen was responsible for the formation of complexes in these gold nephropathy patients with rheumatoid arthritis. However, when the kidneys were stained with antibody to this ubiquitous antigen, it was not possible to stain the antigen. So it's a very important hypothesis but it still has to be proved.

QUESTION: In the paper from Finland, how did they get the kidney material from which to elute the antibody?

RESPONSE: They got it by surgical biopsy, relatively large samples.

QUESTION: On the general business of immune complexes being found in the region of the tubular basement membrane and giving rise to interstitial nephritis, is there any correlation between that and the histologic type of lupus you get? I don't know whether you go along with the idea originally put forward that there are at least four histologic types of lupus. There might be more than that. Let's just say that there's a type where you have no changes, a type where you have mesangial increase only, the type where you have focal glomerulonephritis, the type where you have extra-membranous deposits, the type where you have diffuse proliferation and wire loops. What I'm saying is that there were four in the original description, but you can go on adding as many as you like. Is there any correlation between those histologic types and the likelihood of getting complexes in the tubules?

RESPONSE: Yes, I think that probably the most important factor is the severity of the disease and presumably the extremely large amount of complexes which are present in the circulation of these patients. Usually it is a tubulointerstitial nephritis mediated by immune complexes--presumably DNA and anti-DNA complexes, perhaps some other types of complexes--associated with the diffuse proliferative glomerulonephritis which is the most severe variety of glomerulonephritis.

QUESTION: But only with that?

RESPONSE: Well, usually only with that. There is a recent report of a patient who developed a transient renal failure as a consequence of lupus tubulointerstitial nephritis which was not associated with severe glomerular pathology. There were only minimal changes with minimal mesangial fluorescence. Perhaps we have the formation of a different type of antigen-antibody complex which, as a consequence of physicochemical characteristics, may have a propensity to localize in tubulointerstitial tissue.

COMMENT: We had another case of lupus nephritis that started some years ago with distal tubular acidosis and then calcinosis. After three or four years, I don't remember exactly, she started to menstruate and she developed lupus nephritis. She died because of that. She had diffuse proliferation and a tubulointerstitial nephritis. It was a completely different picture from the one that you are talking about.

COMMENT: This is the reason I asked my first question: was there any positive immunofluorescence in this case?

RESPONSE: No. Not in this case.

COMMENT: If it had been positive, it would have explained the interstitial nephritis.

COMMENT: I would like to present the tubulointerstitial lesions we observed in lupus nephritis. These are our findings in 38 cases of lupus nephritis with different glomerular lesions: 13 with membranous proliferative glomerular lesions, 8 with focal and segmental glomerular lesions, 8 proliferative endocapillary glomerulonephritis, 5 endo- and extra-capillary glomerulonephritis, 2 extramembranous glomerulonephritis and 2 minor abnormalities. Tubulo-interstitial lesions were present in 77% of the membranoproliferative cases, 50% of the segmental and focal type, 25% of the proliferative endocapillary type, and 100% in the few cases with endo- and xtra- or extramembranous glomerulonephritis, and one out of the two cases with minor abnormalities. In 33 cases studied by immunofluorescent techniques, 8 out of these 23 cases had some kind of positive tubulointerstitial deposits. That means about 24%.

MODERATOR: Is this all settled? If so, we shall have the last question.

QUESTION: Did anyone look at this patient's urine when she had TB? Did anyone stain the biopsy for acid-fast bacili?

RESPONSE: Yes, but there were no abnormal findings.

MODERATOR: We must adjourn now. Thank you.

PART TWO

NUTRITIONAL ASPECTS OF RENAL DISEASE

HIGHLIGHTS
RELATION OF CELL METABOLISM TO NUTRITIONAL STATE

Jack Metcoff, M.D.

Dept. Pediatr.,Biochem. and Molecular Biol., Univ. Okla. Health Sci. Ctr., Okla. City, Okla. 73190,USA

In severe protein-calorie malnutrition (PCM) in children (Kwashiorkor and/or Marasmus) cellular energy metabolism is impaired. Using muscle biopsies or circulating leukocytes for cell studies, PCM is characterized by accumulation of cell Na, with reduction of K and Mg. Cell metabolite levels, associated with utilization of glucose and with turnover of the citric acid cycle, are reduced. The electrolyte changes are related to simultaneous changes in cell metabolite levels. Activities of some regulatory enzymes in the glycolytic and citric acid cycle pathways are impaired. The inhibition of pyruvate kinase, for example, represents an allosteric effect related to the high Na level in the cell. Cell energy levels are reduced and appear to limit the effectiveness of the Na pump. Plasma amino acid levels and amino acid uptake by cells are abnormal. Phagocytosis by leukocytes is impaired and this is related to impaired glycolysis and depressed hexose monophosphate shunt activity. Death in PCM is associated with exaggeration of the cell metabolic abnormalities leading to a breakdown in cell energy production. Recovery is associated with improvement in cell substrate and energy levels.

We have shown that maternal nutritional status and leukocyte metabolism at midpregnancy are closely related. In this instance the maternal leukocyte is used as a model to study the effect of nutrition on rapidly dividing and growing cells, including fetal cells. Our hypothesis holds that some interaction of nutrients regulates the metabolism of all replicating, maturing cells. Ten metabolic characteristics of the circulating granulocyte were used as dependent variables for the metabolic cell model while plasma levels of 13 nutrients, including trace minerals (TM), and 18 free amino acids (AA's) were used as independent variables in the same blood sample to characterize the nutrient microenvironment. Significant correlations ($p < 0.05$) were found between each of the leukocyte enzyme activities (Pyruvate kinase, adenylate kinase, phosphofructokinase, glucose-6-P-dehydrog), protein (^3H leucine) and RNA (^3H uridine) synthesis and cell levels of ATP and ADP with interactions between the levels of the trace minerals, Zn, Cu, and Fe with levels of certain amino acids. The correlations suggest that the cell activity may be modulated by the trace mineral-amino acid interaction. Further, the data provide evidence, in the complex multivariable system existing in vivo in humans, that specific metabolic activities in the cell are related to interactions of nutrients in the surrounding microenvironment.

These observations emphasize that nutritional states imply effects on cell metabolism. Nutritional imbalances or deficits are expressed at the cellular level by interrelated changes in cell electrolytes, energy metabolism, amino acids and protein synthesis. The impact of malnutrition on critical, vital functions of the cell apparently determines the effects on growth and/or survival.

REFERENCES

1. Metcoff, J.: Cellular energy metabolism in protein-calorie malnutrition. In Olson, R.E. (ed.): Protein-Calorie-Malnutrition. New York: Academic Press, 1975, p. 65.

2. Waterlow, J.C. and Alleyne, G.A.O.: Protein malnutrition in children: advances in knowledge in the last 10 years. Adv. Protein Chem. 25:117, 1971.

3. Patrick, J. and Golden, M.: Leukocyte electrolytes and sodium transport in protein-energy malnutrition. Amer. J. Clin. Nutr. 30:1478, 1977.

4. Felig, P. and Wahren, J.: Protein turnover and aminoacid metabolism in the regulation of gluconeogenesis. Fed. Proc. 33:1092, 1974.

5. Metcoff, J., Costiloe, P., Sandstead, H., et. al.: Relation of cell metabolism to interactions of nutrient levels in the plasma microenvironment. Abstr., Fed. Proc. 38:708, 1979.

6. Douglas S.D. and Schopfer, K.: The phagocyte in protein-calorie malnutrition - a review. In Suskind, R.M. (ed.): Malnutrition and the Immune Response. New York: Raven Press, 1977, p. 231.

7. Delaporte, C., Jean, G., and Broyer, M.: Free plasma and muscle amino acids in uremic children. Amer. J. Clin. Nutr. 31:1647, 1978.

WATER AND ELECTROLYTES IN MALNOURISHED AND UREMIC CHILDREN

Gaston Zilleruelo, M.D. and José Strauss, M.D.

Div. Pediatr. Nephrol., Dept. Pediatr., Univ. Miami Sch. Med., Miami, Fla. 33152, USA

The following review presents general concepts about water and electrolyte homeostasis, with particular emphasis on malnourished children and children with chronic renal failure.

WATER AND ELECTROLYTE HOMEOSTASIS

General Concepts

Volume and composition of extracellular fluid (ECF) in terrestrial mammals are threatened constantly by entry of widely varying amounts of water and solutes. The major role of the kidney as an excretory organ is to maintain balance and integrity of body fluids by returning to the external environment the substances which are not needed.

One of the most jealously guarded constants of ECF is its total volume. Under normal circumstances, the kidney compensates for salt and water overload or deficit with great precision, thereby insuring ECF volume stability within narrow limits. The main energy expenditure of the kidneys is for tubular reabsorption of the major extracellular ions; sodium is the dominant ion and key solute in ECF. Homeostatic control of sodium is intimately linked with that of water.

Potassium is the dominant and key solute of the intracellular fluid (ICF). About 91% of total body potassium is located in ICF (1½% is in ECF, 7½% in bone). Potassium plays an important role in physiological and biochemical mechanisms (nerve and muscle tissue excitability, carbohydrate and protein enzyme activation, and acid-base balance). Although potassium is handled all along the nephron, the distal tubule is most involved in its secretion. This tubular secretory mechanism is dependent upon delivery of sodium to the distal tubule, presence of aldosterone, and intracellular pH.

Factors involved in maintaining steady control and urinary excretion of sodium, potassium and water include glomerular filtration rate, glomerulotubular balance, peritubular forces (hydrostatic and oncotic pressures in peritubular capillaries), renin-angiotensin-aldosterone system, antidiuretic hormone (ADH), and natriuretic factors or hormones (Table 1). The homeostatic control of ECF volume depends upon renal tubular reabsorption of sodium, mediation by the renin-angiotensin system, and the adrenal cortical secretion of aldosterone which has a direct action on the distal tubule sodium transport.

ECF volume is regulated by urinary excretion of both sodium and water, whereas ECF osmolality is regulated by only water excretion. The most important mediator in water excretion is ADH. Three fundamental processes seem to be involved in the renal control of water (Fig. 1):

a. *delivery* of filtrate to the ascending limb of Henle's loop,
b. *separation* of water from electrolytes and urea in the ascending limb,
c. *controlled* reabsorption of water in the collecting duct under the influence of ADH.

The action of ADH involves the synthesis of cyclic 3-5 AMP with consequent alteration in water permeability of the luminal and lateral plasma membranes of the distal tubule and collecting duct.

Table 1. Factors Influencing Renal Salt and Water Control

- Glomerulotubular balance
- Peritubular forces (hydrostatic and oncotic pressure)
- Renin-angiotensin-aldosterone system
- Antidiuretic hormone
- Natriuretic factor or hormone

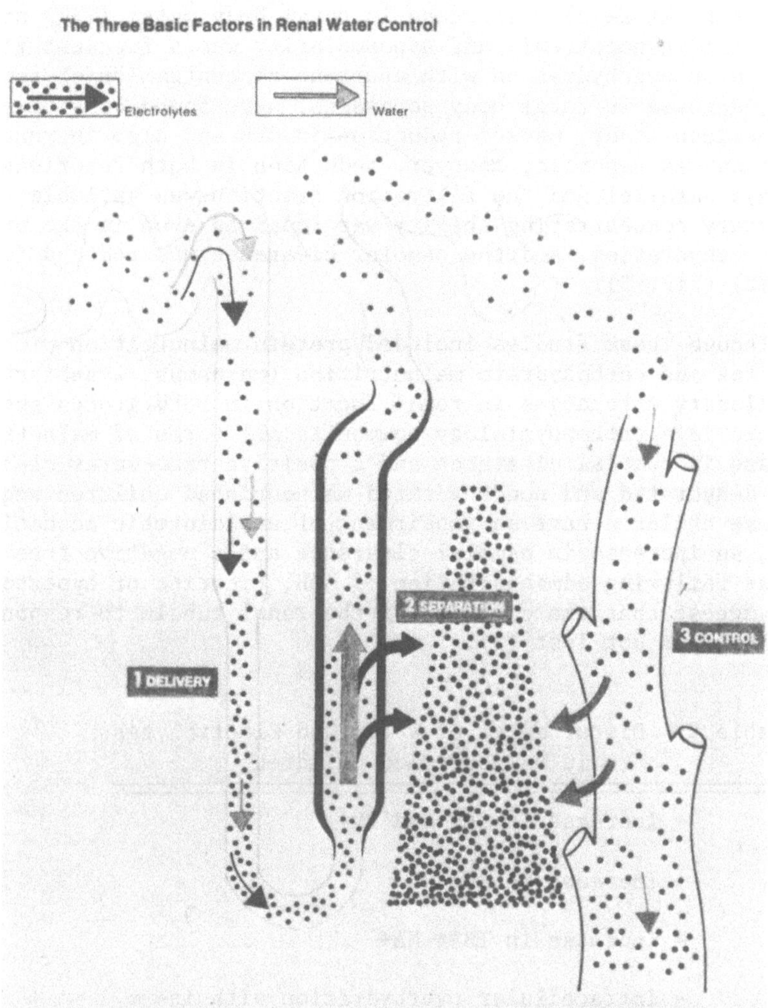

FIG. 1. Fundamental processes involved in the renal control of water. (From Goldberg, M.: Water control and the dysnatremias. In Bricker, N.S. (ed.): The Sea Within Us: Clinical Guide to Fluid and Electrolyte Imbalance. Chicago: Science and Medicine, 1975, p. 20, with permission).

WATER AND ELECTROLYTES IN MALNOURISHED CHILDREN

The kidney's basic function in maintaining homeostasis of water, sodium and potassium, is altered by chronic malnutrition. The effect of severe protein-calorie malnutrition on renal functions (mainly water and electrolyte metabolism) in children has been investigated in classic studies of Jamaican (1) and Mexican (2) children (Table 2). Increase in total body water (TBW) and ECF with mild hyponatremia and hyposmolarity was a frequent finding. Intracellular overhydration with aberrant concentration of sodium in ICF and decrease in total body potassium, were found consistently. In the Mexican study, marked reduction in GFR and also in renal plasma flow was reported; however, reduction in both functions was not always parallel and the filtration fraction was variable (Fig. 2). Urinary concentrating ability was impaired even in the presence of dehydration, and the osmolar clearance was reduced in both groups (2) (Fig. 3).

Although these studies included protein malnutrition with and without fat and carbohydrate malnutrition (marasmus, kwashiorkor), the similarity of changes in renal function in both groups suggests that there is a pathophysiology common to all forms of malnutrition. A decrease in osmolal clearance and a positive free-water clearance in both dehydrated and nondehydrated malnourished children suggest that these children have an impairment of antidiuretic mechanisms. However, an increase in osmolal clearance and a negative free water clearance following administration of ADH, nicotine or hypertonic saline suggest that the capacity of the renal tubule to respond to some stimuli is not lost (3).

Table 2. Disturbances of Water and Electrolytes in Malnourished Children

- Increase in TBW and PV*
- Increase in ECF
- Increase in TB** NA+
- Intracellular overhydration with increase in intracellular Na+ and decrease in K+
- Decrease in TB K+
- Normal or mild hyponatremia
- Mild hypokalemia

*Plasma volume
**Total body

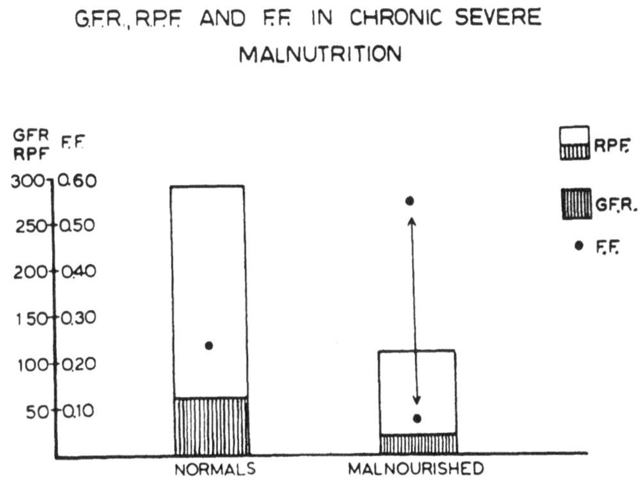

FIG. 2. Renal function in chronic severe malnutrition. (From Gordillo, G., Soto, R.A., Metcoff, J. et al.: Intracellular composition and homeostatic mechanisms in severe chronic infantile malnutrition. III. Renal adjustments. Pediatr. 20: 303, 1957, with permission).

In a study of 23 malnourished infants, the impairment in urinary concentrating ability was progressive and correlated with the degree of malnutrition (Fig. 4) (4); distal tubule response to ADH was dose related (Fig. 5) (5). In those patients whose malnutrition was corrected, the response to vasopressin was especially noteworthy, suggesting the reversibility of changes after protein repletion (3).

What are the mechanisms responsible for the renal functional changes observed in malnourished children? There is no single explanation for the water and electrolyte disturbances; one theory is based on the kidney's inability to excrete water (6). Since the diet of many malnourished patients consists entirely of liquids, abnormal accumulation of fluid may lead to hypotonicity. It also may result from release of endogenous water from cell catabolism, depletion of protein or recurrent stool loss of water and sodium (7). Edema, due to increased total body sodium, would follow a decreased renal sodium excretion ability (6).

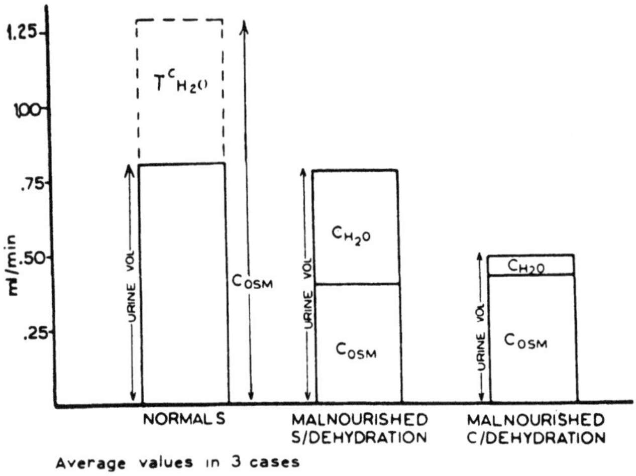

FIG. 3. Renal water handling in malnourished children with and without dehydration. (From Gordillo, G., Soto, R.A., Metcoff, J. et al.: Intracellular composition and homeostatic mechanisms in severe chronic infantile malnutrition. III. Renal adjustments. Pediatr. 20: 303, 1957, with permission).

Expansion of ICF may be a consequence of chronic ECF hypotonicity. Thus, the excretion of a relatively hypotonic urine can be interpreted as a defense against excessive dilution of solutes in body water, and the reduction of GFR may be interpreted as an effort to sustain body water (8).

At the cytoplasmatic level, malnutrition produces a disturbance which generally narrows the flexibility of renal and cellular responses to superimposed events such as dehydration or overhydration. It has been suggested that in severe malnutrition, the intracellular dilution of potassium and enzyme systems or cell substrates leads to further impairment of energy production and results in higher intracellular sodium and lower potassium (8). Thus, this sequence of events would increase depletion of intracellular potassium and make even more scarce the available energy required for active sodium transport.

To explain the concentrating defect of malnourished children, several mechanisms have been postulated (Table 3): 1) *inability to respond to ADH at the renal tubule level* (9). Against this

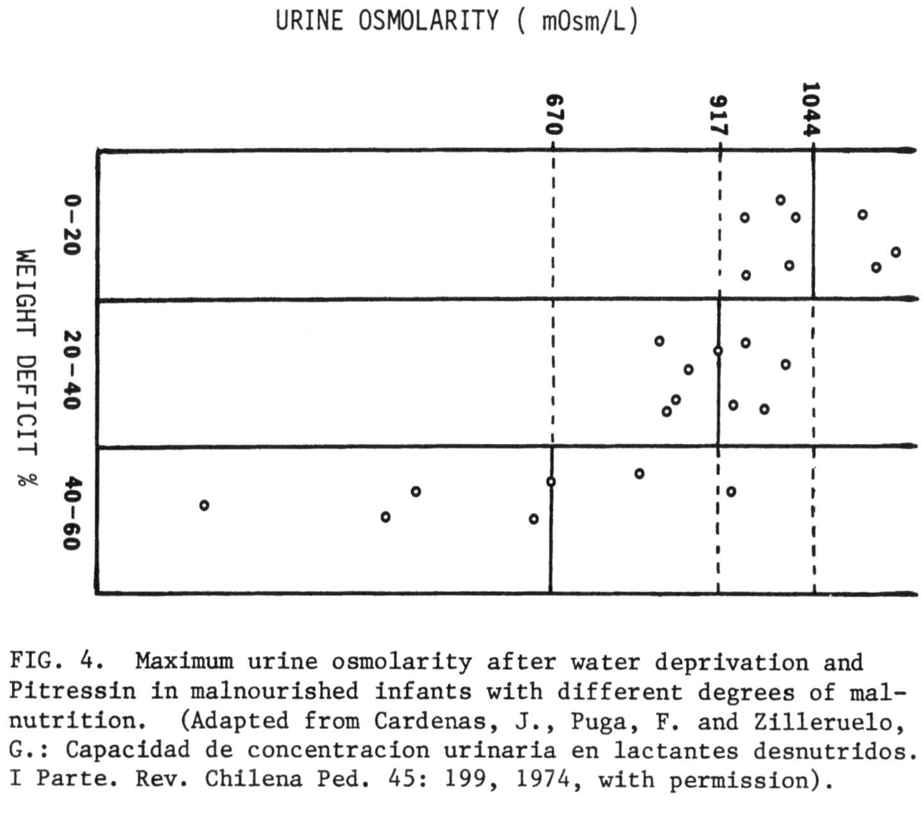

FIG. 4. Maximum urine osmolarity after water deprivation and Pitressin in malnourished infants with different degrees of malnutrition. (Adapted from Cardenas, J., Puga, F. and Zilleruelo, G.: Capacidad de concentracion urinaria en lactantes desnutridos. I Parte. Rev. Chilena Ped. 45: 199, 1974, with permission).

hypothesis is the fact that the response of the renal tubule to ADH is adequate at a higher ADH serum level (5); these children have no important microscopic changes in the renal medulla. Also, recovery after protein repletion is against this theory. 2) *Impaired sodium transport in the loop of Henle.* This seems to affect both the concentrating and diluting mechanisms; however, the diluting capacity is well preserved in these patients and sodium reabsorption is adequate during low sodium intake (3). 3) *Augmented vasa*

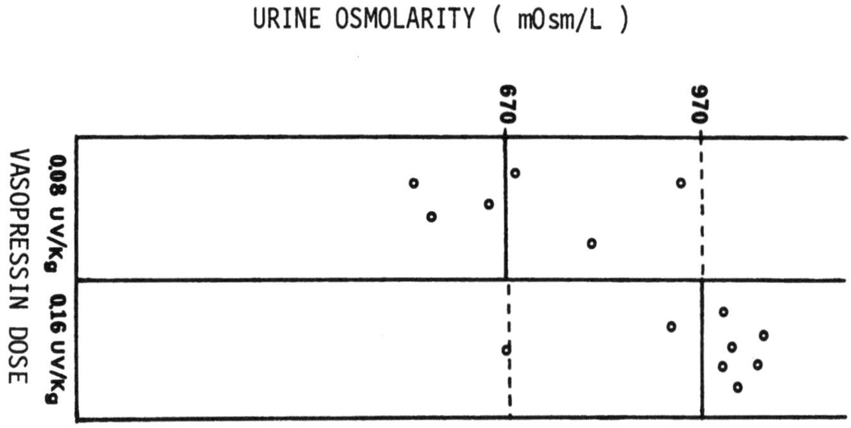

FIG. 5. Maximum urine osmolarity in severe chronic malnutrition after different doses of Pitressin. Note the significant rise in urine osmolarity ($p < 0.01$) when the dose of Pitressin was increased from 0.08 UV/kg to 0.16 UV/kg. (Adapted from Cardenas, J., Puga, F. and Zilleruelo, G.: Capacidad de concentracion urinaria en lactantes desnutridos. II Parte. Rev. Chilena Ped. 45: 205, 1974, with permission).

recta blood flow. This would lead to an impaired countercurrent mechanism. Anemia present in most of these patients possibly could result in higher vasa recta blood flow. However, without correcting the anemia and with protein repletion, the concentration defect subsided; also, rapid correction of the anemia with transfusions did not correct the concentrating defect (3). Patients without anemia also have the concentrating defect (3). 4) *Increased solute output per nephron (osmotic diuresis)*. Against this mechanism is the fact that total solute output should decrease as GFR decreases without a concomitant decrease in nephron population.

Table 3. Theories Proposed to Explain Defect of Concentrating Ability in Malnutrition

1.	Decreased free water clearance
2.	Lack of ADH or decreased tubular response
3.	Impaired Na+ transport in loop of Henle
4.	Increased vasa recta blood flow
5.	Increased solute load per nephron (osmotic diuresis)
6.	Potassium depletion
7.	Protein depletion (decreased urea concentration)

5) *Severe potassium depletion.* This selectively impairs concentrating ability in both man and experimental animals. In young adult men after a deficit of 150-200 mEq of potassium, the maximal attainable urine osmolarity fell rapidly within 10 days (Fig. 6a) (10). At a deficit of 400 mEq of potassium or more, the urine was almost isotonic. There was a good correlation between degree of potassium depletion and decrease in urinary maximal osmolality (Fig. 6b). Potassium deficiency reduces sodium content of the medulla (11), and impairs mitochondrial function in the outer medulla (12). Some evidence suggests that it also may alter the adenyl cyclase system response to vasopressin (13), and induce excessive prostaglandin secretion (14). 6) Finally, *decreased urea concentration in the renal medulla.* This interferes with the urinary concentrating ability of these children (15). A dramatic increase in maximal urine concentration was seen 4-5 days after urea administration (16). Protein repletion usually takes several days/weeks because the positive nitrogen balance impedes an increase in urinary nitrogen. Improvement in concentrating ability correlated well with urinary nitrogen excretion (Fig. 7) (3).

A new explanation for the decreased GFR and concentrating ability has been proposed for adolescents with anorexia nervosa syndrome (AN) (17). These patients have many findings in common with malnutrition including reduced GFR and impaired urinary concentrating capacity of renal origin; still, the absence of anemia or protein depletion suggests a different pathophysiology. An alteration in water permeability of the capillary wall has been suggested (18). According to this hypothesis, certain catabolic states (fasting, AN) alter the molecular composition of the capillary wall, and water permeability decreases. This, then, leads to edema forma-

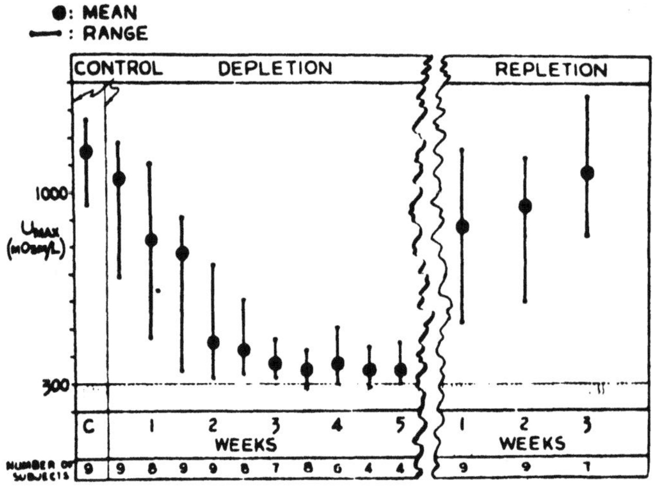

FIG. 6a. Maximum urinary concentration in normal young men subjected to potassium depletion. (From Rubini, M.: Water excretion in potassium-deficient man. J. Clin. Invest. 40: 2215, 1961, with permission).

tion through a reduced fluid reabsorption from the interstitium to the venous side of capillaries. The concentrating capacity of the kidney would be altered because of reduced water permeability in the collecting duct and/or vasa recta. It has been proposed that the renal function abnormalities demonstrated are the result of an adaptive mechanism which decreases GFR and RPF in order to reduce tubular reabsorption and thus minimize energy consumption.

WATER AND ELECTROLYTES IN CHILDREN WITH CHRONIC RENAL FAILURE (CRF)

As chronic renal disease progresses, several functional adaptations occur in the surviving nephrons. Changes in body composition in relation to water and electrolytes in CRF patients are summarized in Table 4. TBW is increased, largely due to excess ECF and higher lean body mass. In the majority of these patients, ICF/body weight is reduced. While exchangeable sodium is increased (19), total exchangeable potassium is decreased (20). These changes are not confined to patients with End Stage Renal Disease (ESRD), are most marked after prolonged treatment with low protein diets, and closely resemble those found in protein-calorie malnutrition (19,21). These changes in body composition can be reversed by hemodialysis or renal transplantation (22,23).

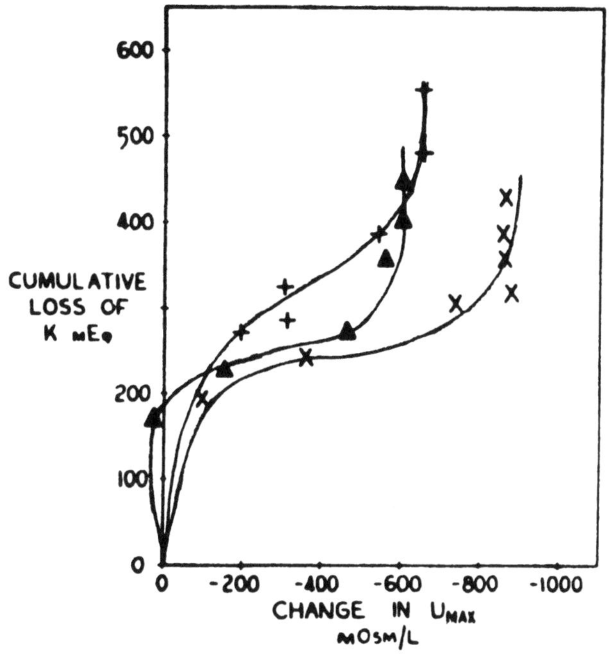

FIG. 6b. Relation of maximum urinary concentration (U max) to cumulative deficit of potassium in potassium depleted subjects. (From Rubini, M.: Water excretion in potassium-deficient man. J. Clin. Invest. 40: 2215, 1961, with permission).

Inability to concentrate urine is consistently present in CRF patients (24). A major factor responsible for this loss of concentrating ability seems to be the increased osmotic load in the remaining nephrons; still, other factors also play a role since reduced solute load does not necessarily improve urine osmolality. There is evidence that the tubules respond less to adequate circulating concentrations of ADH (25); this could be influenced by the presence of uremic toxins which interfere with the action of cyclic 3-5 AMP, alterations in the anatomical architecture of renal tubules or of peritubular capillaries or by changes in calcium metabolism (26).

Derangements in water and sodium homeostasis are interrelated. A classic example of the adaptation of renal function to CRF is the change that occurs in sodium excretion in order to maintain sodium balance as the nephron population diminishes. Thus, the amount of salt a single nephron must excrete increases with each permanent reduction of GFR. For many years it has been known that CRF patients have an impairment of normal ability to conserve sodium and excrete sodium-free urine. However, in most patients plasma sodium is maintained within normal limits despite marked reduction in GFR. Since 1950 (27), it has been accepted that plasma sodium concentration is maintained in a steady state by reduction in tubular reabsorption. This seems to be a physiological adaptation to prevent sodium retention rather than the fortuitous effect of damaged tubules unable to reabsorb as much sodium as before. This change in nephron function in uremia constitutes the central feature of what Bricker has labeled "the magnification phenomenon" (28).

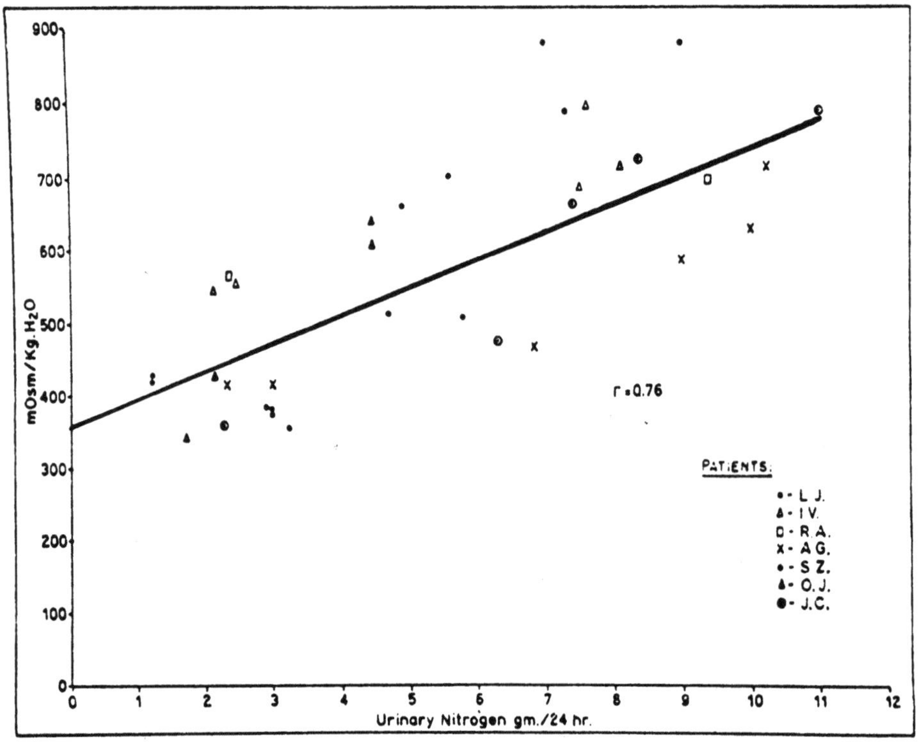

FIG. 7. Relation of urine osmolarity and 24 hrs. urinary nitrogen excretion. (From Klahr, S., Tripathy, K., Garcia, F.T. et al.: On the nature of the renal concentrating defect in malnutrition. Am. J. Med. 43: 84, 1967, with permission).

It has been suggested that adaptation to a progressive decrease in functional nephron units produces a natriuretic response per nephron which is inversely proportional to GFR, and occurs when there is no decrease in sodium in the diet (Table 5) (29). Other evidence supports the view that a natriuretic factor or hormone plays the dominant role (30). There seems to be an increase in synthesis and release of this factor, and an enhanced responsiveness of residual nephrons due to the uremic state (Fig. 8) (31).

Table 4. Disturbances of Water and Electrolytes in CRF

- TBW is increased
- ECF is increased (↑ lean body mass)
- Decrease in ICF
- Exchangeable Na+ is increased
- Total exchangeable K+ is low
- Changes are reversed by HD* and TX**

*Hemodialysis
**Transplantation

It has been proposed that this obligatory excretion of sodium could be a consequence of the adaptive process necessary to maintain sodium balance (32). A slow, stepwise reduction of dietary sodium intake reversed this adaptation, and patients with far advanced GFR ultimately were able to regain their capacity to reduce urine sodium excretion to very low levels (32).

Some evidence suggests that aldosterone also is of physiological importance in the control of urinary sodium, potassium and water excretion in CRF patients (33). These results show an aldosterone-induced enhancement of sodium reabsorption during sodium restriction.

Potassium homeostasis, maintained largely by regulation of renal potassium excretion, changes in CRF patients. Potassium balance may be maintained by increased renal potassium excretion per nephron and increased gastrointestinal secretion, particularly colonic (34).

Table 5. Magnification Phenomenon

Na+ Intake/Day	GFR	Na+ Excretion/Day
7 g NaCl	120 ml/min	1/200 Na+ filtered
7 g NaCl	2 ml/min	64/200 Na+ filtered

Adapted from Bricker, N.S. and Fine, L.G.: The trade-off hypothesis: Current status. Kidney Int. 13 (Suppl. 8) S-5, 1978.

Since plasma potassium is poorly correlated with body potassium stores, especially in acidosis, several techniques have been used to estimate body stores of potassium in renal disease. These include measurement of potassium in red cells, leukocytes, muscle and other cells, as well as measurement of total exchangeable potassium (K42-K43) by radioisotope dilution and total body potassium (TBK) by whole body counting of the natural isotope K40 (35).

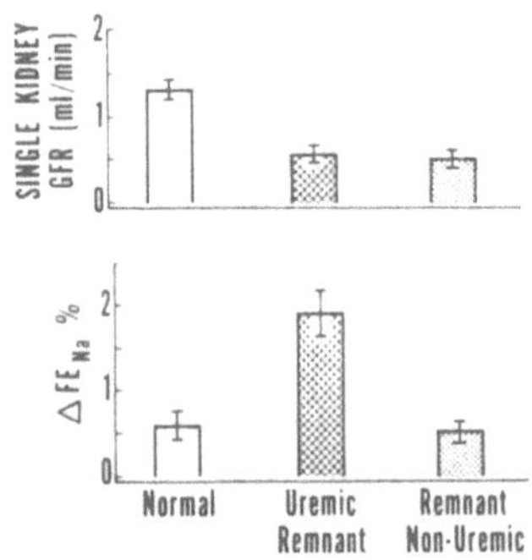

FIG. 8. Effects of the same amount of natriuretic factor on fractional sodium excretion (FE_{Na}) in normal, uremic remnant and non-uremic remnant kidney. (From Fine, L.G. and Danovitch, G.M.: Physiological adaptations in uremia: Recent advances in the understanding of sodium homeostasis in chronic renal failure. In Strauss, J. (ed.): Pediatric Nephrology: Renal Failure. New York: Garland STPM Press, 1978, vol. 4, p. 123, with permission).

Total exchangeable potassium is reported as decreased or normal in CRF (20). However, TBK measured in nondialyzed patients with CRF is normal (22). This apparent inconsistency could be explained if equilibration between radioactive and native potassium was incomplete or if the exchangeable potassium was a smaller fraction of TBK in CRF than in healthy subjects (36).

The distribution of potassium within the body, at least between exchangeable and nonexchangeable fractions, differs in patients with CRF and in normal subjects (35). A number of factors may contribute to this difference: diet, duration of uremia, type of renal disease, duration and frequency of dialysis, and intracellular dilution due to accumulation of sodium and water in CRF.

In summary, we have reviewed basic concepts about the changes observed in malnutrition and uremia and the adaptive mechanisms suggested. Although the increase in knowledge about the role of the kidney in these situations is impressive, we are far from understanding all the mechanisms involved.

Many of the changes observed are common to both malnutrition and uremia. As suggested by Bricker in his "trade off" hypothesis for uremia (29), nothing in nature is free. The body pays a price for the remarkable renal function adaptation that occurs in these two entities. The major "trade off" is loss of flexibility in the kidney's capacity to handle wide variations in the balance of water and electrolytes.

REFERENCES

1. Alleyne, G.A.: The effect of severe protein calorie malnutrition on the renal function of Jamaican children. Pediatrics 39: 400, 1967.

2. Gordillo, G., Soto, R.A., Metcoff, J. et al.: Intracellular composition and homeostatic mechanisms in severe chronic infantile malnutrition. III. Renal adjustments. Pediatrics 20: 303, 1957.

3. Klahr, S., Tripathy, K., Garcia, F.T. et al.: On the nature of the renal concentrating defect in malnutrition. Am. J. Med. 43: 84, 1967.

4. Cardenas, J., Puga, F. and Zilleruelo, G.: Capacidad de concentracion urinaria en lactantes desnutridos. I Parte. Rev. Chilena Ped. 45: 199, 1974.

5. Cardenas, J., Puga, F. and Zilleruelo, G.: Capacidad de concentracion urinaria en lactantes desnutridos. II Parte. Rev. Chilena Ped. 45: 205, 1974.

6. Waterlow, J.C. and Alleyne, G.A.: Protein malnutrition in children. Adv. Protein Chem. 25: 117, 1971.

7. Metcoff, J., Janeway, C.A., Gamble, J.L. et al.: Hypotonicity and intracellular edema in severe chronic malnutrition with recurrent diarrhea. Am. J. Dis. Child. 92: 462, 1956.

8. Metcoff, J., Frenk, S., Gordillo, G. et al.: Intracellular composition and homeostatic mechanisms in severe chronic infantile malnutrition. IV. Development and repair of the biochemical lesion. Pediatrics 20: 317, 1957.

9. Macaron, C., Schneider, G. and Ertel, N.H.: The starved kidney: A defect in renal concentrating ability. Metabolism 24: 457, 1975.

10. Rubini, M.: Water excretion in potassium-deficient man. J. Clin. Invest. 40: 2215, 1961.

11. Buckalew, V.M., Ramirez, M.A. and Goldberg, M.: Free water reabsorption during solute diuresis in normal and potassium depleted rats. Am. J. Physiol. 212: 381, 1967.

12. Finkelstein, F.O. and Hayslett, J.P.: Role of medullary Na-K-ATPase in renal potassium adaptation. Am. J. Physiol. 229: 524, 1975.

13. Beck, N., Reed, S.W. and Davis, B.B.: Inability to concentrate urine in potassium depleted kidney due to impaired cyclic AMP system in renal medulla. In Proceedings of American Society of Nephrology. Washington, D.C., 1973, p. 9.

14. Kunan, R.T. and Stein, J.H.: Disorders of hypo- and hyperkalemia. Clin. Nephrol. 7: 173, 1977.

15. Levinsky, N.G., Berliner, R.W. and Preston, A.S.: The role of urea in the urine concentrating mechanism. J. Clin. Invest. 38: 751, 1959.

16. McCance, R.A., Crowne, R.S. and Hall, T.S.: The effect of malnutrition and food habits on the concentrating power of the kidney. Clin. Sci. 37: 471, 1969.

17. Fohlin, L.: Body composition, cardiovascular and renal function in adolescent patients with anorexia nervosa. Acta Pediatr. Scand. (Suppl.) 268, 1977.

18. Aperia, A., Broberger, O. and Fohlin, L.: Renal function in anorexia nervosa. Acta Pediatr. Scand. 67: 219, 1978.

19. Coles, G.A.: Body composition in chronic renal failure. Qtr. J. Med. 41: 25, 1972.

20. Berlyne, G.M., Van Laethem, L. and Ben Ari, J.: Exchangeable potassium and renal potassium handling in advanced chronic renal failure in man. Nephron 8: 264, 1971.

21. Coles, G.A., Peters, D.K. and Jones, J.H.: Albumin metabolism in chronic renal failure. Clin. Sci. 39: 423, 1970.

22. Boddy, K., King, P.C., Lindsay, R.M. et al.: Total body potassium in nondialyzed and dialyzed patients with chronic renal failure. Br. Med. J. 1: 771, 1972.

23. Blaufox, M.D., Lewis, E.J., Jagger, P. et al.: Physiologic responses of the transplanted human kidney. Sodium regulation and renin secretion. N. Engl. J. Med. 280: 62, 1969.

24. Platt, R.: Structural and functional adaptation in renal failure. Br. Med. J. 1: 1313, 1952.

25. DeWardener, H.E.: Polyuria. In Black, D.A.K. (ed.): Renal Diseases. Oxford: Blackwell Scientific Publications, 1962, p. 566.

26. Tannen, R.L., Regal, E.N., Dunn, M.J. et al.: Vasopressin-resistant hyposthenuria in advanced chronic renal disease. N. Engl. J. Med. 280: 1135, 1969.

27. Platt, R.: Sodium and potassium excretion in chronic renal failure. Clin. Sci. 9: 367, 1950.

28. Bricker, N.S., Fine, L.G., Kaplan, M. et al.: "Magnification phenomenon" in chronic renal disease. N. Engl. J. Med. 299: 1287, 1978.

29. Bricker, N.S. and Fine, L.G.: The trade-off hypothesis: Current status. Kidney Int. 13 (Suppl. 8) s-5, 1978.

30. Bricker, N.S., Schmidt, R.W., Favre, H. et al.: On the biology of sodium excretion: The search for a natriuretic hormone. Yale J. Biol. Med. 48: 293, 1975.

31. Fine, L.G. and Danovitch, G.M.: Physiological adaptations in uremia: Recent advances in the understanding of sodium homeostasis in chronic renal failure. In Strauss, J. (ed.): Pediatric Nephrology: Renal Failure. New York: Garland STPM Press, 1978, vol. 4, p. 123.

32. Danovitch, G.M., Bourgoignie, J. and Bricker, N.S.: Reversibility of the "salt losing" tendency of chronic renal failure. N. Engl. J. Med. 1: 14, 1977.

33. Schrier, R.W. and Regal, E.M.: Influence of aldosterone on sodium, water and potassium metabolism in chronic renal disease. Kidney Int. 1: 156, 1972.

34. Hayes, C.P., McLeod, M.F. and Robinson, R.R.: An extrarenal mechanism for the maintenance of potassium balance in severe chronic renal failure. Trans. Assoc. Am. Phys. 80: 207, 1967.

35. Letteri, J.M., Ellis, K.J., Asad, S.N. et al.: Serial measurement of total body potassium in chronic renal disease. Am. J. Clin. Nutr. 31: 1937, 1978.

36. Boddy, K., King, P.C., Lindsay, R.M. et al.: Exchangeable and total body potassium in patients with chronic renal failure. Br. Med. J. 1: 140, 1972.

SERUM NUTRIENT ALTERATIONS IN CHRONIC RENAL DISEASE

Lewis A. Barness, M.D.

Dept. Pediatr., Univ. So. Fla. College Med., Tampa, Fla. 33612, USA

Serum nutrient alterations represent a balance between ingestion, excretion and utilization. Among the functions of the kidney, one of the longest and best recognized is that of excretion. In children with renal disease, excretion of certain metabolic products is limited. Especially significant is the increase in the serum of metabolic nitrogen compounds, hydrogen ion, organic acids, phenols, phosphate, potassium, sodium, chloride and water. In contrast, in those with renal tubular disease, excessive losses may occur, particularly of phosphate, bicarbonate, sodium, chloride, potassium, and water. Amino acids may be retained in glomerular or lost in tubular disease and this loss is responsible for so-called urinary amino-acidopathies. Secondary serum alterations may occur, such as lowered serum calcium and increased parathormone in the presence of phosphate retention. Other minerals, vitamins, and energy may also be excreted, depending on the type of disease.

When glomerular filtration is reduced, nitrogen products (Table 1) are retained. Uric acid may reach toxic levels. Phenols, indoles and amines may be responsible for some toxic signs, including, but not limited, to the central nervous system. Serum lipids, particularly triglycerides, are frequently elevated in chronic renal disease. There is an increase in atherosclerosis in chronic glomerular disease and these may be related. Not only is excretion of triglyceride decreased but also changes in metabolism may be responsible for triglyceride elevation. Serum phosphate rises, potassium may reach toxic levels, and pH falls as hydrogen ion is retained (Table 2). Though sodium and water are retained, serum sodium may be normal or low since volume is expanded. With failure

Table 1. Glomerular Disease - Nitrogen Retention

Urea	Trimethylamines
Ammonia	Methylguanidine
Creatinine	Guanido-Succinic Acid
Uric Acid	Phenols

to ingest sufficient foods and calories, serum calcium falls, amino acids are low, vitamin D is decreased, parathormone is increased, and other vitamins and minerals may be deficient (Table 3). Conversely, phosphate may initiate the onset of hyperparathyroidism and the decrease in serum phosphate. If persistent, renal osteodystrophy, bone pain, and central nervous system alterations follow. Pyridoxine levels have frequently been found to be low and zinc levels may be decreased. After prolonged renal disease, serum proteins fall.

With renal tubular disease, especially renal tubular acidosis, hydrogen ion is retained. Serum sodium, potassium and calcium are decreased because of urinary losses. While all blood chemistries must be monitored, potassium requires especially careful determination. Low serum potassium is associated with heart and muscle abnormalities but correction of other electrolyte and pH abnormalities may be almost impossible without serum potassium which approaches the normal. In some forms of tubular disease phosphate is low due to little reabsorption. Urea nitrogen is frequently normal or low as excessive water may be excreted. Serum chloride may be elevated as in hyperchloremic renal tubular acidosis (Table 4), or may be low in those with excessive excretion of sodium (1). Amino acids and sugar may be excreted in excess, and serum levels decreased though rarely to the extent of producing symptoms. Secondary hypoparathyroidism does not usually occur in this group (2) but hypophosphatemia and growth failure are marked (3,4,5). Alkaline phosphatase is usually elevated. In these, craniotabes and cranial changes of rickets do not usually occur, but the lower extremities develop deformities of rickets.

Table 2. Glomerular Disease - Retention

Nitrogen	
Hydrogen	Chloride
Organic acids	Water
Phosphate	Magnesium
Potassium	
Sodium	Lipids

Table 3. Glomerular Disease - Deficits

Calories
Calcium
Vitamin D, B6
Zinc
Amino Acids
Protein

One of the most striking renal diseases is the nephrotic syndrome. Water and electrolytes are retained but serum determinations frequently show few changes from normal. Sodium and chloride may be slightly decreased. With low serum albumin, total calcium is decreased but ionized calcium is usually normal. Lipids, cholesterol, and lipid carrying proteins are elevated. With successful treatment these usually return to normal levels.

Certain serum alterations are directly related to drug treatment. Many diuretics cause electrolyte losses as well as water (Table 5); prednisone may increase energy losses as well as electrolyte changes (Table 6), and any drug used may lead to retention and toxicity. Constant monitoring is necessary for each of these to avoid iatrogenic disease.

Serum changes remain a sum of intake, output, and metabolism. Diet, parenteral administration, medicines, and natural processes can influence their levels in the presence of excretory defects, whether these be too great or too little. Departure from normal serum levels is a signal that something is wrong though the nature or site of the wrong is not specified. Furthermore, changes in serum levels of certain products may be a signal for the type of investigation needed.

Table 4. Tubular Disease - Losses

Sodium
Potassium
Phosphate
Bicarbonate
Glucose
Amino Acids
Water
(Chloride)

Table 5. Diuretics

Water
Sodium
Potassium
Chloride
Bicarbonate

Serum changes, while they are indicative of progress of the disease, unfortunately represent only an incomplete understanding of underlying processes. It is the latter which need correction before health is possible.

Table 6. Cortisone Derivatives

+	-
Sodium	Potassium
Chloride	Vit. C
Water	Glucose
	A.A.

REFERENCES

1. Holliday, M.A., Chronic Renal Disease: In Pediatric Nutr. Handbook. Am. Acad. Pediatr., Chicago, 1979, p. 202.

2. Lewy, J.E., Cabana, E.C., Repetto, H.A., Canterbury, J.M. and Reiss, E.: Serum parathyroid hormone in hypophosphatemic vitamin D resistant rickets. J. Pediatr. 81: 294, 1972.

3. Stickler, G.B. Growth failure in renal disease: Pediatr. Cl. N. Am. 23: 885, 1976.

4. Beale, M.G., Salcedo, J.R., Ellis, D. and Rao, D.D.: Renal Osteodystrophy, Pediatr. Cl. N. Am. 23: 873, 1976.

5. Chan, J.C.M. and Hsu, A.C.: Vitamin D and Renal Diseases. In Barness, L. (ed.): Advances in Pediatr. 27: 117, 1980.

HIGHLIGHTS

PLASMA AND MUSCLE FREE AMINO ACID ALTERATION IN UREMIC CHILDREN

Michel Broyer, M.D., G. Jean, M.D., C. Kleinknecht, M.D., A.M. Dartois, M.D., and F. Gros, M.D.

Serv. Nephrol. Pediatr., Hôpital Necker Enfants - Malades, Paris, France

Simultaneous assessment of plasma and muscle free amino acids (AA) has been performed in children in order to obtain more information about metabolic disturbances presumably related to growth retardation. Plasma and muscle were sampled after an overnight fast and amino acids were measured by ion exchange chromatography with five step lithium buffers.

A first study concerned 8 children in severe chronic renal failure (creatinine clearance < 10 ml/min/1.73 m^2). The plasma nonessential AA pool was significantly increased as well as proline, OH proline, glycine, citrulline, ornithine ($p < 0.01$), and taurine, asparagine, glutamine, and methionine ($p < 0.05$), but some essential AA such as valine and tryptophane, were decreased ($p < 0.01$). Tyr/phe and val/gly ratios were both depressed and 1 and 3 CH3 histidine were present in all patients. Muscle essential and nonessential AA were increased and all AA tended to be higher than controls except for tyrosine. Cellular/extracellular gradients were either increased (serine, glutamic acid, methionine, ornithine, arginine) or decreased (aspartic acid, alanine) by uremia.

In a second study plasma and muscle AA were analysed in four groups of children with different levels of renal failure in order to determine the stage of renal insufficiency for which AA alterations appear and their eventual relationship with growth velocity and nutritional factors. Mean plasma creatinine of the group one to four was, respectively, 1.3, 2.3, 3.3 and 4.9 mg/100 ml Significant but different alterations of plasma and muscle AA pattern were found in the four groups of patients. Alterations were already present in the first group which exhibited a decrease of plasma valine, threonine, phenylalanine, tryptophane, alanine, and tyrosine, and an increase of citrulline and aspartic acid while in muscle alanine and valine were reduced but glutamine, arginine, and ornithine were increased. These alterations became generally worse with renal failure for tyr/phe ratio and 3-methylhistidine and a significant increase of muscle total AA content was noted only in group IV. Group III patients (creatinine 3 to 4 mg/100ml) had nevertheless the greatest number of individual AA alterations and the lowest val/gly ratio; this group of patients also had higher protein intake than group II and group IV. No relationship was found between energy or protein intake and plasma or muscle AA.

Normal or accelerated growth velocity was associated with lower muscle AA content and the pattern of muscle AA was more related with growth rate than with the level of renal failure. In contrast, plasma AA alterations are not so informative.

These results could mean that muscle AA determination is of critical importance in the detection of children at risk for growth retardation or for comparison of several therapeutic approaches for improving growth velocity.

A number of factors have been supposed to cause plasma and muscle AA alterations in uremia:

1. energy-protein malnutrition, but in this study protein intake was close to or above the recommended dietary allowance.
2. reduced kidney metabolism, as kidney normally adds some AA (serine, alanine, threonine, etc.) which are decreased in plasma and muscle, and removes some others (glutamine, glycine, arginine, etc.) which are increased.
3. reduced protein synthesis and/or accelerated catabolism as an effect of uremic toxicity or other factors.
4. specific enzymatic alterations such as decrease of phenylalanine oxydase or arginine synthetase activity.
5. alteration of cell membrane transfer and/or hormone-fuel relationship.
6. alteration of albumin binding of some amino acids (e.g. tryptophane).

The relative importance of these different factors and their clear understanding remain to be established.

PANEL DISCUSSION

Moderator: José Strauss, M.D.

Div. Pediatr. Nephrol., Dept. Pediatr., Univ. Miami Sch. Med., Miami, Fla. 33152, USA

COMMENT: The question of reference is, again, dependent upon what you think about. For example, if one thinks that protein synthesis is dependent upon concentration of relative aminoacids, then the concentration relationship becomes important. But it may not be dependent upon concentration; it may be dependent upon certain enzyme activities with vast excesses of substrate, serum concentration; overdoses may not be important. There is one thing to say for the ratio and that is that if the ratio excludes the independent division so that if one is concerned with phenilalanine and valine for example, they are both divided by the same thing, that is to say water content and the water cancels out. So, the relationship of each to the other is at least stabilized by the ratio; that is also arbitrary. I just wanted to comment about one more thing. I did not mean to imply that measurement of plasma values is useless. Of course they are not useless. They are invaluable, but what I did want to emphasize is that the plasma value by itself is not going to tell you the whole story. High plasma potassium could mean that a lot of potassium is coming out of the cells or it could mean that not enough potassium is going into the cells or it could mean that not enough potassium is excreted or that too much has been given. So, unless one knows what the actual direction of the metabolism is in the cell, the blood level itself is difficult to interpret. All of us get around that because we make a guess as to what the clinical situation is accounting for a particular plasma level that we measure. I just want to emphasize that sometimes that guess *is* a guess and may be very inaccurate unless you have some better idea about what's going on in the cell. Plasma levels should not be discarded; they should just be looked at, as Dr. Gamble used to say, with a certain grain of salt.

QUESTION: I was wondering whether you have compared uremia with other pure metabolic disturbances or even with another acidosis like asthma where all kinds of changes occur in terms of essential or non-essential aminoacids and other conditions, like stress situations which may include cortisone treatment. Are the changes similar to those seen in uremia?

RESPONSE: Uremia is a peculiar combination of two phenomena. One is the acidosis which accompanies uremia which is a cellular destructive phenomenon. The other is an inability to excrete which is the retention phenomenon. In diabetic ketoacidosis we have measured urinary aminoacids and they are extremely high and we think this is due particularly to the acidosis because this immediately goes down as soon as the pH goes up. We have found in acidosis in general that especially the essential aminoacids are low. But this is also the kind of data that we were shown today. In the uremics when they were acidotic - at least the ones who did not recover any growth I think there is a similarity from the acidosis standpoint. The same thing is true about cortisone. Cortisone is a cellular destructive phenomenon especially related to the gluconeogenic aminoacids. So the gluconeogenic aminoacids are the ones that are most decreased in cortisone administration.

QUESTION: For those of us who don't think about aminoacids day in and day out it is difficult to get the drift of what is happening. I wonder if you could summarize in some way for us the results of your work. I hope that's not too broad a question.

MODERATOR: I gather from the practical point of view. Is that what you would want? In other words, would you recommend administration of aminoacids - essential or non-essential - to patients with chronic renal failure?

RESPONSE: I think you have to be very cautious before giving general recommendations because this study is more or less preliminary regarding infusion of aminoacids.

I think we will later on be preparing a paper for the book, so we will take that opportunity to discuss further this point. But from our results it is clear that muscle content of aminoacids moves toward the normal range after six weeks of infusion. So, I feel that it would be better for the patients. But I could not for a moment recommend for a given patient because it was a very short study and it is not a definitive demonstration of its usefulness.

MODERATOR: Today's presentations, as you know, deal mainly with the physio-chemistry and tomorrow we will go into the treatment more actively but this is an important question and it is important to keep in mind that there are no definitive results, yet.

COMMENT: Thinking of the metabolic alterations in the uremic patient, I would like to ask one of the panelists if he has a study of the tissues like liver, kidney, or brain in terms of composition with aminoacids infusion.

RESPONSE: We are planning to study those tissues in a manner similar to what has been presented to you on the leukocytes. Currently, we know very little on that subject.

RESPONSE: Tomorrow I will talk about the influence of dialysis and aminoacid infusion on cell composition and functions. I don't want to repeat myself. I should say that if one reviews the literature, it is amazing the conclusions that have been drawn from extraordinarily limited studies. Most of us in trying to assess the question you asked about aminoacid infusion being beneficial might have to conclude from the literature that it may very well be beneficial, but without certainty. That's pretty extraordinary to try to find an answer under such limited experience. That's one of the troubles - that all of us have a limitation as to what we can measure and how many patients we can study. The nature of the circumstances is such that one is forced to draw some kind of conclusions. When you draw these conclusions, no matter how much you qualify them, they are going to be interpreted in a way which may or may not be correct. Though I think that some people's positions are absolutely correct, it's too early to say what the possible benefits are for aminoacid infusions in patients with uremia. It seems reasonable and even probable that some benefits can be attained as far as restoring composition is concerned. We can show some benefits as far as restoring metabolism. But, I'm still forced to say that it seems reasonable but the data are not very strong.

MODERATOR: At the risk of asking a question which may need to be answered tomorrow, in relationship to dialysis, how easily removed are those aminoacids? If you were to infuse them prior to or during the dialysis procedure, would you still have enough circulating aminoacids to make it worthwhile? Or if you eventually were to recommend because of your results or anybody else's, that it is desirable, when would you think the infusion should be done in relationship to dialysis?

RESPONSE: In our study we infused aminoacids during the last hour of dialysis and we checked the aminoacid loss with and without an aminoacid infusion and there's not a big difference between the two approaches. We calculate the volume of infusion as a function of the increase in losses during the infusion. To my way of thinking, it is easier to infuse aminoacid during dialysis than at any other time.

QUESTION: Did you correlate plasma aminoacid level with protein electrophoresis - different levels of protein?

RESPONSE: No, we did not correlate that.

QUESTION: I was wondering if that might give some information about catabolism or anabolism of proteins related to aminoacid levels.

RESPONSE: We checked for transferrin, albumin and fractions of complement and we didn't find, in the twenty children who were in the study of early stages of uremia, an increase in these proteins. So, we didn't check the rest of the proteins.

QUESTION: I would like to also ask whether you have measured insulin/glucagon ratios in fat and lean uremic animals.

RESPONSE: No. We haven't done that. Of course there are probably important modifications in carbohydrate metabolism in those animals. You have to be cautious before interpreting those results. It's a complex matter.

MODERATOR: We have talked about calcium and phosphorus metabolism. What about vitamin D metabolites? Are they altered with decreased GFR?

RESPONSE: Yes, they are, but somebody is going to be discussing this later on. Yes, they are markedly altered.

MODERATOR: You would not want to comment on the tissue pH stimulus here? The answer is "no". Very good. We are among very careful people!

RESPONSE: I'm afraid I will be wrong.

MODERATOR: What about the role played by acidemia in chronic diarrhea? You mentioned some examples where correction of the acidemia leads to striking improvement in the growth rate. What about other conditions?

RESPONSE: Diarrhea sometimes can be very beneficial in all the abnormalities that I mentioned as far as the glomerular diseases are concerned with retention. The gut is a good dialysis system and was one of the earliest systems used to get rid of some of the nitrogen metabolized and some of the fenoles. We have all seen children in whom the diarrhea has been corrected and the uremia becomes worse. Part of this is related to the reduced excretion of metabolites. The acidosis correction that I was talking about was not uremia. I was talking about that in terms of tubular disease. People in California, Michigan, and Minnesota have all shown that in some kids with chronic renal tubular disease manifested by acidosis, hypophosphatemia followed the administration of phosphate and the correction of acidosis with an increase in protein breakdown. I was not talking about uremia when I mentioned that.

MODERATOR: Because the role of acidosis or acidemia is argued back and forth in terms of growth retardation, many question the role played by a low blood pH in terms of growth impairment. I believe that what they say is that these may be concomitant findings but are not necessarily related to one another. Could you comment on that?

RESPONSE: I would agree. I think that we have enough evidence now - enough clinical experience - to say that acidosis by itself is not one of the major factors causing growth retardation. I think that twenty or thirty years ago we all assumed that the acidotic nephritic was not going to grow because of the acidosis. And that if you had normal growth, you could not have very severe kidney disease. We've all burned with this concept and now recognize that this is not a good concept.

COMMENT: An observation we made about the acidosis in some tubular acidosis is that if we corrected the acidosis, at least we corrected also the loss of calcium - the hypercalciuria. If we don't correct the hypercalciuria, we don't get a good growth curve.

COMMENT: I think we have a lot of questions regarding the things that have been expressed this morning but they still don't have answers. I wonder if someone can comment about a study just finished in Venezuela of about 88 uremic patients; 25% of them were children. I did EEG studies on all of them and I found things very interesting - at least to me - without getting all the answers. Some of the patients even if they were very uremic, if their clinical conditions were okay, they had normal EEG patterns. If some of the patients with lower serum concentration had very bad clinical conditions, the EEG patterns were very bad. But, as an average, what we saw was that when the urea nitrogen was over 350 mg/dl, most of the EEG's registered were bad. So, some of the patients were dialyzed, of course; some of the patients were treated with conservative methods. I remember I had two patients with serum creatinine of 51 mg/dl. One of them was a 17-year-old who used to work as a cook ten hours a day until she came to the hospital. While she had "normal" clinical conditions - her EEG registered almost normal - when she entered the hospital she needed the whole range - dialysis and whatever. Her EEG patterns were very bad then. I wonder if you have any comments about this.

MODERATOR: May I clarify one figure you gave. Is that the BUN or urea?

RESPONSE: Urea. U.N. I'm sorry, blood urea nitrogen, BUN.

COMMENT: I am fascinated by that experience and congratulate you for exploring it. I have no good, solid answer for it. It calls to mind the fact that many years ago we were interested in the electro-encephalographic pattern in nephrotics. If one examined the EEG's in nephrotic children at the time they were maximally edematous, they had strikingly abnormal EEG's with general flattening and other features that went along with their very regressed clinical condition. With diuresis their EEG was normal. I would wonder in this situation whether one was not dealing with alteration both in brain cell metabolism and most especially in brain water.

MODERATOR: What happens with the EEG after the BUN goes down? We tend to see those problems right at the time of the dialysis of patients who have had such high BUN's. We haven't had one that high - but when they go over 100 or so - 150 mg/dl - we start seeing convulsions if we dialyze the patients too aggressively and lower the BUN too rapidly.

RESPONSE: We have been aware of the previous work on electro-encephalographic studies post-dialysis. What happens is what you just said. Probably, you lowered the BUN levels too rapidly. We did have some patients who had very abnormal weights in the EEG studies. Whatever treatment we did - transplant or dialysis, or some of them dietary treatment for a short period - when they improved clinically, the EEG patterns improved also. And if they deteriorated further after 2 months, 3 months, again the waves were very abnormal.

COMMENT: I don't have any explanation but I was wondering if the girl who was a cook with a creatinine of 51 mg/dl worked in a Chinese restaurant, would she spit monosodium glutamate?

QUESTION: I would like to go back to one of the papers presented. Did you say that the total intracellular water was decreased in renal insufficiency?

RESPONSE: Yes, some studies have shown that.

COMMENT: I would like to know if it's a decrease of the total mass, etc. or is it only a question of hydration? The electrolyte question is very interesting. What is the work behind your assumption?

RESPONSE: The way I interpreted those values or statements is a proportional reduction in intracellular compartment in proportion to the increase in the extracellular fluid. So we are talking about proportional changes compared to the weight of the patient. You may be right. There may be certain reasons to think that even intracellular space could be increased - thinking of accumulation of urea, for instance - that would shift also water to the intracellular compartment. But, in proportion, there is a larger increase in the extracellular than in the intracellular compartment.

COMMENT: You bring two possibilities: either decrease of the total mass of tissue or increase in intracellular fluid content. This hasn't been done. It would be so easy to study that, just by comparing intracellular versus extracellular water and second, by weight and wet weight muscle.

COMMENT: I was going to ask my colleague here, whom I expect has measured this, to comment.

RESPONSE: Yes, we have assessed sometimes extracellular and intracellular water by different means. They gave us the picture of a condition which may very well have an increase in intracellular water at some period if the patient is overloaded with water. If the patient is overloaded with water and we take care of it so that we do not give too large an amount of water, there is a decrease of intracellular water relative to the decrease in lean body mass in the uremic state.

COMMENT: I'd also like to add that an increase of intracellular water has got to depend on the relative quantity of solute that's available for expanding intracellular space. Of course, urea which moves across the cell membrane does not make a big difference one way or the other. But sodium, if it accumulates in the cells, will expand intracellular volume. So, I suppose the circumstance in uremia would be a function of whether or not there was a marked increase of intracellular sodium vis a vis the expansion of volume. Osmotic equilibrium is going to be maintained, of course, one way or the other. The relative hydration of the sodium molecule apparently is the factor that with its lattice structure determines the relative quantities of water available.

COMMENT: I am not very happy because you are discussing factors which go to the opposite side. If you have sodium accumulation you should have an increase of water.

RESPONSE: That's what I am saying.

COMMENT: I have been told that there is a relative decrease of intracellular water.

RESPONSE: I was speaking of an increase in intracellular water. That is correct.

COMMENT: May I add something. Some years ago we studied intracellular and extracellular fluids in patients during dialysis, performing muscle biopsies before and after dialysis. At the same times that the muscle biopsies were obtained, total body measurement by inulin space and variation of total water and chloride space were determined. Just after the dialysis session there was a tremendous increase in intracellular water and a decrease to very low levels in extracellular water. And within 10-12 hours the difference went in the other direction: extracellular water increased and intracellular water decreased. So, there is not only one answer to your question; it depends on the moment in relationship to the dialysis treatment, on the time of the last dialysis and the next dialysis, and on the water balance. So, there is no contradiction, as such, between the stated increase in intracellular water of some studies and the stated decrease in the same variable of other studies. It depends on the moment the patients were studied.

COMMENT: I would like to emphasize what was just said. There is no contradiction. This is a dynamic process. What happens will depend upon the degree of renal failure and the type of renal disease. Some of them will have much more of an increase in total body sodium than the other types of renal disease with the same GFR. So, we cannot say that it is a fixed relative decrease in intracellular fluid. There is also one important difference in the malnourished and the uremic patient. As we heard this morning, in malnutrition you definitely have an increase in intracellular sodium while this has not been shown as conclusively in uremic patients. I do not know for what reason but total body sodium - total exchangeable sodium - is defintely increased but not always do you have a parallel increase in the intracellular sodium.

QUESTION: Do you accept this explanation?

RESPONSE: Yes.

MODERATOR: I think it's good to bring questions into the open and when there are inconsistencies in what we have perceived we go back to the sources and discuss among ourselves, constructively. This is what the seminar is supposed to be for. Thanks to you all for a good discussion period.

NUTRITIONAL ASPECTS OF CHRONIC RENAL DISEASE IN CHILDREN

George Christakis, M.D. and Anthony Kafatos, M.D.

Div. Nutri., Dept. Epidem. and Publ. Health, Univ. Miami Sch. Med., Miami, Fla. 33152, USA

Assessment of the nutritional status of a child with chronic renal disease involves the triad of clinical investigation utilized in any medical problem: historical review, physical examination, and laboratory studies. The child with renal disease, however, presents a special clinical challenge which can be approached from three aspects:

1. Documenting the nutritional status of the patient, and perhaps the mother, prior to as well as during the clinical onset of the disease.
2. Determining the specific pathogenetic effects of the renal disease which alter the nutritional status of the patient as the natural history of the disease evolves into its progressively severe clinical manifestations.
3. Assessing the influence that the therapeutic regimen may have in contributing to the nutritional status of the patient.

Obtaining these data collectively and periodically represents a real challenge, but would contribute to an understanding of the disease process and its total clinical impact and management.

THE NUTRITIONAL HISTORY

An initial approach can be a retrospective and prospective evaluation of the patient's dietary pattern. This would appear to be particularly useful in persons at high risk of malnutrition, such as children whose teenage mothers may have been suboptimally nourished during pregnancy, were delivered prematurely, failed to thrive and who were also at high risk of developing congenital anomalies, including those of the genitourinary system. It is also possible that careful dietary history may reveal nutritional factors associated with later renal disease. For example, it has been hypothesized that the mineral content of the drinking water in Greece, perhaps in association with hypovitaminosis A, may contribute to the considerable prevalence of bilateral nephrolithiasis which is a major cause of later chronic renal failure in both children and adults.

The dietary history can uncover malnutrition of selected types in children with renal disease. One study revealed that despite adequate protein and calorie intake, intakes of vitamin A, folic acid and vitamin C were 68% of the recommended dietary allowances (1). These deficiencies could have been uncovered and prevented with a timely dietary history. If an already malnourished child develops chronic renal disease, the patient's response to the disease, as well as the physician's approach to therapy may well be different from that of an optimally nourished child.

PATHOGENETIC EFFECTS OF RENAL DISEASE ON NUTRITIONAL STATUS

The second area of concern in nutritional assessment is documentation of the impact of renal disease on nutritional status. Uremia itself induces a wide spectrum of nutritional and metabolic effects, first by further deepening preexisting anorexia, then by making prescribed dietary intake a real chore to the young patient, who may fail to meet macro- and micronutrient requirements. However, nutritional insult is added to injury when a second mechanism compounds poor dietary intake: the specific effects on micronutrient metabolism imposed by uremia itself. Thus decreased serum zinc may result from redistribution of the body pool as well as decreased intake of protein (4). Folic acid deficiency may also result from anion inhibition of folate transport into cell membranes (5). Indeed, folic acid absorption from the GI tract may be decreased by concomitant zinc deficiency. Cellular uptake of potassium is decreased by uremia, and low serum vitamin C and B_6 levels have also been detected in uremic children (6,7).

Additional pathogenetic factors associated with chronic renal failure which can compromise nutritional status are:

1. Anorexia, decreased calorie and nutrient intake, acidosis, chronic hypersomolarity, potassium, phosphate, zinc, pyridoxine, ascorbic acid and folate deficiency.
2. Osteodystrophy
3. Decreased somatomedin
4. Abnormal glucose tolerance
5. Chronic infection
6. Retention of metabolites

7. Anemia
8. Steroid therapy

The above factors contribute to malnutrition in the child with chronic renal failure. However, patients may manifest micronutrient excesses such as hyperlipidemia, elevated phosphate levels and hypervitaminosis A.

The skillfully conducted nutritional review of systems, often omitted in the medical history, and the choice of appropriate laboratory determinations will further assist the renal team in tracing the clinical evaluation of the disease and plotting the best therapeutic course for the patient (Table 1). For example, the child or parent may affirm symptoms of specific micronutrient deficiencies and should be asked (3):

1. Has hair fallen out spontaneously, suggesting severe protein-calorie malnutrition or hypervitaminosis A?
2. Have the child's gums bled when teeth are brushed, which may indicate low serum vitamin C, or impending uremia?
3. Is the tongue sore or sensitive to hot beverages? This may suggest nutritional anemias due to deficiency of one or more micronutrients such as iron, folic acid, riboflavin, niacin, zinc, pyridoxine and ascorbic acid.
4. Is the child anorexic? This constitutes a significant clinical event in the uremic or nonuremic child with chronic renal disease. This may be due to mental depression, changes in taste induced by uremia or zinc deficiency, impaired appetite due to psychological and/or metabolic factors. Hypertriglyceredemia, hypoglycemia and hyperinsulinemia which may occur in chronic renal disease, influence the hypothalamic nuclei which regulate hunger and satiety.
5. Does the patient exhibit fatigue, malaise or apathy, which may reflect effects of amino acid deficiencies and/or imbalances on central nervous system functions? Tyrosine deficiency affects norepinephrine synthesis; micronutrient deficiencies may also affect other neurotransmitter precursors. In addition, thiamin, riboflavin, niacin, folic acid, zinc, magnesium, iron, as well as hypoglycemia and hypervitaminosis A, may contribute to central nervous system and behavioral changes per se.

These examples illustrate how an organized nutritional review of systems can assist in elucidating the pathogenesis and clinical course of chronic renal failure. The nutritional review of systems, in conjunction with the dietary history can also contribute to the clinical management of renal disease.

To establish a rational basis for nutritional therapy, it is

Table 1. Examples of History Questions Related to Nutritional Diagnoses*

Symptom	Nutrient Deficiency or Excess to be Considered
Hair becomes thin, coarse, falls out or changes colors	Protein
Slowed speech, "thickened tongue", dysphagia	Iodine
Poor night vision, especially at twilight hours, eyes feel dry	Vitamin A
Gums bleed or skin ecchymoses occur easily	Vitamin C
Tongue sore, sensitive to hot beverages (due to filiform and/or fungiform atrophy), impaired taste, poor appetite	Nutritional anemias: iron, folic acid, riboflavin, niacin, zinc
Lips burn (due to cheilosis)	Thiamin
Fatigue, malaise, apathy, mental depression	Nutritional anemias (iron, folic acid), electrolytes (potassium and sodium), protein, hypoglycemia; multiple vitamin (especially B vitamins) and mineral deficiencies
Tingling, numbness, "burning" of hands or feet (due to polyneuritis)	Thiamin, Riboflavin
Personality changes, hyperexcitability	Niacin; electrolytes, hypoglycemia, magnesium
Headache	Hypoglycemia, hypervitaminosis A
Blurred vision (optic neuritis)	Alcohol excess, B Vitamin deficiencies
Low back pain	Folic acid, B_{12} and osteoporosis related to protein, calcium and fluoride deficiencies

Table 1 (continued)

Exertional dyspnea, congestive heart failure, angina	Hyperlipidemias, aggravation of preexisting coronary heart disease by anemia; thiamin deficiency
Dry, scaly skin	Linoleic acid, arachidonic acid
Diarrhea	Lactose intolerance, gluten sensitivity, niacin
Stools which do not float	Fiber
Pica (compulsive eating of ice, earth, laundry starch, wall plaster)	Iron
Anorexia	Thiamin, zinc, neoplasms, especially GI; onset of anorexia nervosa; depression
Fatigue, malaise, lethargy, bone pain, headaches, insomnia, night sweats, hair loss	Hypervitaminosis A
Hypercalcemia and renal damage, anorexia, nausea, weight loss, children: failure to thrive	Hypervitaminosis D
Ataxic gait	B_{12}, Thiamin

*Adapted from The Journal of the Florida Medical Association, April 1979, Vol 66, No. 4.

desirable to assess not only the independent effects of dietary intake and the disease itself, but also the therapeutic modalities as they may influence the nutritional status of the patient; this is the third area of concern in nutritional assessment.

INFLUENCE OF THERAPEUTIC REGIMEN ON NUTRITIONAL STATUS

Dialysis has profound effects on nutritional status including: 1) loss of serum transferrin, 2) decreased serum valine and tyrosine, increased glycine, and a decrease in the essential amino acid nonessential amino acid ratio from 0.66 (normal) to 0.44, and 3) decreased serum potassium, folacin, vitamin C, B_6, zinc and iron, the latter through blood loss during dialysis (8).

Prolonged use of prednisone results in:1)calcium malabsorption, by decreasing calcium transport, 2) retarded growth, by decreasing growth hormone release, 3) negative N balance, and 4) sodium retention (9).

Immunosuppressive agents such as azathioprine and cyclophosphamide induce macrocytosis. Hydralazine and penicillamine decrease serum B_6, possibly via increased excretion.

Children with chronic renal failure and uremia fortunately can survive to adulthood. It is therefore important that they achieve satisfactory physical and psychomotor growth and development for which optimal nutrition is necessary. Renal failure delays growth when the glomerular filtration rate decreases below 30%-50% of normal (10). The effects of the decreased GFR depend on the child's age; growth retardation will be much more severe in infants and adolescents when the growth rate is maximum. Nutritional deprivation during infancy may also affect psychomotor development because brain cell multiplication takes place and is almost completed by the end of the first year of life (11).

ASSESSMENT OF NUTRITIONAL STATUS (3,7)

The nutrition laboratory plays a key role in detecting micronutrient deficiencies before they progress to flagrant physical signs. Table 2 outlines useful laboratory determinations.

Table 2. The Biochemical Assessment of Nutritional Status in Chronic Renal Failure

1. Protein
   - Albumin, Pre-albumin
   - Essential/Non-essential A.A. Ratio
   - Hydroxyproline Index
   - Urinary N (BUN, Creatinine)
   - Transferrin
   - Nitrogen Balance Studies
2. Vitamins
   - B_1, B_2, B_6, C, Folic Acid
   - Vitamin A, D
3. Minerals
   - Fe, TIBC, Zn, Mg
4. Lipids
   - Cholesterol, Triglycerides, Lipoprotein Electrophoresis
5. Electrolytes
   - K^+, Ca^{++}, Na^+, Cl^-, $PO_4^=$, Mg^{++}

Dietary Evaluation

The child with chronic renal failure also requires detailed and frequent evaluation of nutrient intake (Table 3). Vital nutrients in chronic renal failure such as calorie, protein (animal and vegetable), carbohydrate, fat, pyridoxine, folic acid, iron, zinc, potassium, calcium and phosphate should be regularly evaluated. This evaluation should be done qualitatively and quantitatively.

Quality of food intake can be detected by:

a. Questionnaires documenting food habits and choices (the socioeconomic status and the ethnic background of the family are important).
b. Frequency of foods used in a week will indicate food preferences and habits.
c. Knowledge the family and child have about nutrition in relation to renal disease.
d. Food allergies, pica, and coexisting diseases.
e. Medications administered which may interact with nutrient intake.
f. Vitamin and mineral supplement intakes.

Quantity of nutrient intake can be evaluated through:

a. The 24-hour dietary recall taken by the dietitian at every clinic visit. This is the easiest method of evaluating nutrient intake. It has the disadvantage of relying on the mother's and child's memory; daily variations of food intake can also be missed.

Table 3. Special Application of Dietary History in Chronic Renal Failure

1. "Background" dietary history of patient and family
2. Patient and family attitudes and mores toward food
3. Perception and cognition level of dietary instructions
4. Analysis of clinical records
5. Food preparation methods which decrease nutrients
6. Problems with food cost
7. Patient's awareness of salt and fluid intake

b. Weekly food records kept by the mother will have the advantage of detecting daily variations in food intake. In order to obtain accurate records, the mother must be highly motivated to be able to closely monitor the child's activities and food intake. Periodic evaluation of food intake by weekly food records can be useful in helping to assess the clinical course of most children.

The caloric and nutrient intake from both the 24 hours' dietary intake and the weekly food records can be analyzed by using food composition tables. Computer analysis of the individual dietary recalls gives more rapid and complete evaluation of the dietary intake, including amino acids, vitamins and minerals.

Anthropometric Evaluation

Body size, as assessed by weight, height, and skinfold thickness, is clearly related to food intake and utilization. Rapid growth during infancy, childhood and adolescence requires frequent and accurate evaluation during these years. The frequent evaluation of growth rate is far more important in children with chronic renal failure in comparison to healthy children because of the serious impact of renal diseases on growth.

The most practical and easily obtainable anthropometric measurements are the following:

1. Weight
2. Height or length
3. Weight to height ratio
4. Head circumference
5. Chest circumference
6. Head-to-chest circumference ratio
7. Left mid-arm circumference
8. Triceps and subscapular skinfold thickness
9. Left mid-arm muscle circumference

The muscle circumference is calculated by subtracting the skinfold thickness from the mid-arm circumference. The muscle circumference will indicate muscle wasting while the skinfold thickness will indicate caloric reserves. The measurement of head circumference will indicate brain growth; it is important that it be determined in infants and preschool children. Measurements obtained are plotted on growth charts.

The interpretation of anthropometric findings in children should be based on serial observations rather than measurements at one point in time.

Normal growth can occur after renal transplantation but may often be limited by steroid therapy.

Evaluation of Skeletal Growth

Skeletal maturity is assessed by the appearance of ossification centers in the wrist, elbow and ankle, and comparison to available standards. Measurement of cortical thickness at the middle of the diaphysis of the metacarpal bones may be more accurate. Increased bone resorption leads to decreased cortical thickness. The effectiveness of therapy with vitamin D and calcium can also be evaluated by this method.

Evaluation of the Teeth

The use of carbohydrate supplements and sticky sweets in the diet increase risk for dental caries. At times amino acid supplements and ketoacids are given in syrup solutions to enhance palatability and may also contribute to dental problems.

CLINICAL SIGNS AND SYMPTOMS OF MALNUTRITION IN CHILDREN WITH CHRONIC RENAL FAILURE

Children with chronic renal failure often do not obtain adequate amounts of calories and protein because of decreased dietary intake, through excessive urinary losses, or following dialysis. They will be in negative nitrogen balance and start consuming their body carbohydrate, fat and protein stores for energy. A rapid downhill course will lead to kwashiorkor, the most common features of which are:

1. Growth failure
2. Edema
3. Mental changes (apathy)
4. Hepatomegaly (fatty infiltration)
5. Hair changes (fine, dull, brittle, reddish color, easily pluckable)
6. Dermatosis (hyperkeratosis, hyperpigmentation)
7. Anemia
8. Reduced subcutaneous fat
9. Anorexia
10. Muscle wasting
11. Weakness, fatigue

Table 4 presents the differential clinical status of children with kwashiorkor and chronic renal failure. Most symptoms and signs are the same in both, with the exception that blood pressure is decreased in kwashiorkor and increased in chronic renal failure. The differential nutritional and metabolic status of kwashiorkor and chronic renal failure is presented in Table 5. Vitamin A is usually increased in chronic renal failure and low in kwashiorkor, while potassium, phosphate, magnesium, triglycerides and cholesterol are low in kwashiorkor and increased in late chronic renal failure. Table 6 summarizes the differential hormonal status of kwashiorkor and chronic renal failure. Insulin and growth hormone are decreased in kwashiorkor and increased in chronic renal failure while somatomedin and thyroid hormone are low in both conditions.

Besides protein-calorie malnutrition, the most common deficiencies in children with chronic renal failure are:

1. *Folate*, presenting with pallor, aphthous stomatitis, glossitis and painful tongue.
2. *Pyridoxine*, presenting with blepharitis, nasolabial seborrhea, glossitis, peripheral neuropathy, symmetrical sensory and motor deficits (especially in the lower extremities), and drug resistant convulsions and dementia.
3. *Vitamin C*, recognized clinically by interdental gingival hypertrophy, gingivitis, perifollicular petechiae, purpura, ecchymoses due to capillary fragility, cortical hemorrhages of bone visualizable on x-rays, subperiosteal hematoma, intradermal petechiae, epiphyseal enlargement and intramuscular hematoma.
4. *Riboflavin*, the most common clinical signs of which are circumcorneal capillary injection, angular blepharitis, nasolabial dyssebacea, cheilosis, angular stomatitis, magenta colored tongue, atrophic lingual papillae and fungiform papillary hypertrophy.
5. *Niacin* presents with gingivitis and a scarlet, raw fissured tongue with atrophic lingual papillae. The skin is erythematous with increased pigmentation, desquamation and vascularization. Scrotal dermatitis, dementia and diarrhea are other characteristics of niacin deficiency.
6. *Vitamin D and Calcium* deficiencies almost always occur in children with chronic renal failure. The clinical signs are hypotonia, epiphyseal enlargement, rachitic rosary, delayed fusion of fontanelles in infants with chronic renal failure, craniotabes, bowed legs, cranial bossing, deformities of the thorax and osteomalacia.

Table 4. Differential Clinical Status of Kwashiorkor and Chronic Renal Failure

Sign	Kwashiorkor	Chronic Renal Failure
Edema	+	-, + late, or in nephrosis
Diarrhea	+	+
Infection	+	+
Anorexia	+	+
Apathy	+	+
Blood Pressure	↓	↑
Cardiomyopathy	+	+
Growth	↓	↓
Physical Activity	↓	↓
GFR	↓	↓
Body K+	↓	↓
Muscle mass	↓	↓
Body fat	↓	↓
Intolerance to Cold	↑	↑

7. *Fluoride* is characterized by increased dental caries and osteoporosis.
8. *Zinc*, presenting with anorexia, ageusia, growth retardation, hypogonadism and delayed sexual maturation, skin rash, and hyperkeratosis. Many enzymes are known to be zinc dependent. Enzymes involved in protein synthesis such as ribonuclease are zinc dependent. Therefore, zinc deficiency decreases protein synthesis and may be another factor contributing to negative nitrogen balance in children with chronic renal failure.

CONCLUSION

Nutritional assessment is important in every child. However, the child with chronic renal failure requires much more intensive and detailed evaluation of nutritional status. Early correction of excessive or deficient nutrients following nutritional evalua-

Table 5. The Differential Nutritional and Metabolic Status of Kwashiorkor and Chronic Renal Failure

	Kwashiorkor	Chronic Renal Failure
Albumin	↓	±; ↓ in nephrosis
Pre-albumin	?	N or ↑
Transferrin	↓	↓
N-balance	↓	↓
A.A. E/Non-E	↓	↓
Thiamin, Riboflavin	↓	±
Vitamin A	↓	↑
Folic Acid	↓	↓
Iron	↓	↓
B6	↓	↓
Zinc	↓	↓
Acidosis	↑	↑
K+	↓	↑ (late)
$PO_4^{=}$	±↓	↑
Na+	↑	↑
Ca++	↓	↓
Mg++	↓	↑
Vitamin D	±↓	↓
Osmolality	N	↑
Triglycerides	↓	↑
Blood sugar	↓	↓
Cholesterol	↓	↑

tion will have a significant impact on physical and psychomotor development. With more optimal nutritional status, the child with chronic renal disease can hope to have an improved course.

Table 6. Differential Hormonal Status of Kwashiorkor and Chronic Renal Failure

Hormone	Kwashiorkor	Chronic Renal Failure
Insulin	↓	↑
Somatomedin	↓	↓
Growth Hormone	↓	↑
Thyroid Hormone	↓	↓

REFERENCES

1. Kage, M.: Mineral metabolism during dialysis. In Koishi, H. and Yasumoto, K. (eds.): X International Congress of Nutrition (Kyoto, Japan, Aug., 1975), 1976, p. 295.

2. Broyer, M., Kleinknecht, C., Gagnadouy, M.F. et al.: Growth in uremic children. In Strauss, J. (ed.): Pediatric Nephrology: Current Concepts in Diagnosis and Management. New York: Garland Press, 1978, Vol. 4, p. 185.

3. Christakis, G.: How to make a nutritional diagnosis without really trying. A. Adult nutritional diagnosis. J. Fla. Med. Assoc., Vol. 66, 1979, p. 349.

4. Burch, R.E. and Sullivan, J.F.: Clinical and nutritional aspects of zinc deficiency and excess. Symposium on Trace Elements. Med. Clin. N.A. 60: 4, 1976.

5. Jennete, J.C. and Goldman, I.D.: Inhibition of membrane transport of folates by anions retained in uremia. J. Lab. Clin. Med. 86: 834, 1975.

6. Stone, W.J., Warnock, L.G. and Wagner, C. Vitamin B_6 deficiency in uremia. Am. J. Clin. Nutrit. 28: 950, 1975.

7. Holliday, M.A., McHenry-Richardson, K. and Portale, A.: Nutritional Management of Chronic Renal Disease. Med. Clin. N. Am. 63: 945, 1979.

8. Kluthe, R. and Schaeffer, G. Nutrition and nutritional status in regular dialysis treatment patients. In Koishi, H. and Yasumoto, K. (eds.): X International Congress of Nutrition (Kyoto, Japan, Aug., 1975), 1976, p. 297.

9. Lewy, J.E. and New, M.E.: Growth in children with renal failure. Am. J. Med. 58: 65, 1975.

10. Broyer, M., Kleinknecht, C., Loirat, C. et al.: Growth in children with long-term hemodialysis. J. Pediatr. 84: 642, 1974.

11. Kafatos, A.G.: How to make a nutritional diagnosis without really trying. B. Pediatric nutritional diagnosis. J. Fla. Med. Assoc., Vol. 66, 1979, p. 356.

Appendix. Tests Performed by Nutrition Division Laboratory

Test	Author	Principle	Apparatus
Albumin (serum, micromethod)	Doumas, B.T. & Biggs, H.G. Standard Methods of Clin. Chem. Acad. Press, New York, V. 7, 1972.	The absorbance of a dye (bromcresol green) is increased in the presence of serum albumin This increase in absorbance is directly proportional to the concentration of albumin.	UV-visible spectrophotometer, with an automatic sampler, pump and recorder.
Thiamin (RBC, micromethod)	Brin, M. et al.: J. Nutri. 71, 273, 1960.	A functional test of nutritional adequacy of thiamin. Hemolyzed whole blood samples are incubated with an excess of ribose-5-phosphate, and in both presence and the absence of excess thiamin pyrophosphate. The ribose-5-phosphate utilized, or sedoheptulose-7-phosphate produced, are measured.	same as above
Riboflavin (RBC, micromethod)	Glatzle, D., et al.: Int. J. Vitam. Nutri. Res. 40: 166, 1970.	A functional test of nutritional adequacy of riboflavin. During riboflavin deficiency, the activity of erythrocyte glutathione reductase is lowered, but can be returned to normal level by the in vitro addition of the coenzyme, FAD. The enzyme activity is estimated by measuring the oxidation of $NADPH_2$.	same as above

Pyridoxine (RBC, micromethod)	Cheney, M., et al.: Am. J. Nutri. 16: 337, 1965.	A functional test of nutritional adequacy of pyridoxine. During pyridoxine deficiency, the activity of erythrocyte glutamate-pyruvate transaminase is lowered, but can be returned to normal level by the in vitro addition of the coenzyme-pyridoxal phosphate. The rate of decrease of NADH absorption is directly proportional to the enzyme's activity.	same as above
Ascorbic Acid (plasma, micromethod)	Bessey, O.A. et al.: J. Biol. Chem. 168: 197, 1947.	Ascorbic acid is oxidized to dehydroascorbate by Cu ions. The 2, 4-dinitrophenylhydrazine derivative is dissolved in concentrated H_2SO_4 and the absorbance of the red-orange product is measured.	UV-visible spectrophotometer
Vitamin A, B-carotene (plasma, micromethod)	Neeld, J.B. and Pearson, W.W.: J. Nutri. 79:45, 1963.	Carotene is the precursor of vitamin A and is usually determined along with the vitamin. The proteins in the serum are precipated with alcohol and the carotene and vitamin A extracted with petroleum ether. Carotene is determined directly by its absorbance at 450 nm. Vitamin A is determined by the reaction with trifluoroacetic acid to give a transient blue color. Since carotene also produces some color with the reagent, a correction must be made.	UV-visible spectrophotometer

Triglycerides (serum, micromethod)	Dept. of HEW Manual of Lab Operations. Lipid Res. Clinics Program. Vol. 1. Pub. No. (NIH) 75-628.	Extracted serum is saponified with alcohol and KOH to glycerol and followed by oxidation and condensation reactions to produce a fluorescing compound.	Technicon Autoanalyzer II
Cholesterol (serum, micromethod)	Dept. of HEW Manual of Lab Operations. Lipid Res. Clinics Program. Vol. 1. Pub. No. (NIH) 75-628.	Extracted serum is reacted with the Lieberman-Buchard color reagent and color is developed at 60°C. The absorbance is read at 630 nm.	same as above
Iron (serum, micromethod)	Yeh, Y.Y. and Zee, P.: Clin. Chem. 20: 360, 1974.	Serum is treated with tricholoroacetic acid to precipitate protein. The sample is diluted with deionized water and its iron content is measured.	atomic absorption spectrophotometer with a graphite furnace
TIBC (serum, micromethod)	Yeh, Y.Y. and Zee, P.: Clin. Chem. 20: 360, 1974	Transferrin is saturated by exogenous ferric ions and the excess iron is removed. The protein is then precipitated, the sample diluted and the iron content measured.	same as above
Free Glycerol (plasma)	Kreutz, F.H.: Klin. Wschr. 40:362, 1962	Uses Sigma test kit - eliminates unspecific DP(HN) oxidoreductases by scanning scanning	UV spectrophotome-
Urea Nitrogen (urine plasma)	Fearon, W.R., Friedman, H.S.: Anal. Chem. 25: 662, 1953.	Adaptation of Fearon diacetyl monoxime method	Same as above

Free Fatty Acids (plasma)	Novak, M.J.: Lipid Res. 6, 431, 1965.	Long chain fatty acids complex with Co++ and Ni++. Adapted for use with radioactive tracers	liquid scintillation
Ketone Bodies (plasma)	Persson, B., Scand. J. Clin. Lab. Invest. 25: 9, 1969.	B-hydroxybuetyrate and acetoacetate determination after precipitating plasma proteins.	UV spectrophotometer

NUTRIENT REQUIREMENTS

Lewis A. Barness, M.D.

Dept. Pediatr., U. So. Fla. College Med., Tampa, Fla. 33612, USA

Aggressive nutritional treatment is frequently necessary in the management of children with chronic renal disease. Failure to provide adequate calories and nutrients may aggravate the signs, symptoms, and secondary effects of renal disease (Table 1). Nutritional therapy is frequently difficult not only because losses may be excessive, but also because a sick child may be anorexic. Children with renal disease in particular may be depressed, just not hungry, or may vomit and have diarrhea. As a result, protein metabolism is decreased. Often, the physician is limited to correcting the detected chemical errors; and correction of one serum abnormality may produce another. Many secondary errors, particularly those related to hormonal deficits or excesses, and especially those related to secondary messengers cannot be approached with present knowledge. Dehydration, overhydration, electrolyte imbalance, acidosis, and hypertension are common. Osteodystrophy, rickets and central nervous system abnormalities occur. Least understood is the growth failure and the many factors causing this in children with chronic nephritis.

Nutrient requirements of a normal growing child have been determined by observing the needs of populations and by balance studies. Many of these requirements need modification in some children with renal failure, due to decreased ability to excrete, increased losses, or increased metabolism (Table 2).

Water requirements are of prime concern. Too little water results in dehydration and worsening renal function (1). Too much water results in edema and also in worsening renal function. Water requirements can be met by daily weighing, or by careful measurement of 24 hour urine volume and adding about one-half estimated

Table 1. 2° Effects of Renal Disease

Decreased protein catabolism
Dehydration
Overhydration
Electrolyte imbalance
Acidosis
Hypertension
Osteodystrophy
Rickets
CNS
Growth failure

insensible water loss. The other half of insensible water loss is supplied by the water of oxidation of foods.

Sodium requirement is next in importance (2). Low sodium leads to dehydration, hypotension, impaired potassium exchange and decreased renal function. Excess sodium leads to edema, water retention, heart failure, and hypertension. Sodium requirements can be estimated by measuring 24 hour urine losses; determining serum sodium provides information for rapid correction of deficits or excesses. Deficits can be corrected by enteral or parenteral intake. Salt tablets may not dissolve and should not be used. Excesses can be relieved by potent diuretics such as furosemide. Minimum requirements for sodium are 1-3 mEq/kg with several times this dose in salt losers.

Because effect of potassium can be rapid, potassium requirements are best estimated from serum levels. High potassium foods, potassium sparing diuretics such as spironolactone or triamterene, or low-sodium diets leading to further potassium retention, should

Table 2. Concerns

Water
Sodium 1-4 mEq/kg/day
Chloride 1-6 mEq/kg/day
Potassium 1-4 mEq/kg/day
Protein 0.6-1.1 g/day
Phosphate 0.4-1 g/day
Calcium 0.5-1 g/day
Vitamin D 1 μg/day (400 U/day)
Magnesium 0.1-0.5 g/day
Iron 10-20 mg/day
Calories
Bicarbonate

be used with caution. In the presence of alkalosis or chloride deficiency, chloride salts should be used. In renal tubular disease with acidosis, potassium acetate or phosphate is preferred. Requirements are 1-3 mEq/kg with supplements adjusted for losses.

Protein requirements do not differ greatly from normal minimal requirements. About 0.6-1.1 g/kg/day can be given plus allowance for urinary losses (2,4). Giordano (3) and Giovanetti (4) suggested that a diet containing only essential amino acids would force the use of urea and other nitrogenous products. A diet in which the protein is of high biological value such as egg protein is useful in supplying these essential amino acids. There may be an advantage to using ketoacids of the essential amino acids. Theoretically, and in animal experiments, urea and ammonia were decreased with substitution of these ketoacids for one-half the amino acids (5).

Retention of phosphate results in decreased serum calcium, increased parathormone, and osteitis fibrosa cystica. Rickets may also occur. Serum phosphate can be lowered by using low phosphate foods and by inhibiting absorption of phosphate by giving aluminum hydroxide gel. 1,25 dihydroxycholecalciferol, 1-3 μg/day helps raise serum calcium and may relieve bone pain and osteodystrophy. Calcium supplements, 1-3 g/day, may be given by mouth. Serum calcium should be monitored as hypercalcemia leads to further renal deterioration. In contrast to calcium, magnesium is usually retained. Magnesium containing cathartics should be avoided. In those forms of renal disease characterized by phosphaturia, supplemental phosphate must be supplied. Phosphate supplements, when isotonic, produce little diarrhea. Associated rickets is improved, but 1,25 dihydroxycholecalciferol is also beneficial. Anti-convulsants affect vitamin D metabolism, and may increase need for vitamin D metabolites.

Iron stores may be depleted. Iron may be given by mouth. If not absorbed, intramuscular iron can be given. Androgens may stimulate hematopoiesis.

Caloric intake should be maintained at as near normal levels as possible. Deficient calories results in tissue breakdown and increased catabolism. Excessive calories may produce vomiting or diarrhea. High fat, high carbohydrate diets should make up most of the intake. If oral feedings are not tolerated, 10% glucose solutions with intralipid 1-2 g/kg are available. Caloric intake should approach 100 cal/kg/day the first year of life, plus about 100 calories per year of life to age 14.

Acidosis associated with uremia probably is best not treated with bicarbonate, unless the pH is less than 7.1. Bicarbonate not only may increase cerebral acidosis with deterioration of cerebral function, but excessive amounts of sodium may be given with further compromise of the electrolyte status. With acute elevation of serum potassium, however, bolus sodium bicarbonate treatment may be necessary. In contrast, those with chronic renal tubular acidosis appear to benefit from chronic administration of sodium bicarbonate. In these, 6-10 mEq/kg/day has been associated with better growth than in those remaining persistently acidotic.

If symptomatic deficiency of folic acid, zinc, vitamin C or other minerals or vitamins develops, they should be supplied in therapeutic doses.

Those not tolerating these requirements, or those in whom oral or parenteral modifications result in insufficient correction of deficits or excesses can be aided by dialysis. Dialysis fluids can supply electrolytes, minerals and calories. More experience is needed to determine the usefulness and feasibility of supplying amino acids via peritoneal dialysis. Consideration should be given to the desirability of supplying only essential amino acids, to further reduce, through utilization, ammonia and urea; also keto-acids of the essential amino acids should be well absorbed through the peritoneum, again theoretically reducing ammonia and urea.

Supplying calories, protein and trace elements can result in an active child. Unless some element is at a critically toxic level, slow correction over a period of days generally results in a more satisfactory return to homeostasis than rapid correction. Many children have performed well with their abnormal chemistries for long periods. Proper nutrition support requires a sanguine attitude, encouragement, and help from dietitians or nutritionists.

REFERENCES

1. Ing. T.S. and Kark, R.M.: Renal Disease. In Schneider, H.A., Anderson, C.E. and Coursin, D.B.: Nutritional Support of Medical Practice. Harper, 1977, p. 367.

2. Holliday, M.A.: Chronic Renal Disease. In Pediatric Nutrition Handbook, Am. Acad. Pediatr., Chicago, 1979, p. 202.

3. Giordano, C.: Use of exogenous and endogenous urea for protein synthesis in normal and uremic subjects. J. Lab. Clin. Med. 62: 231, 1963.

4. Berlyne, G.M., Shaw, A.B. and Nilwaraugkur, S.: Dietary treatment of chronic renal failure: Experiences with a modified Giovanetti diet. Nephron 2: 129, 1965.

5. Walser, M., Coulter, A.W., Dighe, S. et al.: The effect of keto-analogues of essential amino acids in severe chronic uremia. J. Clin. Invest. 52: 678, 1973.

HYPERLIPIDEMIA SECONDARY TO RENAL DISEASE

Guido O. Perez, M.D. and Sung Lan Hsia, M.D.

Depts. Med., Dermatol., Biochem., Univ. Miami Sch. Med. and Vet. Adm. Med. Center, Miami, Fla. 33125 USA

Hyperlipidemia is a common metabolic complication in patients with chronic renal failure. In view of the association of hyperlipidemia with atherosclerosis, and the greatly increased incidence of atherosclerosis among uremic patients, the study of lipid metabolism in chronic renal failure has drawn much attention. A brief review of current literature and the results of some of our recent studies are presented in this paper.

ATHEROSCLEROSIS IN UREMIA

Analyses of the causes of death of patients on maintenance hemodialysis have shown a high prevalence of atherosclerotic events (1,2). A recent report, however, has pointed out that pre-existing hypertension, metastatic calcification, diabetes mellitus and hyperlipidemia may be the cause for the apparent increase in atherosclerosis in regularly dialyzed patients (3). The thesis that dialysis patients carry a higher than normal risk for accelerated atherosclerosis remains unproven and can only be established with carefully designed prospective studies.

HYPERLIPIDEMIA

Most studies have shown increased triglyceride levels while serum cholesterol is normal or decreased in uremia (4-6). The lipoprotein electrophoretic pattern usually corresponds to that of Type IV hyperlipoproteinemia. These lipid abnormalities are commonly thought to promote or contribute to the early development of ischemic heart disease.

The etiology of hypertriglyceridemia in uremia has not been definitely elucidated. It has been suggested that this abnormality may be due, at least in part, to increased hepatic synthesis of very low density lipoproteins (VLDL) mediated by increased plasma levels of hormones such as insulin, growth hormone, glucagon and parathyroid hormone.

The insensitivity of peripheral tissues to insulin in uremia and the resultant hyperinsulinemia could lead to increased hepatic synthesis of VLDL. Two recent studies, however, showed fasting insulin levels within the range of normal in non-diabetic uremic patients (5,7). Furthermore, glucose loading has not been found to affect triglyceride levels in these patients (8).

Another postulated cause of increased triglyceride production in uremia is abnormally high growth hormone levels (9). In a recent study, however, no correlation was found between fasting triglyceride and growth hormone levels in dialysis patients (5). The possible role of hyperglucagonemia and hyperparathyroidism (10,11) in the pathogenesis of uremic hypertriglyceridemia remains undefined.

LIPOPROTEIN LIPASE ACTIVITY

Plasma post-heparin lipolytic activity (PHLA), an indirect measurement of tissue lipoprotein lipase and capacity for triglyceride removal, has been shown to decrease in uremia, and on that basis it has been postulated that a defect in VLDL catabolism may be the main cause of hypertriglyceridemia in these patients (4). Most studies have shown a decrease in adipose tissue lipoprotein lipase (10). Other studies (12) have shown that hepatic lipoprotein lipase is also reduced in patients with chronic renal failure and it has been shown that both patients on peritoneal dialysis and hemodialysis have impaired ability for triglyceride removal leading to hypertriglyceridemia (13). Moreover, Ibels et al. (7) have shown that triglyceride clearance was low in uremic patients evaluated after an infusion of a triglyceride emulsion.

The cause of reduced PHLA in uremia remains under active investigation. There may be inhibitors present in uremic serum (14, 15) or possibly the function of a particular activator such as insulin (16) or apolipoprotein CII (17) is impaired. It has been shown recently that administration of parathyroid hormone to rats results in an acute depression of adipose tissue lipoprotein lipase (11). Repeated administration of heparin could play a role in the decreased levels of PHLA seen in dialysis patients; however, hyperlipidemia has also been described in patients on peritoneal dialysis who do not receive systemic heparin regularly (18).

A recent study in uremic rats showed that lipoprotein lipase activity did not differ in heart, diaphragm and adipose tissue from that in control animals (19). On the other hand, serum from acutely uremic rats significantly inhibited tissue lipoprotein lipase. Similar findings have been reported in experiments using sera from patients with chronic renal failure (15). These findings make it unlikely that a quantitative defect of lipoprotein lipase is present in uremia, and suggest that the decreased clearance of triglyceride-rich lipoproteins from the circulation may be due to an inhibitor. Recent experience with hemofiltration (20) has shown that serum lipid levels decrease during therapy suggesting that the putative inhibitor of lipoprotein lipase is of medium molecular weight (500-5000 daltons).

EFFECTS OF DRUGS AND ASSOCIATED DISEASES

A pronounced increase in serum triglyceride levels has been noted when rather high dosages of an androgen preparation, dromostanolone, was administered to dialysis patients (21). It is possible that the widespread use of androgen compounds further enhances the lipid abnormalities manifested by uremic patients. Similarly, propanolol therapy for hypertension has been associated with increases in serum triglyceride levels (22).

Hyperlipidemia and accelerated atherosclerosis are particularly common among patients with diabetes mellitus and/or the nephrotic syndrome. Since many of these patients develop chronic renal failure, the combined effect of the original disease and uremia on plasma lipid levels may cause a wide spectrum of lipid abnormalities.

EFFECTS OF DIALYSIS AND TRANSPLANTATION

The lipid abnormalities of uremia are not corrected by dialysis (23,24) and may persist following successful renal transplantation (5-7). Following renal transplantation, serum lipid levels are quite variable and hypercholesterolemia is more common and hypertriglyceridemia less so than in the uremic group. Thus, Types IIa, IIb and IV occur with equal frequency. The abnormalities have been attributed to obesity, prednisone, and impairment of graft function. Moreover, PHLA has been found to be decreased in allograft recipients that have some degree of renal impairment.

CHOLESTEROL METABOLISM

Cholesterol metabolism in uremia has not been systematically evaluated perhaps because serum cholesterol concentrations are generally normal. The possibility that acetate loads delivered to the patients during dialysis could be used for the synthesis of cholesterol seems unlikely on the basis of recent observations (25).

There is recent evidence suggesting that the efflux of cholesterol from the arterial wall may regulate the process of atherogenesis. Several investigators have presented data indicating that a reduction of plasma high density lipoproteins (HDL) may be associated with decreased clearance of cholesterol from the arterial wall (26-29). According to recent studies, after tissue cholesterol is picked up by HDL, it is esterified by lecithin-cholesterol acyl transferase (LCAT) (30). The cholesteryl esters are then transferred from HDL to VLDL which eventually takes them to the liver for disposal. In addition, HDL partially inhibits uptake and internalization of low density lipoproteins by arterial smooth muscle cells (31). These findings may account for the well-known negative correlation between plasma concentrations of HDL and the risk of clinically evident atherosclerosis (26).

It has been proposed that LCAT may play an important role in regulating lipoprotein catabolism and preventing cholesterol from accumulating in peripheral tissue (30). Serum LCAT activity and cholesteryl ester clearance were recently determined in patients with chronic renal failure (32). The activity of the enzyme was determined by using the serum of each patient both as a source of enzyme and as a substrate ("intrinsic activity") and by using a standard substrate ("extrinsic activity") in order to ascertain the presence of inhibitors in serum. Both activities were found to be significantly lower in chronic uremic patients than in controls.

LIPOPROTEIN ABNORMALITIES

In patients with chronic renal failure, HDL cholesterol has been found to be lower, and HDL triglycerides higher than controls matched for serum lipid levels (17,33,34). In addition, their apolipoprotein AI levels were found to be normal (17,33) while apolipoprotein CII was decreased and apolipoprotein E was increased (17). Thus, it appears that in addition to hypertriglyceridemia, the uremic state exerts an effect on HDL composition.

Since LCAT catalyzes the formation of cholesteryl esters by promoting the transfer of the acyl group from lecithin to cholesterol in HDL, it is possible that the low HDL cholesterol levels in uremic patients are related to the above mentioned abnormality of LCAT in uremia.

The possibility that HDL apolipoproteins of uremic patients may have a decreased affinity for cholesterol was recently evaluated (35) using a method developed by Hsia et al. (36) (vide infra).

SERUM CHOLESTEROL BINDING RESERVE (SCBR) IN RENAL DISEASE

Hsia et al. (36) observed that the human serum is capable of solubilizing a measurable amount of exogenous cholesterol in addition to its cholesterol content. This amount has been designated serum cholesterol binding reserve (SCBR). Further studies showed that SCBR could be accounted for by the cholesterol-solubilizing capacity of VLDL and HDL. It was postulated that SCBR may be an index of the capacity of the serum lipoproteins in facilitating cholesterol efflux from the arterial wall, therefore, individuals with decreased SCBR would be at higher risk for developing atherosclerosis. Consistent with this postulate were findings of decreased SCBR in patients who suffered premature myocardial infarction (36), and in patients with adult onset diabetes (37).

SCBR was evaluated in two groups of renal patients, those with the nephrotic syndrome (38) and those on chronic hemodialysis (35).

Nephrotic Syndrome

Twenty-two non-uremic patients (14 men and 8 women) ages 19 to 70 years (mean ± SE, 47 ± 3) were studied. Serum creatinine concentration was below 2 mg/100 in all but two patients. Clinical diagnosis of the nephrotic syndrome was made on the basis of a 24 hour urinary protein determination exceeding 3 g. Histologic examination of renal tissue obtained by percutaneous renal biopsy was available in 19 cases. The remaining 3 subjects had chronic diabetes mellitus and were presumed to have diabetic nephropathy. Mild to moderate hypertension was present in 8 cases.

Controls were 21 hyperlipidemic men, between 35 and 59 years of age. Their serum cholesterol levels were above 250 mg/100 ml and serum triglycerides above 150 mg/100 ml. None had signs or symptoms of diabetes mellitus or nephropathy.

Fifteen of the 22 nephrotic patients had serum triglyceride levels above 160 mg/100 ml, but the average value was not significantly different from that of 21 control subjects (Fig. 1). Serum cholesterol levels exceeded 250 mg/100 ml in all but three patients. The mean value was significantly higher ($P < 0.005$) than that of control subjects. SCBR in patients with the nephrotic syndrome was significantly lower ($P < 0.001$) than that of controls (nephrotics 75 ± 6 mg/100 ml; controls 102 ± 6 mg/100 ml).

Because mean serum cholesterol and triglyceride levels in the nephrotic patients were not the same as those of controls, we used covariant analysis to adjust the mean SCBR values. The differences between the adjusted means (nephrotics 79; controls 98 mg/100 ml) remained statistically significant ($P < 0.02$).

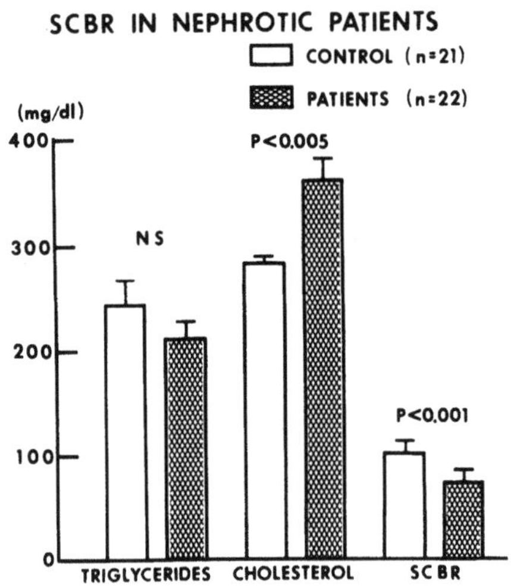

FIG. 1. Serum lipid levels and SCBR of nephrotic patients and controls.

Multiple regression analysis revealed that the SCBR values in controls tended to increase with increasing serum cholesterol values (SCBR = 36 + 0.18 cholesterol + 0.05 triglycerides), while the opposite was the case in the nephrotic group (SCBR = 89 - 0.092 cholesterol + 0.009 triglycerides).

Patients With Chronic Renal Failure On Maintenance Hemodialysis

Eighty-three patients (59 men and 24 women) between the ages of 25 and 75 years receiving maintenance hemodialysis from 3 months to 11 years were evaluated. Ten patients had diabetes mellitus. All were oliguric with an endogenous creatinine clearance of less than 5 ml/min. Each patient was undergoing hemodialysis for approximately 5 hrs, three times a week, using the Cordis-Dow No. 4 Hollow Fiber Artificial Kidney or standard coils. Twenty of the patients were receiving androgen therapy (fluoxymesterone 30 mg/day). All were prescribed 1 g protein/kg body weight and were sodium and potassium restricted according to clinical need. All patients were taking standard dialysis medications, including a water soluble vitamin preparation, oral iron and aluminum hydroxide. None of the patients, except for those taking insulin and androgens, were receiving medications known to affect lipid or endocrine metabolism. Likewise, none of the patients had liver disease, endocrinopathy other than diabetes mellitus, primary hyperlipidemia or the nephrotic syndrome.

Control subjects were participants in the Miami Multiple Risk Factor Intervention Trial (MRFIT) Program (n = 149). They were white men between the ages of 35 and 59, who were placed in the upper 10% of the estimated risk for coronary heart disease by the combination of cigarette smoking habit, serum lipid levels and diastolic blood pressure.

The patients and controls were separated into normolipidemic and hyperlipidemic (serum cholesterol $\geq$ 250 mg/100 ml and/or triglycerides $\geq$ 160 mg/100 ml) subgroups. The results of SCBR and HDL-cholesterol (HDLC) in 53 patients (40 men and 13 women) are shown in Figure 2.

In the 40 men on chronic hemodialysis, serum cholesterol was 180 $\pm$ 7 mg/100 ml and triglycerides 176 $\pm$ 18 mg/100 ml. The SCBR in both hyperlipidemic and normolipidemic men on maintenance dialysis was not different from that of controls. HDLC, however, was significantly lower ($P < 0.005$) in hyperlipidemic dialysis patients than in controls, while the values in the normolipidemic patients were not different from control values. Because none of the controls were older than 59, the data were analyzed after excluding 8 patients older than that age. The mean SCBR of the group (combining normolipidemic and hyperlipidemic patients) was 98, which was not different from the value of 100 for the whole group. SCBR values of the 10 diabetic patients undergoing hemodialysis (60 $\pm$ 6 mg/100 ml) were, however, significantly lower than those in non-diabetic patients and controls ($P < 0.001$). This finding is in agreement with our previous finding of decreased SCBR in diabetes mellitus (37).

The results in women demonstrated lower HDLC values in normolipidemic patients than in controls, who were 27 hospital employees with no evidence of renal, endocrine or cardiovascular disease. However, SCBR levels were not different. There were not enough hyperlipidemic control women to make meaningful statistical comparisons.

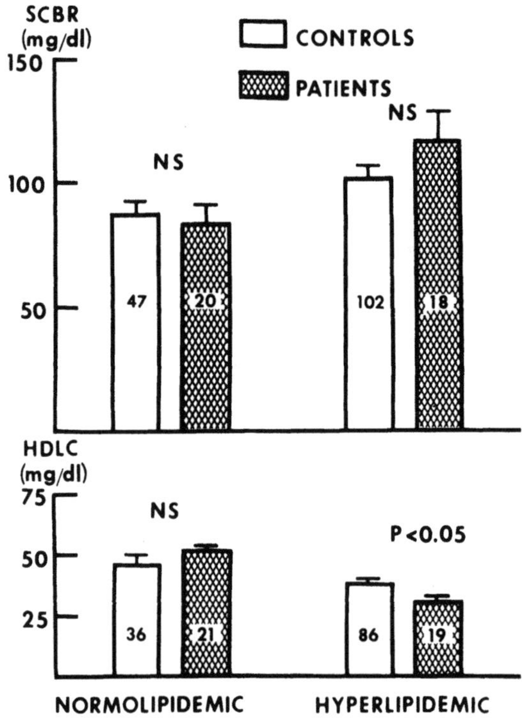

FIG. 2. SCBR and HDLC in normolipidemic and hyperlipidemic men on hemodialysis.

The lack of difference in SCBR between the hemodialyzed patients and controls is in contrast with the significantly lower SCBR in patients with nephrotic syndrome. The significance of these findings needs to be clarified in future studies.

The relationship between HDLC and triglyceride levels is shown in Figure 3. The negative correlation between HDLC and triglycerides has been previously observed in other hyperlipidemic states; however, its mechanism has yet to be elucidated.

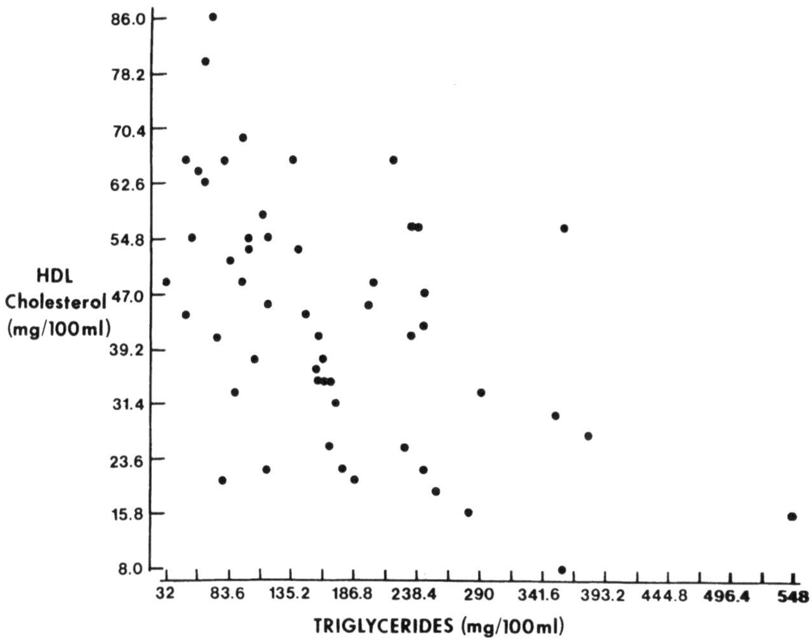

FIG. 3. Correlation between HDLC and serum triglycerides in dialysis patients.

RATE OF CHOLESTEROL TRANSFER (RCT) IN UREMIC PATIENTS ON CHRONIC HEMODIALYSIS

Although a number of lipid abnormalities have been identified in patients with uremia, their accelerated atherosclerosis has not been satisfactorily explained. It is significant that these patients develop severe atherosclerosis in the absence of elevated serum cholesterol levels.

Since several abnormalities in HDL exist in uremia, it is possible that some of these abnormalities may impair the normal function of HDL in removing cholesterol from the arterial wall.

Recent studies have shown that after the HDLC is esterfied by LCAT, the esters are transferred to VLDL and LDL (39). Nestel et al. (40) injected HDL labelled with (^{3}H) cholesterol into 3 healthy men and followed the disappearance of the label from HDL and appearance in VLDL and LDL. They estimated the rate of the flux of cholesterol from HDL to VLDL and LDL to be between 148 and 168 mg of cholesterol per hour.

It can be calculated from these data that the amount of cholesterol transported via this pathway in 24 hours in an average man is between 3.5 and 4.0 g. Since in vivo, HDLC maintains a steady level, presumably, this amount of cholesterol is removed daily from peripheral tissues by HDL, then transported via VLDL and LDL to the liver for disposal.

In our laboratory, we have developed a simple method to measure the transfer of cholesterol from HDL to VLDL and HDL, in vitro. The method requires the incubation of a small serum sample (0.5 ml) at 37° C under constant mixing to allow the transfer to take place. The cholesterol content in HDL is measured before and after the incubation, after the removal of VLDL and LDL by precipitation with heparin and manganese chloride. The difference in HDLC represents the amount of cholesterol transferred during the incubation. We have found that the transfer proceeds at a nearly linear rate for 4 hours, then levels off. The RCT is calculated from the data after 4 hours of incubation, and is expressed in mg of cholesterol transferred per hr per 100 ml of serum.

We determined RCT of 40 patients (29 men and 11 women) with chronic renal failure. Their clinical characteristics and treatment were the same as those of the dialysis patients as described before. Controls were 14 healthy men who were hospital workers in the age range of 41 to 60 years (mean ± SE 47.8 ± 3.4 years) and 78 blood donors (55 men and 23 women) at the local blood bank. Ages of the blood donors ranged from 17 to 58 years (mean ± SE 29.6 ± 1.4 years for men and 33.0 ± 2.5 years for the women). None of the controls had clinically manifest atherosclerosis or renal disease.

RCT values of the 29 uremic men and 11 uremic women are compared with those of control men and women in Figure 4. The mean ± SE of RCT of dialyzed men and women were 1.85 ± 0.24 and 1.84 ± 0.30 mg per hour per 100 ml of serum, respectively. These values were significantly lower ($P < 0.001$ in both cases) than the control values (4.51 ± 0.35 and 3.54 ± 0.40 mg/hr/100 ml for men and women, respectively). Six of the dialyzed men but none of the controls had zero RCT value, i.e., a total lack of the ability for cholesterol transfer.

The lipid levels of the male patients and controls are shown in Table 1. It is seen that the patients had significantly lower HDLC levels and were older than the controls. These differences were taken into consideration and RCT values of 11 patients and 41 controls having HDLC in the range of 30 to 65 mg/100 ml (mean ± SE 44.0 ± 3.2 and 44.8 ± 1.3 mg/100 ml, respectively) were compared. RCT values of the patients (mean ± SE 2.61 ± 0.86 mg/hr/100 ml) were again significantly lower ($P < 0.039$) than those of the controls (3.58 ± 0.89 mg/hr/100 ml). When 18 patients were

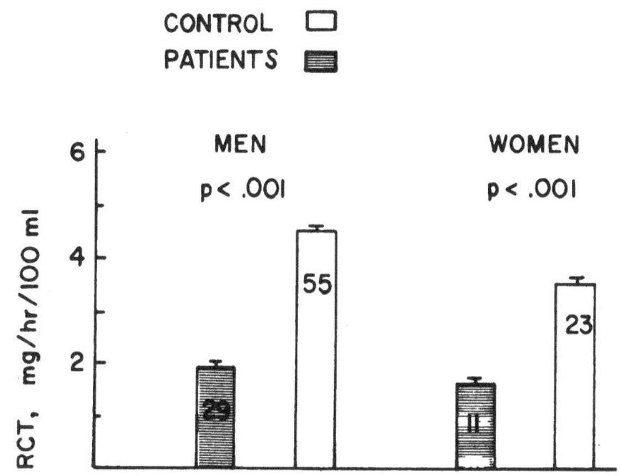

FIG. 4. Comparison of RCT between patients on chronic hemodialysis and controls.

matched with 14 controls for age (41 to 60 years, mean ± SD 51.8 ± 1.4 and 53.4 ± 1.2 years, respectively), RCT values of the patient (1.82 ± 0.33 mg/hr/100 ml) were also significantly lower (P < 0.003

Table 1. Comparison of mean ± SE of lipid levels and age in hemodialyzed men and controls

	SC (mg/100 ml)	TG (mg/100 ml)	HDLC (mg/100 ml)	Age (yrs)
Hemodialyzed men (n = 29)	151.4 ± 7.7	146.6 ± 19.5	30.3 ± 2.5	50.4 ± 2.1
Controls (n = 59)	167.9 ± 5.4	122.5 ± 7.8	51.6 ± 2.0	29.6 ± 1.4
P Value	.082	.368	<.001	<.001

SC = serum cholesterol; TG = triglycerides; HDLC = high density lipoprotein cholesterol.

than those of controls (5.14 $\pm$ 0.88 mg/hr/100 ml). Because of the small sample size, a more detailed analysis for the women was not feasible.

These results indicate that the uremic patients had impaired ability for cholesterol transport. An impaired ability of HDL to pick up cholesterol from peripheral tissues could result in decreased HDL cholesterol levels, and subsequently decrease RCT. Our data further showed that the decreased RCT in the uremic patients could not be totally accounted for by their lower HDL cholesterol levels, as patients matched with controls for HDL cholesterol levels also had significantly lower RCT. Whatever causes the decreases in RCT in uremia, the outcome of the defect in cholesterol transfer could enhance the accumulation of tissue cholesterol and accelerate atherosclerosis.

REFERENCES

1. Lowrie, E.G., Lazarus, J.M., Mocelin, A.J. et al.: Survival of patients undergoing chronic hemodialysis and renal transplantation. N. Engl. J. Med. 288: 864, 1973.

2. Linder, A., Charra, B., Sherrard, D.J. et al.: Accelerated atherosclerosis in prolonged maintenance hemodialysis. N. Engl. J. Med. 290: 697, 1974.

3. Burke, J.F., Francos, G.C., Moore, L.L. et al.: Accelerated atherosclerosis in chronic dialysis patients - Another look. Nephron 21: 181, 1978.

4. Bagdade, J.D., Porte, D., Jr. and Bierman, E.L.: Hypertriglyceridemia: A metabolic consequence of chronic renal failure. N. Engl. J. Med. 279: 181, 1968.

5. Ibels, L.S., Simons, L.A., King, J.O. et al.: Studies on the nature and causes of hyperlipidemia in uremia, maintenance hemodialysis and renal transplantation. Q.J. Med. 44: 601, 1976.

6. Bagdade, J.D., Casaretto, A. and Albers, J.: Effects of chronic uremia, hemodialysis and renal transplantation on plasma lipids and lipoproteins in man. J. Lab. Clin. Med. 87: 37, 1976.

7. Ibels, S.L., Reardon, M.F. and Nestel, P.J.: Plasma postheparin lipolytic activity and triglyceride clearance in uremic and hemodialysis patients and renal allograft recipients. J. Lab. Clin. Med. 87: 648, 1976.

8. Dombeck, D.H., Lindholm, D.D. and Vieira, J.A.: Lipid metabolism in uremia and the effects of dialysate glucose and oral androgen therapy. Transactions ASAIO 13: 150, 1973.

9. Kaye, J.P., Moorhead, J.F. and Willis, M.R.: Plasma lipids in patients with chronic renal failure. Clin. Chim. Acta. 44: 301, 1973.

10. Henck, C.C., Ritz, E., Liersch, M. et al.: Serum lipids in renal insufficiency. Am. J. Clin. Nutr. 31: 1547, 1978.

11. Bagdade, J., Yee, E. and Pykalisto, O.J.: Parathyroid hormone and triglyceride transport: Effects on triglyceride secretion rates and adipose tissue lipoprotein lipase in the rat. Horm. Metab. Res. 10: 443, 1978.

12. Mordasini, R., Frey, F., Flury, W. et al.: Selective deficiency of hepatic triglyceride lipase in uremic patients. N. Engl. J. Med. 297: 1362, 1977.

13. Cattran, D.C., Steiner, G., Fenton, S.S.A. et al.: Hypertriglyceridemia in uremia and the use of triglyceride turnover to define pathogenesis. Transactions ASAIO 20: 148, 1974.

14. Boyer, J.L. and Scheig, R.L.: Inhibition of post-heparin lipolytic activity in uremia and its relationship to hypertriglyceridemia. Proc. Soc. Exp. Biol. Med. 134: 603, 1970.

15. Murase, T., Cattran, D.C., Rubenstein, B. et al.: Inhibition of lipoprotein lipase by uremic plasma: A possible cause of hypertriglyceridemia. Metabolism 24: 1279, 1975.

16. Austin, W. and Nestel, P.J.: The effect of glucose and insulin in vitro on the uptake of triglyceride and on lipoprotein lipase activity in fat pads from normal fed rats. Biochem. Biophys. Acta 164: 59, 1968.

17. Rapoport, J., Aviram, M., Chaimovitz, C. et al.: Defective high-density lipoprotein composition in patients on chronic hemodialysis. N. Engl. J. Med. 299: 1326, 1978.

18. Cattran, D.C., Fenton, S.A., Wilson, D.R. et al.: Defective triglyceride removal in lipemia associated with peritoneal dialysis and hemodialysis. Ann. Intern. Med. 85: 29, 1976.

19. Bagdade, J.D., Yee, E., Wilson, D.E. et al.: Hyperlipidemia in renal failure: Studies of plasma lipoproteins, hepatic triglyceride production, and tissue lipoprotein lipase in a chronically uremic rat model. J. Lab. Clin. Med. 91: 176, 1978.

20. Quellhorst, E., Rieger, J., Doht, B. et al.: Treatment of chronic uraemia by an ultrafiltration artificial kidney - first clinical experience. Proc. Europ. Dial. Transpl. Assoc. 12: 314, 1976.

21. Choi, E.S.K., Chung, T., Morrison, R. et al.: Hypertriglyceridemia in hemodialysis patients during oral dromostanolone therapy for anemia. Am. J. Clin. Nutr. 27: 901, 1974.

22. Brunzell, J.D., Albers, J.J., Haas, L.B. et al.: Prevalence of serum lipid abnormalities in chronic hemodialysis. Metab. 26: 903, 1977.

23. Daubrese, J.C., Lerson, G., Plomteux, G. et al.: Lipids and lipoproteins in chronic uraemia. A study of the influence of regular hemodialysis. Europ. J. Clin. Invest. 6: 159, 1976.

24. Berger, M., James, G.P., Davis, E.R. et al.: Hyperlipidemia in uremic children: Response to peritoneal dialysis and hemodialysis. Clin. Nephrol. 9: 19, 1978.

25. Davidson, W.D., Morin, R.J., Rorke, S.J. et al.: The role of acetate in dialysate for hemodialysis. Proc. 10th Ann. Contr. Conf. Artif. Kidney Prog. NIAMDD, DHEW Publication No. (NIH) 77-1442, 1977, p. 15.

26. Miller, G.J. and Miller, N.E.: Plasma-high-density lipoprotein concentration and development of ischaemic heart disease. Lancet 1: 16, 1975.

27. Stein, Y., Galngeaud, M.C., Fainru, M. et al.: The removal of cholesterol from aortic smooth muscle cells in culture and Landschutz ascites cells by fractions of human high-density lipoprotein. Biochim. Biophys. Acta 380: 106, 1975.

28. Baily, J.M.: Regulation of cell cholesterol content. In Porter, R. and Knight, J. (eds.): Atherosclerosis: Initiating Factors. Amsterdam: Elsevier, 1973, p. 63.

29. Bohdjers, G. and Buorkerud, S.: Cholesterol transfer between arterial smooth muscle tissue and serum lipoprotein in vitro. Artery 1: 3, 1974.

30. Glomset, J.A.: The plasma lecithin cholesterol acyl transferase reaction. J. Lipid Res. 9: 155, 1968.

31. Koschinsky, T., Carew, T.E. and Steinberg, D.: Binding, internalization, and degradation of high density lipoprotein by cultured normal human fibroblasts. J. Lipid Res. 18: 438, 1977.

32. Guarnieri, G.F., Moracchiello, M., Campanacci, L. et al.: Lecithin-cholesterol acyl transferase (LCAT) activity in chronic uremia. Kidney Int. 13: S-26, 1978.

33. Brunzell, J.D., Albers, J.J., Haas, L.B. et al.: Prevalence of serum lipid abnormalities in chronic dialysis. Metab. 26: 903, 1977.

34. Bagdade, J.D. and Albers, J.J.: Plasma high-density lipoprotein concentrations in chronic hemodialysis and renal transplant patients. N. Engl. J. Med. 296: 1436, 1977.

35. Perez, G.O., Hsia, S.L., Christakis, G. et al.: Serum cholesterol binding reserve and high density lipoprotein cholesterol in patients on maintenance hemodialysis. Horm. Metab. Res. (In press).

36. Hsia, S.L., Chao, Y.S., Hennekens, C.H. et al.: Decreased serum cholesterol binding reserve in premature myocardial infarction. Lancet 2: 1000, 1975.

37. Hsia, S.L., Fishman, L.M., Briese, F.W. et al.: Decreased serum cholesterol binding reserve in diabetes mellitus. Diabetes Care 1: 89, 1978.

38. Perez, G.O., Levine, S., Gomez, E. et al.: Serum cholesterol binding reserve in patients with the nephrotic syndrome. Nephron 24: 146, 1979.

39. Chajek, T. and Fielding, C.J.: Isolation and characterization of a human serum cholesteryl ester transfer protein. Proc. Natl. Acad. Sci. U.S.A. 75: 3445, 1978.

40. Nestel, P.J., Reardon, M. and Billington, T.: In vivo transfer of cholesteryl esters from high-density lipoproteins to very low-density lipoproteins in man. Biochim. Biophys. Acta 573: 403, 1979.

ALUMINUM IN CHRONIC RENAL FAILURE: A PEDIATRIC PERSPECTIVE

Martin S. Polinksy, M.D., Alan B. Gruskin, M.D., H. Jorge Baluarte, M.D., James W. Prebis, M.D., and Abdelaziz Y. Elzouki, M.D.

Dept. Pediatr., St. Christopher's Hosp. for Children and Temple Univ. Sch. Med., Philadelphia, Pa. 19133

During the past decade it has been suggested that aluminum may be substantially more toxic to the human body than had previously been thought (1). Much evidence has accumulated implicating aluminum, either directly or indirectly, in the pathogenesis of several forms of progressive central nervous system dysfunction, bone disease, and possibly cardiac and hematologic disturbances. For reasons which will be discussed below patients with renal insufficiency may be at greater risk of developing these sequelae which appear to be associated with an increasingly positive body aluminum balance. Although these problems have been reported almost exclusively in adults, it has become increasingly apparent that pediatric patients may be similarly affected. Consequently, an understanding of the current status of aluminum as a potential toxin is important to those caring for children with chronic renal disease. This paper will review 1) major environmental sources of aluminum, particularly those of importance to patients with chronic renal insufficiency; 2) factors affecting the uptake, distribution, and elimination of aluminum in normal individuals and those with diminished renal function; and 3) the evidence for aluminum toxicity, and its relevance to organ system dysfunction in renal insufficiency.

Supported in part by General Clinical Research Center Grant RR-75 and Hoechst-Roussel Pharmaceuticals.

ENVIRONMENTAL SOURCES OF ALUMINUM

Aluminum is the commonest metal and the third most common element in the earth's crust, of which it comprises 8%. Thus, it is not surprising that aluminum is normally found in most human tissues, the highest levels being in the lung (2). Continued exposure thoughout life appears to be associated with progressive accumulation in some organs, as suggested by the finding at autopsy of significantly higher mean aluminum levels in the brains of patients over 70 years of age as compared to those in a younger group (3).

The environmental sources of aluminum from which increased intake may occur are summarized in Table 1. Major interest in recent years has focused on gastric antacids and the water used to prepare dialysate as sources of aluminum for patients with chronic renal failure; these will be discussed in greater detail below. The extent to which the other sources listed may represent a significant risk to renal patients has yet to be determined.

Table 1. Potential Sources of Increased Body Aluminum Burden*

1. Aluminum-containing phosphate-binding gels, antacids (4)

2. Water treated by alum precipitation (5,6), water supply derived from watershed fed by acid rains

   (a) drinking water
   (b) used for hemodialysis

3. Edible vegetation

4. Aluminum cooking utensils and foil wrap

5. Other sources

   (a) inhalation - aerosolized antiperspirants; aluminum dust; alumina volatilized during coal burning
   (b) cutaneous absorption - astringents (e.g., Burow's solution

*From Reference 1, except where otherwise indicated.

ALUMINUM METABOLISM: FACTORS AFFECTING UPTAKE, DISTRIBUTION, AND ELIMINATION (TABLE 2)

Gastrointestinal Absorption

Plasma aluminum levels increase following both acute and chronic oral administration of aluminum-containing antacids to normal and uremic man and laboratory animals (4,7-11). Gorsky et al. (7) demonstrated that only a small, but variable percent of aluminum was absorbed (2.1-24.4%; mean 14.4%) after chronic ingestion of pharmacologic doses of antacid; yet, these quantities were sufficient to produce daily aluminum balance during the period of study. This apparent discrepancy was attributed to the limited aluminum-excretory capacity of the kidneys which, nonetheless, constitute the major route by which absorbed aluminum is eliminated from the body, even in the presence of reduced glomerular function (see below). A day-to-day variability in gastrointestinal aluminum absorption has been observed and attributed to normal variations in intestinal motility (7).

Gastrointestinal absorption of aluminum has also been demonstrated indirectly in normal volunteers by an increase in daily

Table 2. Factors Affecting Body Aluminum Balance

A. Uptake
   1. Gastrointestinal absorption
      (a) quantity of aluminum ingested
      (b) intestinal motility
      (c) parathyroid hormone
   2. Parenteral acquisition: aluminum concentration of dialysate
B. Distribution
   1. Plasma protein binding
   2. Parathyroid hormone-enhanced tissue uptake
C. Elimination
   1. Excretion
      (a) biliary
      (b) renal
   2. Gastrointestinal secretion

urinary aluminum excretion, from less than 50 μg to greater than 500 μg after two days of oral loading (12). In addition, whole blood aluminum levels have been shown to correlate significantly with the estimated quantities of aluminum ingested by dialysis patients in the form of phosphate-binding gels (13). Similarly, serum aluminum levels are higher in dialyzed and non-dialyzed patients receiving phosphate-binding gels when compared to those for whom they were not prescribed (11). Mean blood aluminum levels for several groups of normal adult controls have recently been reported and range from 3.7 to 28 μg/l (Table 3). Comparable data for children are not currently available.

Parathyroid hormone (PTH) excess augments the gastrointestinal absorption of aluminum. Rats given PTH extract and fed aluminum chloride show enchanced uptake and parenchymal tissue deposition as compared to those fed identical amounts of aluminum but given no PTH (9). This effect is reversible following discontinuation of PTH administration (18). Significant correlations have also been demonstrated between serum levels of PTH and those of aluminum in whole blood and in hair (13). These observations suggest that patients with chronic renal insufficiency may be at greater risk for developing toxic sequelae due to the parenchymal accumulation of aluminum absorbed from orally ingested phosphate-binding gels, since many have some degree of secondary hyperparathyroidism.

Parenteral Acquisition of Aluminum

Water may also contribute to body aluminum burden. Water treated by alum (aluminum sulfate) precipitation may contain metal concentrations as high as 1200 μg/l (19) unless further treated to remove ionic contamination by deionization or reverse osmosis. Although patients with chronic renal insufficiency may acquire some aluminum from drinking water, they are exposed to far greater volumes of water during each dialysis (approximately 120 liters/ 4-hour treatment, at a dialysate flow rate of 500 ml/min). Kaehny et al. (20) have shown that aluminum is transferred across the

Table 3. Blood Aluminum Levels in Normal Controls

Serum/Plasma Aluminum, μg/l	Reference
28 ± 9	14
24.3 ± 8.4	14a
23.2 ± 7.3	15
12.0 ± 4.0	16
6 ± 3	4
3.72 ± 1.2	17

dialyzer membrane from dialysate to blood; this transfer occurs *into* the patient even when blood aluminum levels exceed those of dialysate. Moreover, aluminum is dialyzed *out* of blood with great difficulty, although it is readily added. These findings may be explained by the recent observation that aluminum in blood is highly protein-bound (21). The ultrafiltrable fraction has been found to vary between 10 and 40% and to decrease with decreasing total plasma aluminum concentration; at levels appreciably below 200 μg/l most plasma aluminum is protein-bound (22).

Other studies have documented a relationship between specific tissue aluminum burdens and the duration of exposure to high aluminum-containing dialysate. In the patients with dialysis encephalopathy (see below) reported by McDermott et al. (19) and Alfrey et al. (23), the aluminum levels in brain gray matter correlated significantly with duration of dialysis (19,23). Elliott et al (24) have shown plasma aluminum to be significantly related to the aluminum concentration of the untreated tap water used to prepare dialysate.

Major Routes of Elimination of Body Aluminum

Aluminum introduced into the body parenterally or via the gastrointestinal tract is eliminated by urinary and biliary excretion (4,12,25). Urinary aluminum excretion in normal adults increased to rates 50 times greater than control values during three days of oral loading with aluminum-containing antacids (4). A recent investigation of the urinary and biliary excretion routes in normal and acutely uremic dogs (25) has shown that following parenteral aluminum loading via hemodialysis:

1. biliary aluminum excretion increased significantly but accounted for elimination of only 0.1% of the administered dose;
2. the extent to which biliary excretion rose was not significantly greater in the presence of acute renal failure; and
3. the kidneys provided the major route for aluminum elimination, with 37% of the total load excreted by eight hours post-dialysis.

Thus, patients with chronic renal insufficiency may develop an increasingly positive body aluminum balance because of diminished or absent renal function in the presence of prolonged exposure to the aluminum in dialysate and/or phosphate-binding gels. It is these patients who should be at greatest risk for developing any toxicity associated with aluminum overload.

TOXIC EFFECTS OF ALUMINUM

A physiologic role for aluminum has not yet been identified, at least to the extent that attempts to produce a deficiency state through restriction of dietary intake have failed (2). Conversely, aluminum may be a biologic poison when present in the body in sufficient quantities, as suggested by observations made over several decades. The principal toxic effects attributed to aluminum are summarized in Table 4.

Table 4. Toxic Effects Attributed to Aluminum

A. Enzyme inhibition

1. Hexokinase
2. Dihydropteridine (dihydrobiopterin) reductase
3. Ferroxidase

B. Aluminum binding to nuclear chromatin. ?Interference with DNA replication/RNA transcription

C. Effects on individual organ systems

1. CNS

   (a) seizures and neurofibrillary degeneration in animals
   (b) inhibition of neuronal microtubule protein subunit aggregation
   (c) disturbed conditioned behavior in animals
   (d) ?interference with transport and storage of catecholamines by cerebral cortical synaptosomes
   (e) clinical disorders:
   - dialysis encephalopathy (dialysis dementia)
   - Altzheimer disease

2. Bone - fracturing dialysis osteodystrophy

3. Cardiovascular

4. Hematologic

5. Respiratory - Shaver disease (26)

6. Phosphate depletion (27) (neuromuscular, skeletal, hematologic effects)

Mechanisms of Aluminum Toxicity

While the mechanisms by which aluminum may exert its toxic effects on cellular metabolism are not yet known, several observations are of interest in this regard. Aluminum has been noted to bind directly to nuclear chromatin (28) and thus may interfere with DNA replication and/or RNA transcription. Ribosomal RNA levels have also been found to be depressed in aluminum-treated neuroblastoma cells (29). Inhibitory effects on isolated enzyme systems have been noted in vitro (30-33), suggesting that aluminum may disrupt cellular function at more than one site. With respect to central nervous system dysfunction, it has also been suggested that aluminum may diminish catecholamine neurotransmitter levels in central adrenergic presynaptic terminals, either by inhibiting their synthesis (31) or their uptake and storage (33-34a). Aluminum has also been shown to inhibit the aggregation of neuronal microtubules in adult rabbit brains in vitro (35), an observation of possible relevance to the pathogenesis of the "neurofibrillary tangles" described in the brains of patients dying with Altzheimer disease (3,36,37).

Aluminum and Neurologic Disease

Evidence that aluminum may be neurotoxic has existed since 1897, when Doellken (38) reported disturbances in central nervous system function and morphology following the systemic administration of aluminum salts to laboratory animals. Its epileptogenic properties were investigated by Kopeloff, et al. (39) who produced seizures in rabbits by applying alum-containing discs directly to the leptomeninges. Since then seizures and neurofibrillary degeneration (neurofibrillary tangles) have been produced in animals following the intracerebral, intrathecal, and subcutaneous administration of aluminum salts (40,41).

Chronic oral administration of aluminum to rats has been shown to affect the acquisition of shuttlebox avoidance, a form of conditioned behavior (42). Aluminum-related behavioral disturbances have also been observed in cats (43a-b).

Perhaps the most incriminating evidence that aluminum may be neurotoxic in man has come from attempts to understand the causes of dialysis dementia (dialysis encephalopathy). This is a syndrome of progressive neurologic dysfunction first described by Alfrey (44) in adults who were stable on maintenance hemodialysis for 3-6 years. Since then other patients have been reported to have developed the syndrome after as few as seven months on dialysis (45). The earliest and most characteristic manifestations of the dialysis dementia syndrome include speech disturbances, mental changes, and an abnormal electroencephalogram, the latter characterized by generalized slowing of the background rhythm with multifocal, paroxysmal discharges of high amplitude delta waves. Electroencephalographic changes have been shown to antedate the clinical onset of disease by several months (46) if screening studies are routinely performed.

The clinical syndrome is heralded by the onset of speech disturbances which have been characterized by dysarthria, dyspraxia, and dysphasia (47). Mental changes have begun insidiously in some, with forgetfulness, decreased ability to concentrate, and changes in affect. In others, a delirium or toxic psychosis may occur acutely during dialysis. Ultimately, progressive dementia becomes apparent. Motor disturbances are seen, including asterixis, myoclonus, apraxia, facial grimacing, tremor and twitching. Seizures, either focal or generalized, are also characteristic. The disturbances usually first appear during dialysis and disappear during the interdialytic period; later on they become persistent. Secondary hyperparathyroidism is usually present, as it often is in association with severe chronic renal insufficiency, and may be pathogenetically related to this disorder (see below).

Response to therapy has generally been poor. Diazepam therapy improves seizure control, electroencephalographic abnormalities, and the movement and speech disorders (44,46,48). Increased dialysis time has failed to produce improvement, as would be expected with most other neurologic disturbances associated with uremia per se; this is one of the most characteristic features of the syndrome, and best serves to differentiate it from those other disorders. Renal transplantation has also failed to halt disease progression (46). Other therapies have been attempted, generally without success (45,46).

The differential diagnosis of dialysis encephalopathy must include other, commoner causes of neurologic dysfunction in patients with chronic renal failure. Uremic encephalopathy usually responds to adequate hemo- or peritoneal dialysis, and to renal transplantation with establishment of adequate function. Electrolyte and metabolic imbalance (hyponatremia, hypocalcemia, hypo- and hyperglycemia (49)) may produce seizures; phosphate depletion has produced a syndrome of neurologic dysfunction clinically similar to that of dialysis encephalopathy (50), with symptoms usually appearing at serum phosphorus levels below 2 mg/dl in the adult (36). The possibility of a pre-existing neurologic disorder should be considered, especially that associated with familial or hereditary disease. Hypertensive encephalopathy and central nervous system infection (abscess, meningitis, encephalitis) should be ruled out by appropriate studies. Finally, in the dialysis patient who develops seizures or other alterations in mental status, hypotension, dialysis dysequilibrium, intracranial hemorrhage and, rarely, thiamine deficiency (49,51) should be considered in addition to the causes just noted.

The etiology of this dialysis-related encephalopathy remains unknown, although multiple factors have been considered (8). Particular emphasis has been placed on the possible roles of aluminum and PTH in the pathogenesis of the syndrome. The serum aluminum levels of home hemodialysis patients have been shown to correlate with the concentration of metal present in the untreated tap water used to prepare their dialysate (24). Alfrey et al. (23) showed cerebral gray matter aluminum levels to be significantly higher in dialyzed patients with encephalopathy than in those dying of nonneurologic causes; however, these levels were positively correlated with the number of months on dialysis. These finds were subsequently confirmed by McDermott et al. (19), who further demonstrated that it was not the overall duration of dialysis, but duration of therapy with nondeionized, aluminum-rich dialysate which correlated best with mean gray matter aluminum levels. The last observation may explain the different attack rates for dialysis encephalopathy noted in several adult dialysis centers in the U.S. (52). Epidemic occurrences of the encephalopathy in Chicago (6) and Alma, Michigan (5) were temporarily related to the use of alum precipitation in purifying water supplied to the dialysis units in those municipalities, at a time when no in-center deionization units were operational. With the institution of deionization and cessation of alum precipitation, dialysate aluminum levels fell dramatically and no new cases of the encephalopathy occurred. The development of dialysis encephalopathy thus appears to be more closely related to aluminum toxicity than to dialysis per se.

As noted previously aluminum absorbed from the gastrointestinal tract may constitute an additional source of increased uptake for dialysis patients ingesting large quantities of antacids for control of hyperphosphatemia (23). The extent to which aluminum ingestion may be hazardous to patients with chronic renal insufficiency has, however, remained controversial because of the failure of some investigators to establish significant relationships between oral aluminum intake and either tissue levels (19) or the occurrence of dialysis encephalopathy (53). Conversely, Hendricks et al. (13) have shown whole blood aluminum levels to be significantly correlated with the estimated quantity of aluminum ingested by 21 dialysis patients. In addition, several patients with dialysis encephalopathy showed symptomatic improvement following withdrawal of therapy with aluminum-containing phosphate-binders (54). Failure to relate oral aluminum intake per se to body burden or the occurrence of toxic sequelae may be due to 1) noncompliance with prescribed regimens for taking phosphate-binding gels; 2) the concomitant uptake of aluminum from other sources, such as dialysate (19); or 3) variation in the percent of the ingested dose which is absorbed from day-to-day (7).

The secondary hyperparathyroidism of chronic renal insufficiency has also been identified as a potential risk factor for the development of dialysis encephalopathy. PTH in excess can alter brain function in man and laboratory animals (55,56) as manifested by abnormalities in the electroencephalogram and, in humans, by poor performance on cognitive function studies. These disturbances were reversed or prevented by parathyroidectomy. Moreover, two patients with dialysis encephalopathy experienced dramatic improvement in their neurologic symptoms following subtotal parathyroidectomy for severe hyperparathyroidism (46,57). The hormone has also been shown to enhance gastrointestinal absorption of aluminum and its selective deposition in cerebral gray matter (9). Whether PTH is directly toxic to cerebral cortical neurons or acts indirectly by enhancing neuronal aluminum accumulation has yet to be determined.

Aluminum and Unexplained Neurologic Dysfunction In Childhood Uremia

Until recently this syndrome of unexplained encephalopathy remained an adult problem. However, in 1977 five children being treated for progressive renal insufficiency were reported to have developed a syndrome of progressive neurologic dysfunction clinically indistinguishable from that of adult dialysis encephalopathy (58). All of the children had congenital renal disease (hypo- and/or dysplasia) initially diagnosed between 3 weeks and 6½ years of age. At the time of onset of neurologic symptoms they were between 2 and 10 years old, had elevated BUN and creatinine concentrations and glomerular filtration rates (GFR) of 5-10 ml/min/1.73 m^2. Neurologic disturbances in the children differed from those reported in adults only in that they developed prior to their having received any dialysis. Electroencephalograms were abnormal in all five patients, showing progressive slowing and disorganization of the background rhythm and paroxysmal bursts of high amplitude, 2-4 Hz polyspike wave discharges (58).

The encephalopathy in these patients could not be related to pre-existing neurologic disease, hypertension, or electrolyte or metabolic disturbances associated with uremia per se, which was substantiated by failure of hemo- and peritoneal dialysis to effect improvement in the three patients in whom it was attempted. No difference in neurologic status was noted between dialyzed and nondialyzed patients. Likewise, renal transplantation failed to improve the status of two patients with adequately functioning grafts (GFR greater than 50 ml/min/1.73 m^2). Anticonvulsant therapy improved seizure control and myoclonus but did not alter disease progression. (Two patients died and three are currently severely neurologically impaired.)

All of the patients had severe secondary hyperparathyroidism as evidenced by serum PTH levels of 500-2100 pg/ml (normal less than 300 pg/ml), elevated serum alkaline phosphatase concentrations and radiographic changes consistent with osteitis fibrosa. Hyperphosphatemia (serum phosphorus greater than 6 mg/dl) necessitated the continuous oral administration of massive doses of aluminum-containing phosphate-binding gels (240-800 mg/kg/day) for 4-12 months and lesser doses (90-200 mg/kg/day) for 9-62 months, resulting in considerable exposure to exogenous aluminum. All of the patients experienced the onset of neurological deterioration within six months of beginning maximum dose phosphate-binder therapy. Although blood and tissue aluminum levels were unavailable, the clinical course in all five patients was indistinguishable from that described in dialysis encephalopathy, and they all had exposure to the same potential risk factors for the development of aluminum intoxication as have been identified in adults. These observations suggest that the adult and pediatric syndromes may represent the same or similar disease processes.

Additional cases of an unexplained encephalopathy similar to those described above were identified in a recent epidemiologic survey of 96 pediatric dialysis and transplant centers (59). Fourteen of 61 centers (9 U.S.; 5 foreign) reported that 24 of their 728 end-stage renal disease patients had developed an encephalopathy characterized by mental changes (personality disturbances, dementia, regressing of developmental milestones), speech disturbances, seizures, and focal or generalized electroencephalographic abnormalities. None of the cases could be explained on the basis of preexisting neurologic disease, hypertension, dialysis dysequilibrium, or electrolyte or metabolic disorders associated with uremia per se. Nearly 74% of affected children had *congenital* renal disease; in the remaining 26% an acquired etiology was responsible for renal failure. All of the centers reported that patients had received or were receiving aluminum-containing phosphate-binding gels prior to or at the time of appearance of symptoms. Secondary hyperparathyroidism was reported in all but one patient. Thirty-one percent of centers reported that affected patients had not received dialysis prior to onset of symptoms, in contrast to the previously-discussed adult experience. However, the adult encephalopathy has also developed prior to initiation of dialysis, to which it then failed to respond (60).

These results indicate that dialysis, secondary hyperparathyroidism, and aluminum intake are associated with the occurrence of a neurologic syndrome similar to that seen in adults with dialysis encephalopathy, and that the problem in pediatrics is also global in its scope. Most important is the observation that the majority of cases occurred in children with congenital renal disease, consistent with the fact that the nervous systems of these children may ultimately be exposed to the effects of renal insufficiency for a longer time and from an earlier stage of development than is true for those with acquired disease. Since the congenital nephropathies are a major cause of childhood chronic renal insufficiency, the associated problem of progressive and unexplained neurologic dysfunction, particularly the nature of its relationship to aluminum exposure, hyperparathyroidism, and the adult syndrome of dialysis encephalopathy, warrants further study.

Aluminum and Bone Disease

A number of studies strongly implicate bone aluminum accumulation in the pathogenesis of adult renal osteodystrophy, particularly in dialysis patients. Nearly ten years ago Parsons et al. (61) demonstrated a mean 6-fold higher bone aluminum content in Newcastle patients receiving, as compared to those with acute and chronic renal failure not receiving, dialysis. A strong association between aluminum exposure, dialysis encephalopathy, and osteomalacic renal osteodystrophy was subsequently noted in an epidemiologic survey of chronic renal failure patients who were dialyzed at home in several areas of Great Britain (62). A significant correlation between biopsy-proven osteomalacia and cortical gray matter aluminum levels has also been demonstrated by the Newcastle group (19). Alfrey et al. (23) demonstrated markedly elevated aluminum levels in biopsy specimens of trabecular bone from patients dying with dialysis encephalopathy, as compared to control values. More recently, an inverse linear relationship was demonstrated between the aluminum and ash contents of bone specimens from dialysis patients in several U.S. cities (63). Furthermore, bone aluminum correlated directly, and ash content indirectly with duration of dialysis. Aluminum may also be associated with bone disease in patients with normal renal function (12).

That aluminum intoxication may be associated with pediatric renal osteodystrophy remains to be investigated. Findings such as those noted above would have important implications in the management of bone disease in uremic children and adolescents, for whom growth retardation may pose major emotional problems (64). Examination of bone biopsy specimens from children with renal osteodystrophy, both histologically and for aluminum content, are needed to clarify this issue.

Aluminum and the Blood-Vascular System

Aluminum inhibition of myocardial energy production was suggested as the cause of otherwise unexplained acute cardiac death in four patients with dialysis encephalopathy (65). Several patients from the same dialysis unit also developed a progressive anemia which was attributed to aluminum inhibition of "enzymes concerned in haem biosynthesis" (24). These observations remain to be substantiated. Such relationships have not yet been reported in children.

CONCLUSIONS

Although much evidence currently exists implicating aluminum in the pathogenesis of the dialysis encephalopathy syndrome and some forms of renal osteodystrophy, persuasive arguments to the contrary have been put forth (8). Nonetheless, the *potential* neurotoxicity of aluminum should be considered in the management of the metabolic complications of chronic renal insufficiency in children. In an attempt to reduce this potential risk for the development of toxic sequelae related to increased body aluminum burden, a number of recommendations have been made:

1. Dialysate should be prepared from water treated by reverse osmosis or deionization, and the aluminum levels therein monitored frequently and maintained below 10-20 μg/l (5,62);
2. Wherever possible, plasma aluminum levels should be monitored periodically in patients receiving dialysis and/or aluminum-containing phosphate-binding gels;
3. In patients exhibiting clinical and electroencephalographic signs of unexplained or progressive neurologic dysfunction, the presence of elevated plasma aluminum levels (Table 3) should be taken as an indication to consider temporarily discontinuing therapy with aluminum-containing medicinals and to check dialysate for possible sources of contamination (66). The patient should then be followed for a prolonged period of time before renewed contact with major sources of aluminum is permitted, as clinical improvement has occurred up to nine months after discontinuation of phosphate-binding gels (54). Clinical improvement should be taken as evidence that aluminum intoxication was present and no further phosphate-binding gels prescribed;
4. Particular emphasis should be placed on the control of secondary hyperparathyroidism in patients with elevated plasma aluminum levels, especially if unexplained, persistent neurologic dysfunction develops. Severe hyperparathyroidism in such a patient may indicate the need for subtotal parathyroidectomy;
5. The presence of progressive osteodystrophy with fractures in a pediatric patient receiving dialysis should prompt an investigation for possible causes. The presence and severity of osteitis fibrosa and associated secondary hyperparathyroidism should be determined. If the primary lesion identified is rickets or osteomalacia, and phosphate depletion and inadequate therapy with vitamin D metabolites are not found to be responsible (67), an evaluation for possible increased bone aluminum burden is indicated.

Bone biopsy, with determination of trabecular bone aluminum levels (23), may be necessary to establish the diagnosis. (It is emphasized that the concomitant presence of osteitis fibrosa and secondary hyperparathyroidism does not eliminate aluminum intoxication as a factor contributing to the patient's bone pathology, as PTH excess may, as previously noted, enhance skeletal aluminum uptake (9).)

REFERENCES

1. Campbell, I.R., Cass, J.S., Cholak, J. et al: Aluminum in the environment of man. AMA Arch. Indust. Health 15: 359, 1957.

2. Trace Elements in Human and Animal Nutrition (4th Ed.), Underwood, E. (ed.), Academic Press, N.Y., 1977, p. 431.

3. McDermott, J.R., Smith, A.I., Igbal, K. et al: Brain aluminum in aging and Altzheimer disease. Neurol. 29: 809, 1979.

4. Kaehny, W.D., Hegg, A.P. and Alfrey, A.C.: Gastrointestinal absorption of aluminum from aluminum-containing antacids. N. Engl. J. Med. 296 (24): 1389, 1977.

5. Rozas, V.V., Port, F.K. and Easterling, R.E.: An outbreak of dialysis dementia due to aluminum in the dialysate. J. Dial. 2 (5 & 6): 459, 1978.

6. Dunea, G., Mahurkar, S.D., Mamdani, B. et al: Role of aluminum in dialysis dementia. Ann. Intern. Med. 88: 502, 1978.

7. Gorsky, J.E., Dietz, A.A., Spencer, H. et al: Metabolic balance of aluminum studied in six men. Clin. Chem. 25 (10): 1739, 1979.

8. Arieff, A.I., Cooper, J.D. Armstrong, D. et al: Dementia, renal failure and brain aluminum. Ann. Intern. Med. 90: 741, 1979.

9. Mayor, G.H., Keiser, J.A., Makdani, D. et al: Aluminum absorption and distribution: Effect of parathyroid hormone. Science 197: 1187, 1977.

10. Clarkson, E.M., Luck, U.A., Hynson, W.V. et al.: The effect of aluminum hydroxide on calcium phosphorus and aluminum balances, the serum parathyroid hormone concentration and the aluminum content of bone in patients with chronic renal failure. Clin. Sci. 43: 519, 1972.

11. Boukari, M., Rottembourg, L., Jaudon, M-C. et al.: Influence de la prise prolongee de gels d'aluminum sur les taux seriques d'aluminum chez les patients atteintes d'insuffisance renale chronique. Nouv. Presse Med. 7 (2): 85, 1978.

12. Recker, R.R., Blotcky, A.J., Leffler, J.A. et al.: Evidence for aluminum absorption from the gastrointestinal tract and bone deposition by aluminum carbonate ingestion with normal renal function. J. Lab. Clin. Med. 90 (5): 810, 1978.

13. Hendricks, D., Mayor, G.H. and Sanchez, T.V.: Antemortem assessment of aluminum burdens in dialysis patients. (Abst.) Kidney Int. 12: 456, 1977.

14. Gorsky, J.E. and Dietz, A.A.: Determination of aluminum in biologic samples by atomic absorption spectrophotometry with a graphite furnace. Clin. Chem. 24: 1485, 1978.

14a. Clavel, J.P., Jaudon, M.D. and Galli, A.: Dosage de l'aluminum dans les liquides biologiques par spectrophotometric d'absorption atomique en four graphite. Ann. Biol. Clin. 36: 33, 1978.

15. Zumkley, H., Bertram, H.P., Lison, A. et al: Aluminum, zinc and copper concentrations in plasma in chronic renal insufficiency. Clin. Nephrol. 12 (1): 18, 1979.

16. Salvedo, A., Minia, C., Segagni, S. et al: Trace metal changes in dialysis fluid and blood of patients on hemodialysis. Int. J. Artif. Organs 2: 17, 1979.

17. Versieck, J.: Measuring aluminum levels (letter). N. Engl. J. Med. 302: 468, 1980.

18. Mayor, G.H., Sprague, S.M., Hourani, M.R. et al: Parathyroid hormone-mediated aluminum deposition and egress in the rat. Kidney Int. 17: 40, 1980.

19. McDermott, J.R., Smith, A.I., Ward, M.K. et al: Brain-aluminum concentration in dialysis encephalopathy. Lancet 1: 901, 1978.

20. Kaehny, W.D., Alfrey, A.C., Holman, R.E. et al: Aluminum transfer during hemodialysis. Kidney Int. 12: 361, 1977.

21. King, S.W., Willis, M.R. and Savory, J.: Serum binding of aluminum. Res. Clin. Pathol. & Pharmacol. 26 (6): 161, 1979.

22. Elliott, H.L., Macdougall, A.I., Fell, G.S. et al: Plasmapheresis, aluminum, and dialysis dementia. Lancet 2: 1255, 1978.

23. Alfrey, A.C., LeGendre, G.R. and Kaehny, W.D.: The dialysis encephalopathy syndrome. N. Engl. J. Med. 294 (4): 184, 1976.

24. Elliott, H.L., Dryburgh, F., Fell, G.S. et al.: Aluminum toxicity during regular hemodialysis. Br. Med. J. 1: 1101, 1978.

25. Kovalchik, M.T., Kaehny, W.D., Hegg, A.P. et al.: Aluminum kinetics during hemodialysis. J. Lab. Clin. Med. 92 (5): 712, 1979.

26. Shaver, C.G. and Riddell, A.R.: Lung changes associated with the manufacture of aluminum abrasives. J. Indust. Hyg. Toxic 29 (3): 145, 1947.

27. Hypophosphatemia - Medical Staff Conference, University of California, San Francisco, West J. Med. 122: 482, 1975.

28. DeBoni, U., Scott, J.W. and Crapper, D.R.: Intracellular aluminum binding: a histochemical study. Histochemie 40: 31, 1974.

29. Miller, C.A. and Levine, E.M.: Effects of aluminum salts on cultured neuroblastoma cells. J. Neurochem. 22: 751, 1974.

30. Harrison, W.H., Codd, E. and Gray, R.M.: Aluminum inhibition of hexokinase. Lancet 2: 277, 1972.

31. Leeming, R.J. and Blair, J.A.: Dialysis dementia, aluminum and tetrahydrobiopterin metabolism. Lancet 1: 556, 1979.

32. Huber, C.T. and Frieden, E.: The inhibition of ferroxidase by trivalent and other metal ions. J. Biol. Chem. 245 (15): 3979, 1970.

33. Bone, I. and Thomas, M.: Dialysis dementia, aluminum and tetrahydrobiopterin metabolism. Lancet 1: 782, 1979.

34. Colburn, R.W. and Maas, J.W.: Adenosine triphosphate-metal-norepinephrine ternary complexes and catecholamine binding. Nature 208 (5005): 37, 1965.

34a. Kirshner, N.: Uptake of catecholamines by a particulate fraction of the adrenal medulla. J. Biol. Chem. 237 (7): 2311, 1962.

35. Bonhaus, D.W., McCormack, K.M., Major, G.H. et al.: Effect of aluminum on microtubule subunit protein aggregation in vitro and microtubule formation in vivo. (Abst.) Kidney Int. 14: 671, 1978.

36. Crapper, D.R., Krishnan, S.S. and Dalton, A.J.: Brain aluminum distribution in Alzheimer disease and experimental neurofibrillary degeneration. Science 180: 511, 1973.

37. Crapper, D.R., Krishnan, S.S. and Quittkat, S.: Aluminum, neurofibrillary degeneration and Alzheimer disease. Brain 99: 67, 1976.

38. Doellken, V.: Uber die wirkung des aluminium mit besonderer berucksichtigung der durch das aluminum versursachten lasionen in zentralnervensystem. Naunyn-Schmiedebergs Arch. Exp. Path. Pharmak. 40: 58, 1897.

39. Kopeloff, L.M., Barrera, S.E. and Kopeloff, N.: Recurrent convulsive seizures in animals produced by immunologic and chemical means. Am. J. Psychiat. 98: 881, 1942.

40. Klatzo, I., Wisniewski, H. and Streicher, E.: Experimental production of neurofibrillary degeneration: I. Light microscopic observations. J. Neuropathol. Exp. Neurol. 24: 187, 1965.

41. DeBoni, U., Otvos, A., Scott, J.W. et al.: Neurofibrillary degeneration induced by systemic aluminum. Acta Neuropath. (Berl.) 35: 285, 1976.

42. Noordewier, B., Commissaris, R.L., Cordon, J. et al.: Effect of chronic oral aluminum on shuttlebox avoidance behavior in rats. (Abst.) Kidney Int. 14: 682, 1978.

43a. Crapper, D.R. and Dalton, A.J.: Alterations in short-term retention, conditioned avoidance response acquisition and motivation following aluminum induced neurofibrillary degeneration. Physiol. Behav. 10: 925, 1973.

43b. Crapper, D.R. and Dalton, A.J.: Aluminum-induced neurofibrillary degeneration, brain electrical activity and alteration in acquisition and retention. Physiol. Behav. 10: 935, 1973.

44. Alfrey, A.C., Mishell, J.M., Burks, J. et al.: Syndrome of dyspraxia and multifocal seizures associated with chronic hemodialysis. Trans. Am. Soc. Artif. Int. Organs 18: 257, 1972.

45. Mahurkar, S.D., Smith, E.C., Mamdani, B.H. et al.: Dialysis dementia - the Chicago experience. J. Dialysis 2 (5&6): 447, 1978.

46. Burks, J.S., Alfrey, A.C., Huddlestone, J. et al.: A fatal encephalopathy in chronic hemodialysis patients. Lancet 1: 764, 1976.

47. Rosenbek, J.C., McNeil, M.R., Lemme, M.L. et al: Speech and language findings in a chronic hemodialysis patient: a case report. J. Speech Hear. Dis. 40 (2): 245, 1975.

48. Nadel, A.M. and Wilson, W.P.: Dialysis encephalopathy: a possible seizure disorder. Neurology 26: 1130, 1976.

49. Martinez, W.C., Rapin, I. and Moore, C.L.: Neurologic complications of renal failure. In C.M. Edelmann, Jr. (ed.), Pediatric Kidney Disease, Boston, Little, Brown and Company, 1978, p. 417.

50. Pierides, A.M., Ward, M.K. and Kerr, D.N.S.: Haemodialysis encephalopathy: possible role of phosphate depletion. Lancet 1: 1234, 1976.

51. Raskin, N.H. and Fishman, R.A.: Neurologic disorders in renal failure. N. Engl. J. Med. 294 (4): 204, 1976.

52. Favero, M.S.: Epidemiologic investigation of dialysis encephalopathy. Proc. 11th Ann. Contract Conf. Artif. Kidney Chron. Uremia Prog. NIAMDD 11: 206, 1978.

53. Jacobs, C., Brunner, F.P., Chantler, C. et al: Combined report on regular dialysis and transplantation in Europe, VII, 1976. Proc. Eur. Dial. Transpl. Assoc. 14: 3, 1977.

54. Buge, A., Poisson, M., Masson, S. et al: Encephalopathie reversible des dialyses apres arret de l'apport d'aluminum. Nouv. Presse Med. 8 (34): 2729, 1979.

55. Guisado, R., Arieff, A.I. and Massry, S.G.: Changes in the electroencephalogram in acute uremia. Effects of parathyroid hormone and brain electrolytes. J. Clin. Invest. 55: 738, 1975.

56. Cogan, M.G., Covey, C.M., Arieff, A.I. et al: Central nervous system manifestations of hyperparathyroidism. Am. J. Med. 65: 963, 1978.

57. Ball, J.H., Butkus, D.E. and Madison, D.S.: Effect of subtotal parathyroidectomy on dialysis dementia. Nephron 18: 151, 1977.

58. Baluarte, H.J., Gruskin, A.B., Hiner, L.B. et al: Encephalopathy in children with chronic renal failure. Proc. Clin. Dial. Transpl. Forum 7: 95, 1977.

59. Polinsky, M.S., Prebis, J.W., Elzouki, A.Y. et al: The dialysis encephalopathy syndrome in childhood: results of a survey to determine incidence and geographic distribution of cases. (Abst.) Chronic Renal Dis. Conf. NIAMDD, Bethesda, Md., 1980, p. 58.

60. Etheridge, W.B. and O'Neill, Jr., W.M.: The "dialysis encephalopathy syndrome" without dialysis. Clin. Nephrol. 10 (6): 250, 1978.

61. Parsons, V., Davies, C., Goode, C. et al: Aluminum in bone from patients with renal failure. Br. Med. J. 2: 273, 1971.

62. Parkinson, I.S., Ward, M.K., Feest, T.G. et al: Fracturing dialysis osteodystrophy and dialysis encephalopathy: an epidemiologic survey. Lancet 1: 406, 1979.

63. Alfrey, A.C., Hegg, A., Miller, N. et al: Interrelationship between calcium and aluminum metabolism in dialyzed uremic patients. Mineral Electrolyte Metab. 2: 81, 1979.

64. Korsch, B.M., Fine, R.N., Grushkin, C.M. et al: Experience with children and their families during extended hemodialysis and kidney transplantation. Pediatr. Clin. N. Am. 18: 625, 1971.

65. Elliott, H.L., Macdougall, A.L. and Fell, G.S.: Aluminum toxicity syndrome. Lancet 1: 1203, 1978.

66. Flendrig, J.A., Kruis, H. and Das, H.A.: Aluminum and dialysis dementia. Lancet 1: 1235, 1976.

67. Ward, M.K., Feest, T.G., Ellis, H.A. et al: Ostomalacia dialysis osteodystrophy: evidence for a water-borne aetiologic agent, probably aluminum. Lancet 1: 841, 1978.

HIGHLIGHTS

LONG TERM CONSTANT RATE ENTERAL NUTRITION IN CHILDREN WITH RENAL DISEASE

Michel Broyer, M.D., M. Guillot, M.D., A.M. Dartois, M.D., *L. Cathelineau, M.D., *M. Guimbaud, M.D.

Serv. Nephol. Pediatr.,Hôpital Necker Enfants-Malades, Paris, France; *Pouponniere Croix Rouge, Margency, France

Constant rate enteral nutrition (CREN) has been generally used in intensive care units for the treatment of surgical or medical G.I. diseases, especially after large enteral resection. This is a report of the results obtained by long term utilization of CREN in infants and young children affected by nephropathies in which nutritional factors are involved: congenital nephrotic syndrome, severe infantile cystinosis, and chronic severe renal failure.

METHODS

CREN was administered 16 hr/day through polyvinyl naso-gastric catheters of different sizes by means of an eventually portable occlusive pump with careful control of tube position in the stomach; the catheter was changed every 3-4 days. Energy supply was calculated on the basis of the recommended dietary allowance (NRC 1968) for children of the same stature age. Protein intake was calculated on the same basis, taking into account the renal losses of nephrotic syndrome or the risks of uremic toxicity in case of renal insufficiency. Minerals were supplied according to the different situations.

Usual components of the mixture administered this way were, for proteins: modified cow's milk, low sodium milk, low lactose milk, hydrolysed casein and more rarely, colostrum, human milk or beef meat; for fat: vegetable oil, long and middle chain triglycerides; for carbohydrates: maltodextrine, polyglucose, saccharose, glucose, modified starch (cereal).

Congenital Nephrotic Syndrome (CNS)

Four children with CNS of Finnish type, respectively 29, four, one-half and seven months old at the beginning of treatment, received CREN during 15, 32, three and one-half, and 32 months. One of these patients died. The others are surviving and are at this time eight, six, and three years old; 100% mortality rate is expected at two years in this disease. CREN was followed by an increase of plasma albumin in spite of persistent proteinuria. All, except the infant who died, resumed stature growth; one of them caught up four standard deviations for height in one year.

Severe Infantile Cystinosis

Four children suffering from severe cystinosis with frequent vomiting and failure to thrive, respectively seven, 19, 11 and 35 months old at the beginning of treatment, received CREN during 14, 11, 37 and 26 months. All improved in condition and resumed stature growth. In spite of the severity of the disease, they survived and kept a height in the limit of the third or fourth standard deviation. Such cases at the same age usually are below the fifth, sixth, or seventh standard deviation for height.

Chronic Renal Insufficiency

Three children suffering from renal insufficiency also received CREN. The etiology of renal failure was hypoplastic kidneys in one case and neonatal bilateral renal vein thrombosis in two cases. Age at the beginning of treatment was respectively seven, two months and ten days. CREN was administered respectively during 15, 14 and four months.

Renal failure assessed by plasma creatinine varied with time. It worsened in the first case from 205 to 400 μ mol/l but improved in the two others respectively from 305 to 103 and from 530 to 230 μ mol/l; creatinine clearance at the beginning was respectively: 4, 5 and 7 ml/min/1.73 m^2. The general condition of these children improved and stature growth resumed in the first and second cases, the latter with a catch up curve; the third case lost three standard deviations during the first four months of life under CREN.

Comments and Conclusion

No complications related to nasogastric catheter occurred during a total of 203 patient months. Severing from CREN was often difficult but succeeded in two patients with CNS, two with cystinosis and one with renal insufficiency. Several attempts to suppress CREN failed in one patient with CNS, one with cystinosis, and two with renal insufficiency. Negative impact on psycho-affective development has to be considered, but five of these children were able to resume a normal family life, and seem to have no obvious sequelae of this long term enteral nutrition except for several months of refusal of all foods which are not mixed and homogenized. One is receiving CREN at home. Attempts will be made to generalize this approach in the future.

In conclusion, CREN has some precise indications in pediatric nephrology: it is a life-saving procedure in CNS and in cystinosis. In these two diseases as well as in severe renal failure, CREN is also almost always associated with a better growth velocity and could be a valuable tool for avoiding the irreversible height loss currently observed in the first year in patients with some renal diseases.

HIGHLIGHTS

CELL METABOLIC RESPONSES TO AMINO ACID INFUSIONS IN CHRONIC UREMIA

Jack Metcoff, M.D.

Dept. Pediatr., Biochem. and Molecular Biol., Univ. Okla. Health Sci. Ctr., Okla. City, Okla. 73190, USA

There are contradictory reports about whether amino acid supplementation (oral or parenteral) will improve nitrogen balance and carbohydrate utilization, and presumably protein synthesis and energy metabolism, in chronic uremics on maintenance dialysis. The circulating leukocyte is a useful cell model to study the metabolic effects directly. Following 3 control studies at one week intervals, 11 adult chronic uremics on thrice weekly hemodialysis (HD), got 500 ml 10% amino acid infusion (AAI) at the end of each subsequent dialysis for a 3 month period. Blood was obtained pre and post dialysis at intervals and leukocytes isolated. Compared to control periods, after only 12 AAI (1 mo) levels of cell ATP, amino acids GLY, TYR, PHE, and TRP, and protein synthesis (^{3}H-leu incorporation) were improved significantly ($p < .05$), Cell levels of Fl-6P, 3PGA, and 2PGA, but not PYR or lactate, were higher ($p < 0.05$), indicating altered glucose utilization (incubation c 5mM glucose). Multiple regression analysis indicated the improved protein synthesis was associated with simultaneous change in levels of cell ASP, CIT, and PHE and plasma THR, VAL, LEU, TYR, and HIS. Thus AAI in uremics on HD improve cell amino acid balance, protein synthesis and energy levels.

The effect of AAI superimposed on maintenance dialysis contrasts with that of dialysis alone. While protein synthesis and AK activity were improved by dialysis, the effects did not persist for more than a few days. ATP and amino acid levels were further reduced and glucose utilization was not significantly improved. The abnormalities in cell bioactivities in chronic uremia resemble those found in protein-calorie malnutrition. The lack of significant improvement in cell metabolism with dialysis alone strongly suggests that the abberations in cell metabolism in chronic uremia result from malnutrition rather than from accumulation of some uremic "toxin". Apparently, even a relatively short period (1 mo) of supplemental amino acid therapy (by infusion), coupled with dialysis, reorders cell substrates and bioactivity levels, leading to partial correction of malnutrition evidenced by improved cell metabolism.

REFERENCES

1. Feldman, H.A. and Singer, I.: Endocrinology and Metabolism in Uremia and Dialysis. A Clinical Review. Medicine 54:345, 1975.

2. De Fronzo, R.A., Andres, R., Edgar, P. et al.: Carbohydrate Metabolism in Uremia. A Clinical Review. Medicine 52:469, 1973

3. Kopple, J.D., Massry, S.G. and Herdland, A. (eds.): Nutrition in Renal Disease Symposium. Amer. J. Clin. Nutr. 31: Part I, p. 1531; Part II, p. 1744, 1978.

4. Bergstrom, J. and Furst, P.: Uremic Toxins. Kidney Intern. 13 (Suppl. 8): 8, 1978.

5. Bergstrom, J., Furst, P., Noree, L.O. et al.: Intracellular free amino acids in uremic patients as influenced by amino acid supply. Kidney Intern. 7:S345, 1975.

6. Rubenfeld, S. and Garber, A.J.: Abnormal carbohydrate metabolism in chronic renal failure. The potential role of accelerate glucose production, increased gluconeogenesis and impaired glucose disposal. J. Clin. Invest. 62:20, 1978.

7. Metcoff, J., Lindeman, R., Baxter, D. et al.: Cell Metabolism in Uremia. Amer. J. Clin. Nutr. 30:1627, 1978.

PANEL DISCUSSION

Moderator: José Strauss, M.D.

Div. Pediatr. Nephrol., Dept. Pediatr., Univ. Miami Sch. Med., Miami, Fla. 33152, USA

QUESTION: I want to make a couple of comments first. I am really glad that Dr. Barness brought out the important point about the psychological value of nutritional aspects. We can talk all you want about the research, but as far as what goes on after the research, it's very important that we all have our treatment modalities together. When we are talking with the patient, we must remember the psychological value. Also, about studies to be done in the future, as far as drug interactions with dietary intake: since dialysis patients are on so many drugs, it would be very important to study this further. I do have a couple of questions. Do you recommend that these patients be supplemented with zinc even though their zinc levels are normal?

RESPONSE: We have used zinc only when there is either clinical or chemical evidence that zinc deficiency exists. We have not used zinc as a routine, no.

QUESTION: Also, as far as measuring iron stores in these patients. I think there has been some controversy on this. I believe that most dialysis units use ferritin levels. Could you comment?

RESPONSE: We use the ferritin levels to monitor iron.

COMMENT: That's what we use also because other methods do not exactly show the iron stores of these patients.

COMMENT: You might be interested in a drug interaction we have seen-the use of Basaljel with Kayexalate in the production of metabolic alkalosis.

QUESTION: I am puzzled by some of the severe nutritional deficiencies you have shown in some of the children. Are these exceptional cases, cases of parental neglect or from underdeveloped countries? Do you see those right here in South Florida and under what circumstances? I have a question regarding the encephalopathy. Do you think that the rarity of it might make the aluminum hypothesis unlikely?

RESPONSE: First, I am very happy that you brought that up because we should have made it clear that these were examples. They were not cases of patients with renal disease. We, by and large, are nutritional epidemiologists and are not day to day clinical nutritionists (nor do we purport to be). In our review of the literature, these were the deficiencies that were described and our purpose was to use them as illustrations of the physical signs that could be seen with renal failure. We did not nor did we intend to show these as actual patients with chronic renal disease. I am glad that was clarified.

COMMENT: We have seen some children who didn't look quite as bad as the pictures but were on chronic end stage therapy, a couple of transplants which didn't work who were on dialysis, whose parents were unable to purchase some of the dietetic supplements, and who began to look like this. Your question about the encephalopathy: I don't think that the syndrome is as rare as it may sound. The recorded incidence in an adult survey of some of the symptomatology associated with dialysis dementia is somewhere between three and five percent in the adult population. In our particular survey of some 700-800 children, the incidence was somewhere between two and three percent. It may be a question of length of time of exposure. It may also be a question of looking for some of the symptomatology which are rather soft. It may be interpreted in more than one way. I think it's impossible to say. There is probably more of it at least up until the recent switch to reverse osmosis. Certainly, in certain areas of the world it is higher and in others, it is lower.

COMMENT: I would like to take up the issue of psychological evaluation in uremic patients. It is extremely important but it is extremely difficult to do as all of you know. It's particularly true when one is intervening with any kind of therapeutic modality. The problem is to separate the effect of the therapy from the potential psychological effect of the therapy on the patient. I would like to call your attention, if you haven't seen it, to an article which attempts to qualify a series of neurophysiologic as well as psychophysiologic behavioral and cognitive responses in patients undergoing management for chronic renal failure. In discussing this with our behavioral scientists, they say that there are now some newer and additional measures for assessing the cognitive and behavioral performance in patients with chronic disease. This is a field that desperately needs attention by those of us who deal with kidney patients. The sooner we can get effectively involved in such areas the more adequately we will be able to evaluate the psychological impact in the potential approach to our patients.

COMMENT: One of the things we have just begun to do--its value remains to be determined--is to use a new instrument with many flashing lights, etc. called neuro methods which is a computerized EEG sort of thing that looks at 300-400 regions of the brain for which there has been some normative data established. We've begun to look at some of our children with this particular technique. Some people think that you can identify learning problems by EEG techniques independent of other variables. I couldn't agree more that there is a need for looking at the neurologic and psychologic function of the developing child who is uremic. That is just beginning to happen and there is going to be a lot more done in the next decade.

COMMENT: We have been following 250 men with detailed dietary histories for four years in a study of multiple risk factors. These are men in the upper 10% risk for coronary heart disease--hypercholesterolemia, smoking--they do everything wrong! My point is that these are intelligent men; we feel that a group of them, by non-compliance, in a sense may be telling us that the outside world is such a heavy burden they are using potential disease (at least clinically potential) as a way of committing suicide. We also have to face the fact that these children who have something so special about them that they are able to tolerate the disease and everything we do to them also may be giving us the messages about when enough is enough in their own life span.

QUESTION: One of the panelists said that they have taken triceps measurements, etc. Was there any improvement on that and did the patients also feel better, those who received the aminoacid supplementation?

RESPONSE: I can't answer with respect to the triceps measurements yet because we have not properly analyzed them. With respect to the patient's feeling better, yes. I'm not involved with the evaluation of those patients but the Nursing Unit staff, the doctors involved with their care, report that as one of the striking features, the patients feel better. I just want to emphasize again, the fact that if they feel better, we feel better, but it may not be real. It may simply be the result of having provided some additional substance beyond that which is provided by dialysis and other medications and this substance requires a certain amount of devotion and time to get. I think we have to evaluate that very carefully. This is why I would like to get the behavioral scientists involved. I think from the physical point of view, the patients seem to be improved in the sense that they seem to have better tissue weight and are less edematous between dialyses. The impression of the doctors is that they have added tissue which is always a desirable situation but is still suspect.

QUESTION: Is there any recommended treatment for hyperlipidemia? If there is, what are the results of the treatment? Are they encouraging?

RESPONSE: There have been really very few nutritional studies regarding lipid levels of patients on dialysis. The recommended treatment, really based on studies that were carried out on the West Coast, is to limit the amount of total carbohydrate intake. They have shown that reducing the total carbohydrate intake in the diet from 50%-60% of intake to about 25%, they can obtain a significant reduction of triglyceride levels. However, the problem remains: how do you make up the rest of the caloric balance of the patient. The only other new development I am aware of is the study using new drugs. They are really being criticized after results suggesting a high incidence of gall bladder disease and other complications particularly in patients with renal failure because of the high incidence of side effects. I think at the moment the use of these drugs has to be viewed as experimental.

MODERATOR: What about in the nephrotic? A couple of years ago we went into some of the potential problems and disagreements as to whether anti-metabolites or immune suppressors may be less dangerous in the long run than the prolonged use of corticosteroids. It was said that if we were not getting good results in inducing remissions with corticosteroids and because of the prolonged relapses with hyperlipidemia, could this eventually lead to atherosclerotic changes? What are your thoughts on that?

RESPONSE: Well, I think now it's clear that patients with nephrotic syndrome who remain unresponsive to treatment really have the highest incidence of atherosclerotic complications. So, the nephrotic patient who remains proteinuric for many years and remains hyperlipidemic for many years is at significant risk of developing premature atherosclerosis. As I mentioned before, there have been many clinical studies pointing out this relationship. Recently there was a very careful autopsy study at NIH showing significant increase of atherosclerosis in the coronary arteries of nephrotic patients. The problem remains, how to handle this complication since again the use of drugs is even more dangerous in patients with hypoproteinemia. There is a very high incidence of GI ulcers as complications. At this time, I really don't know any way you can really control the severe hypercholesterolemia that these patients have year after year.

COMMENT: I can't contribute any suggestions as far as the hyperlipidemia secondary to renal disease but it might be worthwhile just to mention that the experimental pathologists have shown fat reversal in serum with low cholesterol in the diet. At least as we learn what is possible in non-uremic patients, hopefully this may shed some light on approaches to the uremic patient.

Another thing that some of us feel is still valid, namely, that lowering the serum cholesterol in so-called "normal" populations is in fact associated with reduced incidence of coronary heart disease. What is not at all certain is whether or not in hyperlipidemic patients, reduction by either drug and/or diet is effective in preventing coronary heart disease.

QUESTION: What do the panelists think about the etiological importance of the herpes virus in atherosclerosis? A group of patients without uremia, patients who have arterial coronary disease, had low cholesterol and normal serum proteins. It seems that the herpes virus is important in producing the atherosclerosis. Is it possible that in the nephrotic syndrome there may be a similar situation? Have you looked into that at all?

RESPONSE: I'm not aware of any studies of this relationship in patients with chronic renal failure. There are so many theories about atherosclerosis it would be very hard to make a statement about this. For instance, in uremic patients actually there have been recent studies suggesting that in the aorta the main relation is not only with serum cholesterol. It is also related with serum calcium. Some people claim that so-called uremic atherosclerosis is more related to calcium metabolism or abnormalities in calcium metabolism. There are also other theories about the origin of atherosclerosis. We are just using the lipid theory which we think is the most workable theory of the origin of atherosclerosis.

COMMENT: There has been a study in Middlesex, England, on rats with herpes virus, showing that although cholesterol and calcium have importance, one can produce atherosclerosis with a normal cholesterol and normal calcium-in other words, introducing another etiological factor.

COMMENT: I'm glad you raised this point because it is worth emphasizing that the etiology of atherosclerosis in these patients is multifactorial, that really you can't blame the lipids; you have a number of complications including hypertension, disturbances of carbohydrate metabolism, disturbances of immunity. There is a whole host of abnormalities and probably all of them contribute to the development of atherosclerosis. Actually, a recent editorial by a very well known nephrologist suggests that we should forget about the lipids and other things that we can't do anything about and try to concentrate on controlling hypertension and osteodystrophy which are two things that we can do something about.

COMMENT: We are getting dizzy with these trace metals. We talk about zinc an awful lot, we measure zinc. When you measure zinc and you have normal serum levels in spite of stunted growth, then you give zinc and the child grows. The whole thing is so empirical and at times illogical! We really don't know what we measure these days and what does this represent. We have the same experience in acrodermatitis enteropathica when the serum zinc levels are normal, we give zinc and the child improves miraculously. We have the same thing with rheumatoid arthritis where, in spite of the normal levels of zinc, we give zinc and the symptomatology improves. We have problems with manganese not to do with cholesterol but with chromium and toxic effects. Vitamin B_{12} is measured in plasma but it really doesn't correspond with tissue levels. We have some new information about the lack of really zinc deficiency symptoms in terms of taste changes or anorexia but how it affects personality and learning disability. Is it possible that we have in those nutritional problems clearly two groups of patients-one which presents with a severe deficiency and the other one with the low levels of it but perhaps not measured by us right now? They may come out later on with measurements and emotional problems or behavior problems. What is the best? Is the patient's hair analysis the better representative of measurement of trace metals than plasma levels? A number of laboratories using hair analysis such as Case Western trace metal analyses laboratories where they rely much more heavily on hair analysis than on plasma analysis.

RESPONSE: This brings up a very good point. If I had my own choice I would look for a biochemical effect for each one of these things that you mentioned. For example, instead of measuring B_{12} levels it would be important to measure the methylmalonate excretion because this would not measure a level which may or may not be available to the child but the methylmalonate will have the significance of proving that the pathway is working. Similarly with zinc, I think that an enzyme measurement such as alkaline phosphatase which is down the biochemical pathway would be a much better way of measuring zinc sufficiency or zinc insufficiency. There are some 40 enzymes that are known to require zinc; so, maybe picking up one of these enzymes would be better. I think that the evidence still is confusing about which is the best measurement of zinc. It has been said that there's no relationship between hair zinc, blood zinc, or liver zinc. Some are measuring all three and deciding which one on that particular day is the best measurement. I think that most people now do agree that hair zinc is most reflective of metabolically active zinc.

The kind of enzymes that were mentioned, riboflavin, are much better than getting riboflavin levels. The work of enzymes with thiamine is much better than getting a thiamine level or a thiamine phosphate level. I think we have to look at the biochemical pathways. We can measure biotin by looking at propionate, etc. This is the kind of thing we should be looking for to find development of trace metal defectiveness or adequacy.

COMMENT: I certainly agree with everything that has been said so far. I want to add that trace metals are partially protein bound so that zinc, copper, iron are also found in plasma protein. The apparent concentration of a trace metal will vary as its degree of protein binding in cell transport is related to the amount that is not bound. So, it's another complication.

The comment I want to make is, as I reflect on our state of knowledge with regard to nutrition, slow viruses and other factors, I am led to think of a book a man wrote about 1860. The book deals with the rise of witchhunting in Europe during the early Middle Ages and points out that anything we had seen worth grasping to explain the large problems that society was facing at that time could easily be turned to the item of witchcraft and that a responsible individual could easily be identified as clearly responsible and an invoker of witchcraft. Accordingly, there wasn't a major family in Europe who did not have at least one member burned at the stake but I'm not sure that that altered the society's situation except by reducing the population.

COMMENT: I was thinking along the same lines. To illustrate, for the atomic absorption spectrophotometer, you can purchase lamps that measure most of the elements and if you read some of the trace metal articles, you can see all kinds of things that are being measured-lithium, cadmium, etc. One of the new items in the last year has been vanadium measurement. It's a toy that a number of people have-a toy looking for the disease. I'm sure there's going to be all kinds of trace metal reports. Following a course analogous to the potassium and sodium measurement thirty years ago, it's going to take a decade or so before it reaches its level of competence.

MODERATOR: Changing the subject somewhat, could we hear some comments on the psychosocial effects of nutrition? Some fancy machines, EEG's etc., have been mentioned. We have several powerhouses of social work sitting in the audience. Do you have any comments?

COMMENT: I certainly agree with some of the statements made on the psychological effects of some of the treatments. Our staff has great difficulty in determining how much of the effect is due to medication and treatment and how much to the psychological status that developed before dialysis began. That is a problem which we have every day. I was really interested in the talk about dialysis dementia. Up to this poing we haven't had that experience down here. I wonder why. Is it still possible?

RESPONSE: You are fortunate if you haven't seen it. It may be a question of numbers. One kind of psychosocial aspect, most end stage people have a rather large support system for their patients consisting of social workers, psychologists, school teachers, play therapists, etc. I do agree that in general there has been rather limited investigation of these issues. I don't know if the question is worth going into but it's obviously something about which everybody is concerned. Some of the types of experiences that we've had, we've called positive and negative, we've seen good families practically destroyed by this whole process. On the other hand, we have seen some very disadvantaged families where the group, so to speak, has become the parents for these children who, in a psychosocial sense, have grown and developed because they've had chronic kidney disease. I think a lot depends on where you are coming from and what you are exposed to.

COMMENT: We also find that it has a great deal of significance for treatment in terms of medication. That's been one of our major pushes this past year. We have seen families and children who were extremely non-conforming become very active in our programs and with this kind of support, the patients do better and accept treatment better.

MODERATOR: Dr. Gruskin was brainwashed by Paula Mandel who was beautifully trained by him. Now we have the pleasure of having her in our Unit as our play therapist. It does make a difference in terms of compliance and acceptance of those diets and some other things we do to the patients in the Division; among those "things" is hemodialysis...

QUESTION: From one of the talks yesterday, it seems as though some aminoacids have beneficial effects on certain enzymatic reactions whereas other aminoacids have negative effects, as indicated by a minus sign. Today it was demonstrated to us that five aminoacids were most closely associated with protein synthesis. Therefore, I was wondering if you have been working on infusates containing different proportions of the aminoacids which you have found in all these studies to be the most effective.

RESPONSE: That's a super question. It gets right to the issue. The answer is, we have been thinking about it, but we have not been working at it. The reason we haven't been working at it is because the data are still so tenuous. I offered the particular aminoacids which to date would seem to be most closely associated with protein synthesis only to show the power of the system. Using this kind of approach, I suspect that in due course we will know something about which aminoacids are really the ones that are important. I don't know whether the aminoacids I showed are the last word in terms of protein synthesis. Our data base still is too small for that. But the system does give us promise that there will be a way of getting at that through this approach. Others, I think, have shown that it is possible to alter growth patterms, for example, or alter protein synthesis and brain responses by manipulation of the proportions of aminoacids in the environment surrounding the cell. We think that's probable but I don't know which ones yet. As our data base gets to the point where I am more secure of the results, then we will start actively engaging ourselves in experimentation.

COMMENT: I am very much impressed to hear that in congenital nephrotic syndrome you achieve a positive nitrogen balance by parenteral hyperalimentation. Since they have the same increased catabolism and protein loss, their increased anabolism probably was achieved by getting higher doses of aminoacids. I would like to learn what was the dose, the protein equivalent of the aminoacid mixture. Was it one or two or three g/kg? My second question is: at a time when they could tolerate enteric aminoacid mixture, were they ever given such a mixture? What was the result?

RESPONSE: Regarding the question on parenteral nutrition, we did not use an aminoacid preparation neither casein nor modified cow's milk nor low lactose milk. We increased progressively the quantity of protein up to around 3-4 grams of protein per kilogram of body weight per day. So it is possible to attain anabolism in such patients, giving enough energy, too. You could do both at the same time.

MODERATOR: Could you give us some details as to when you administer your enteral infusions? Was there a specific indication- a patient going into a greater catabolic period or in serum changes? Then, when do you stop infusion?

RESPONSE: It depends, of course, on the problem. In congenital nephrotic syndrome, patients died within the first two years of life; so it was a life saving procedure if continued for at least one year. We tried to discontinue after a time when we felt that the patient was better. In cystinotic patients the indication for its use was the impossibility to continue to use the gastrointestinal tract to give electrolytes and to give a sort of normal energy and protein intake. But is is not decided within days; it is decided within weeks. When there are evidences that it is not possible to continue in the usual way giving supplementation, we were forced to go into enteral alimentation. In some cases we began by total parenteral alimentation. It's in rather exceptional cases.

MODERATOR: When do you discontinue them? When the patients reached what you thought was the maximum growth potential? Was that the only parameter?

RESPONSE: It depends again on the etiology. For cystinotic patients, for example, when we observed that the growth curve was demonstrating a catch-up process, we continued so as to not interrupt this process, for at least one year. Several attempts were made to stop this type of continuous nutrition so we were forced to continue enteral nutrition if our attempts to stop, failed. But we don't have absolute criteria for when to stop.

QUESTION: On the enteral nutrition, in our country it started only in the last five to seven years. Anybody who dares to mention that there is anything other than parenteral nutrition usually gets strung up by their toes. I think there are conditions other than chronic renal disease where a child in particular has a relatively good GI tract but for other reasons such as muscle weakness, severe pulmonary disease, etc., is unable to receive an adequate amount of nutrients, and subsequently gets infections, goes down hill and the cycle goes on. I heard that you were giving it over a sixteen hour period of the 24 hour day. Is that correct?

RESPONSE: Yes.

QUESTION: Which means that you were not, I assume, using the overnight period. Is there any particular reason for that?

RESPONSE: We try to save some hours of the day to give them normal activity and normal feeding of the child. We try to give enteral nutrition during 16 hours and to save the other time.

QUESTION: Did you have any problems with aspiration which is what everybody tells me every time I put a tube down?

RESPONSE: No, we had no such problem.

QUESTION: I wanted to address this question to one of the other panelists. In noticing the substrates along the glycolytic pathway, you had a baseline and after dialysis and after aminoacid infusion. Do you have any normal control neutrophil studies, and how do these fluctuations vary compared to normals?

RESPONSE: If you recall, the first glycolytic flux diagram that I showed related the dialyzed uremics to the normal controls. The base line was normal controls. The second diagram with respect to the aminoacid infusions were made in each individual group of patients, dialysis or aminoacid infusion to their own baselines. The change with respect to aminoacid infusions and normal controls is if there has been improvement in the energy flux compared to the controls. It's closer to the controls.

QUESTION: Have you measured oxygen consumption?

RESPONSE: No, we have not.

QUESTION: What is the significance of those two spikes-those two substrates? What do you feel in terms of improving energy metabolism of the cell? Why is that giving you more ATP?

RESPONSE: Those particular spikes, they are not getting more ATP, I don't believe. The first one suggests that there is less utilization of ATP. The spikes relate to two enzymes that we have found measured. One of them, triose-isomerase may be related to utilization of glycerol and that in turn to triglyceride synthesis. We have not measured it. We should measure it. The other one is related to alphaglycerol phosphate dehydrogenase which in turn ought to be associated with secondary electron transport phenomena. We have not measured those items.

MODERATOR: If you want to measure oxygen consumption, it should be possible to make a suitable electrode.

RESPONSE: I would be very pleased to do that because, as you know, in the leucocyte we have attempted to use oxygen electrodes and the one that was available to us was simply too crude to get any good data. I hope that you would be interested to try it because it would be of some interest. The leucocyte does undergo quite a good oxidative phosphorilation but, of course, not in the same level as you would find in other tissues like liver or kidney.

MODERATOR: In terms of the rearrangement of the aminoacid sequence or levels that would improve the protein synthesis, what do you think is going on? What do you do that induces a change? Could more frequent or continuous dialysis be one approach to a continuous improvement in their metabolic situation?

RESPONSE: With respect to the first question, I think we will know better when we have some more data, but I suspect that what's happening is that we are altering the competitive transport of aminoacids across the cell membrane and that alteration is leading to a new balance between intracellular and aminoacid exchange which in some way is more favorable to protein synthesis. I don't know what that proper balance is nor have we produced it except by the administration of these aminoacids which in some way tell the cells that they ought to take up this one and not that one. Which aminoacids are the ones most responsible, as I mentioned earlier, I also am not sure. But I think that the system of going through a multiple regression procedure with subset analysis is going to tell us that, when we get a sufficiently large data base. At the present, the number of independent variables is so great compared to the sample size that the validity of the analysis has to be questioned. So, I'm not sure. As far as continued dialysis, I think you must be continuing infusion because all these patients have been on dialysis for long periods of time and are reasonably stable as adult dialyzed patients. Some of them have been on dialysis for as short a period of time as weeks and are not stable. Others have been on dialysis for years and are reasonably stabilized. The aminoacid infusion effect I think probably requires time. We will know better when we get to analyze our data completely after 36 infusions which is just an arbitrary period of time as well. There is nothing magical about it. But it should show whether there are some critical changes.

MODERATOR: My question about the dialysis was regarding the period of time the dialysis lasts, four or five hours, then you go for two to three days and you find that at the end of the four-five hours you had a marked improvement which has basically disappeared at the end of the two to three days. If instead of the four to five hours two or three times a week, we did one or two hours every day or if we used continuous pumps, portable systems, or chronic peritoneal dialysis, could more frequent procedures or semi-continuous procedures be beneficial? Obviously you don't have the data but do you have any thoughts on that?

RESPONSE: Well, I am certain it would be another approach. Whether it would offer more, I don't know. It should be tried. It's conceivable that we do some harm with the kinds of dialysis that are carried out. After all we are reducing the cell pool of aminoacids and that, I think, is not a desirable thing to do. Perhaps that wouldn't be as prominent a feature if dialysis occurred for a shorter period of time and at more frequent intervals. I think there are many variations that could be and should be tried. My only criterion, however, is that if there are variations tried, that somebody make the measurements and document them.

MODERATOR: A further point, and I may be stretching your conclusions: could it be that we are using the wrong end-point in deciding when the patient needs dialysis or when not to dialyze a patient that was scheduled to be dialyzed. In other words, now we go by the level of BUN and serum creatinine. Is that a good end-point? It's like the proteinuria in the nephrotic syndrome. Those are handy end-points, easy to document, and accepted subjectively, if you want, by most people. But maybe we need to go one step further and get to more basic measurements as to what the cell is doing and what is changing in a more subtle manner. I would hope that studies like yours would help along these lines.

RESPONSE: I think that's a very good and perceptive comment. We do what is the easiest thing to do. As was said a few minutes ago, when flame photometers came out, everybody measured sodium and potassium. When a chloridometer became available and you didn't have to go through the laborious chloride measurement, there was a rash of papers on chloride activity. Atomic absorption is another. BUN and other simple parameters have been used by doctors for a hundred years and they are very reluctant to give up these easy crutches. They have some clinical relevance but that does not mean that we should forever be stuck with it. So, I am certain that as new insights become available and are relatively easy to measure, they will begin to use them. I would hope that the cell state would be a much better determinant of therapeutic intervention, indeed, for therapeutic intervention and response to it. I am very uneasy about the level of anything. As was mentioned a few minutes ago, to question which level to use is the proper position to be in because you don't really know. A more dynamic measure is required, as may be indicated. I believe that looking at certain cell pathways is going to be one of the ways of approaching it more dynamically.

QUESTION: There are two general statements made. One is that you exercise people with chronic renal disease. They feel better, do better. And, two, if you give some of the vitamin B complex to people, they feel stronger, maybe the muscle mass is better. I'm curious as to whether there has been any aminoacid measurements similar to what you describe done in patients in looking at exercise or the use of vitamin B complexes. I am not aware of any.

RESPONSE: Probably one of the other panelists could answer that better than I. There haven't been many groups that have attempted to look at cell composition with respect to anything. I have been reviewing a number of papers and data on the subject are quite limited. To my knowledge there are no pathway studies or cell composition studies respecting aminoacid composition and protein synthesis with the response to exercise or the administration of vitamin B.

MODERATOR: We must end now. Thank you all.

PART THREE

SYSTEMIC ASPECTS OF RENAL DISEASE

RENAL OSTEODYSTROPHY: PATHOGENESIS, PREVENTION AND TREATMENT

Jacques J. Bourgoignie, M.D.

Div. Nephrol., Dept. Med., Univ. Miami Sch. Med., Miami, Fla. 33101, USA

Renal osteodystrophy is a complex disorder expressing at the musculoskeletal level the metabolic abnormalities of renal disease (1). It is universally present in patients with chronic renal disease and continues to be one of the more difficult problems that confront the clinician charged with the responsibility of managing patients with chronic renal failure. A major difficulty in attempting to adopt a rational approach in these patients' management has been the lack of a complete understanding of the pathogenesis of the deranged skeletal metabolism (2,3). Recently, development of morphometric analysis of bone biopsies, sensitive assays of vitamin D metabolites and parathormone (PTH), specific vitamin D metabolites for experimentation combined with formulation of testable hypotheses, have expanded our understanding of calcium and phosphorus homeostasis in renal osteodystrophy. New therapeutic trends, based on recent pathophysiologic information, can be perceived which have already changed the often dramatic clinical picture seen 10-15 years ago. Treatment of renal osteodystrophy undoubtedly will undergo much refinement within the next five years and its prevention appears as a reachable goal.

This review briefly lists the classical modes of expression of renal osteodystrophy and states our current knowledge of its pathogenesis with particular emphasis on vitamin D and PTH.

Supported by NIH Grant AM19822.

MODES OF EXPRESSION

Clinical

The clinical picture of decreased intestinal calcium absorption, excessive bone resorption and defective bone mineralization that can eventually lead to disabling symptoms of bone pain and pathologic fractures is familiar. Other symptoms include articular pain, muscular weakness and pain (proximal myopathy associated with osteomalacia), pruritis, soft tissue calcification, necrosis and ulcers, tendon rupture, ocular calcifications (4).

Biologic

Serum calcium concentration and intestinal calcium absorption are decreased. Levels of serum phosphorus, magnesium, alkaline phosphatase, hydroxyproline, and parathormone are increased. Circulating levels of vitamin D metabolites are normal (25 OH cholecalciferol) or decreased (1,25 and 24,25$(OH)_2$ cholecalciferol). While radioimmunoassayable levels are increased, calcitonin activity may be normal by biologic assay (2,4).

Radiologic

The incidence of roentgenographic abnormalities of renal osteodystrophy is much more frequent than its clinical manifestations (2, 4), and include:

1. Subperiosteal bone resorption (osteolysis) in small tubular bones of hands and feet, in phalangeal tufts, distal clavicles, pubis, skull. The presence of "brown tumors" (long bones, phalanges, skull, metacarpals, ribs) is rare in uremic osteodystrophy and raises the possibility of primary hyperparathyroidism.
2. Looser-Milkman pseudofractures (woven bone of decreased density) in ischion, ribs, femoral neck, metatarsals, external border of scapula and, later, in long bones and pelvis.
3. Osteosclerosis: Rugger-jersey spine.
4. Metastatic calcifications in soft tissues (periarticular, vascular, mediastinal, pulmonary).

Technetium scanning may be more sensitive than roentgenography to demonstrate uremic bone abnormalities. In one series, abnormal bone activity was observed in 90 percent of chronic hemodialysis patients when bone x-rays were abnormal in only 33 percent (5).

Histologic

The bone presents a picture of increased turnover with:

1. Osteitis fibrosa: increased osteoblastic and osteoclastic activities, increased bone resorption, medullary fibrosis and fibrotic bone (woven osteoid). Some of these manifestations occur early in chronic renal disease; woven osteoid can be present at a GFR of 80 ml/min, while endosteal fibrosis does not appear before GFR has fallen below 30 ml/min (6).
2. Osteomalacia (increased osteoid volume with abnormal mineralization and absent calcification front) is a frequent but late manifestation of renal osteodystrophy and is never severe at a GFR greater than 40 ml/min (6). However, pure osteomalacia is rare, occurring in less than 10 percent of chronically uremic patients (4).
3. Osteosclerosis (increased bone mass as calcified bone plus osteoid bone) is present in 30 percent of patients with chronic renal insufficiency (4).
4. Osteoporosis (decreased bone mass) is never present in chronic renal disease in the absence of heparin or steroid treatment.
5. Finally, bone collagen is defective and immature (4).

PATHOPHYSIOLOGY

The views of Dent (7) on the variable histologic patterns of renal osteodystrophy are presented in Figure 1. Three different patients are illustrated: one with osteomalacia, another with osteitis fibrosa cystica, osteomalacia and osteosclerosis and a third with osteitis fibrosa and osteosclerosis. Osteomalacia predominates in diseases characterized mainly by renal tubular failure or interstitial diseases of the kidney as a result of vitamin D deficiency, while glomerular diseases are complicated by osteitis fibrosa and osteosclerosis as a result of excess PTH. Not everybody agrees with this view nor with the classic separation between the histologic manifestations of renal osteodystrophy due to vitamin D lack and those due to PTH excess. Indeed, although a lack of $1,25(OH)_2D_3$ supposedly is the main pathogenic factor of osteomalacia, the latter is not easily accessible to therapy and is not corrected by administration of $1,25(OH)_2D_3$ only (8). Rather, the metabolisms of both endocrine systems are intimately interrelated.

Many factors contribute to the development of renal osteodystrophy (Table 1). Hyperparathyroidism and vitamin D deficiency, however, are principally responsible for the syndrome.

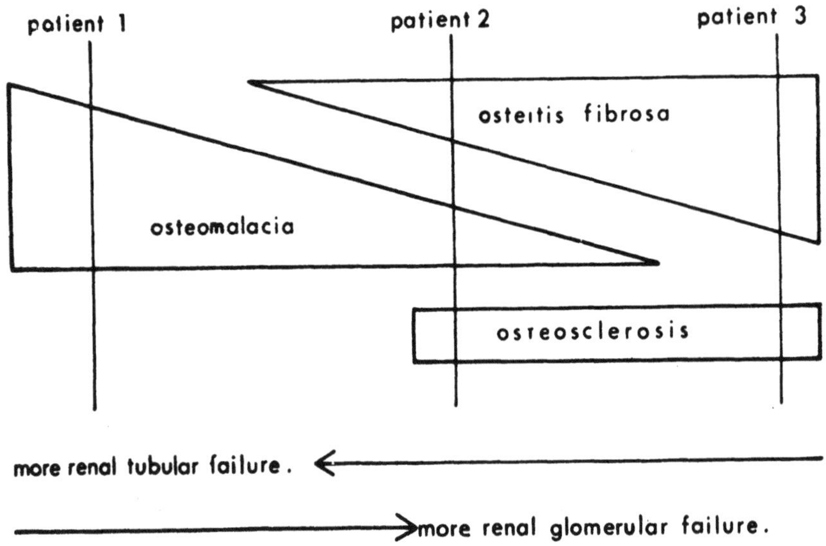

FIG. 1. Schematic illustration of bone manifestations in renal osteodystrophy. Vertical lines indicate the composition of bone disease in 3 hypothetical patients. (From Dent, C.E. and Stamp, T.C.B., Vitamin D, Rickets and Osteomalacia. In: Avioli, L.V. and Krane, S.M. (eds.): Metabolic Bone Disease, Vol. 2, New York: Academic Press, 1978, p. 296).

Hyperparathyroidism

PTH normally functions to maintain serum ionized calcium within narrow limits in the extracellular fluid (9). When serum ionized calcium decreases, the parathyroid glands secrete PTH. PTH then tends to restore eucalcemia directly by increasing calcium resorption from bone and calcium reabsorption by the kidney and, indirectly, by enhancing intestinal calcium absorption through renal stimulation of $1,25(OH)_2D_3$ production. As the level of serum ionized calcium rises, PTH secretion decreases. This feedback loop system between ionized calcium and PTH operates in chronic renal disease (10).

In chronic renal disease, as renal function and glomerular filtration rate (GFR) decrease, the concentration of PTH in blood (iPTH) rises. The more advanced the renal disease, the greater the level of iPTH. Importantly, secondary hyperparathyroidism occurs as an early

Table 1. Pathogenesis of Renal Osteodystrophy

1. Hyperparathyroidism
2. Abnormal Vitamin D metabolism
3. Other factors
   a. Acidosis
   b. Relative deficiency in calcitonin
   c. Aluminum, fluoride, magnesium
   d. Drugs: - steroids, heparin
      - barbiturates, dilantin
      - excess phosphate binding gels
   e. Hypoproteinemic diets poor in phosphorus, calcium and Vitamin D.

manifestation of renal disease and small decreases in GFR are associated with increased levels of iPTH (11) in agreement with the early skeletal abnormalities mentioned above.

A number of factors (Table 2) contribute to the pathogenesis of secondary hyperparathyroidism in advanced renal disease, but no unanimity exists on the initial event leading from a decrease in renal function to hyperparathyroidism in early renal disease (12-17). Several hypotheses with hypocalcemia, at least transient, as a common denominator have been advanced. These theories implicate phosphate retention (18,19), abnormalities in vitamin D metabolism (14,20) or skeletal resistance to PTH (21) as the predominant factor responsible for the development of hyperparathyroidism.

Administration of one gram phosphorus (equivalent to a steak dinner) to normal volunteers results in a progressive increase in serum phosphorus, a reciprocal decrease in ionized calcium and a progressive rise in serum iPTH (22). Thus, the pathogenesis of early secondary hyperparathyroidism has been attributed to phosphate retention (18,19). When GFR decreases, retention of phosphorus occurs that is attended by a reciprocal drop in ionized calcium and secretion of PTH. In this context the increase in iPTH occurs to enhance

Table 2. Pathogenesis of Hyperparathyroidism in Chronic Renal Disease

1. Hypocalcemia
   a. phosphate retention
   b. deficient vitamin D metabolism
2. Bone resistance to PTH
3. Impaired PTH metabolism
4. Decreased sensitivity of the parathyroid glands to calcium
5. Lack of PTH suppression by vitamin D metabolites

urinary phosphate excretion per nephron and restore phosphate balance, thereby returning to normal the concentration of serum phosphorus. In chronic renal disease, daily phosphate balance would be maintained but at the expense of a progressively increasing secre-

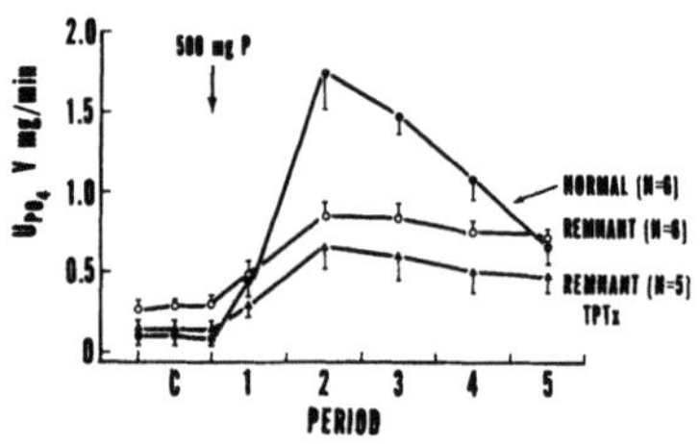

FIG. 2. Urinary excretion of phosphate in six normal dogs (GFR 69 ml/min), six dogs with a remnant kidney and chronic renal insufficiency (GFR 12 ml/min) and five thyroparathyroidectomized dogs with a remnant kidney (GFR 13 ml/min). After three control clearance periods (C) all animals were challenged orally with 500 mg phosphorus and five one-hour clearance periods were obtained (10).

tion of PTH. In dogs with a remnant kidney and chronic renal insufficiency given an oral phosphorus load, the urinary excretion of phosphate is severely blunted and retention of phosphorus ensues (Fig. 2). As a consequence, hyperphosphatemia is augmented leading to prolonged hypocalcemia (Fig. 3) (10).

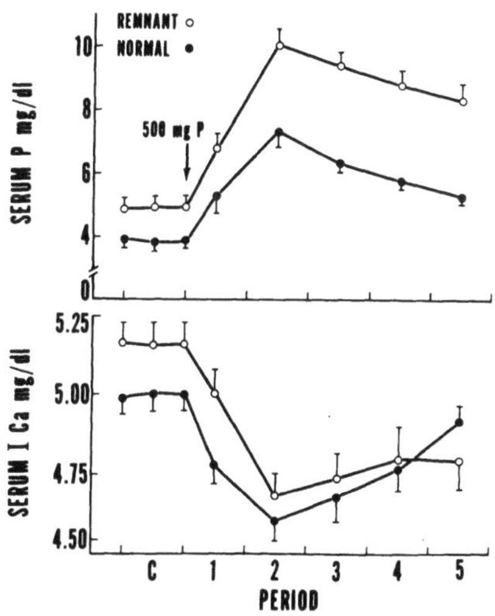

FIG. 3. Changes in serum phosphorus and serum ionized calcium in normal and in remnant dogs after a 500 mg oral phosphorus. Data from animals described in Fig. 2.

This concept, which ascribes a central role to phosphorus retention in the genesis of uremic hyperparathyroidism, is experimentally supported by the observations that dietary phosphorus restriction can prevent the development of hyperparathyroidism or reverse existing hyperparathyroidism in chronic renal insufficiency (23-25). Nevertheless, despite phosphate restriction, dogs with a remnant kidney develop late, albeit mild, hyperparathyroidism (23). It is now also apparent that the bulk of circulating iPTH is not necessary for maintenance of external phosphate balance in uremic dogs with a GFR about 30 percent of normal (26). Even totally parathyroidectomized animals can maintain phosphate homeostasis (27-29) and thy-

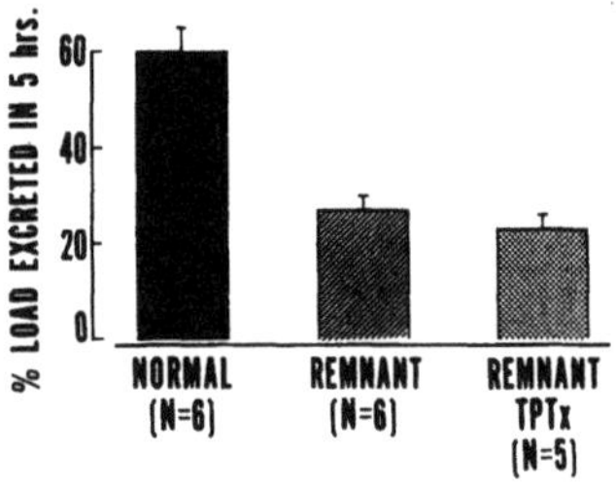

FIG. 4. Net cumulative 5-hr excretion of a 500 mg phosphorus load, expressed as a percent of the load, in normal, hyperparathyroid remnant and thyroparathyroidectomized (TPTX) remnant dogs. The dogs in the different groups are the same as described in Fig. 2. In five hours the normal animals excreted 60 $\pm$ 4.9 percent of the load, the remnant dogs 27 $\pm$ 1.9 percent and the TPTX remnant dogs 22 $\pm$ 6.6 percent. 5-hr phosphate excretion in both groups of remnant dogs was markedly blunted ($p < 0.001$ vs normal group) without significant difference between the remnant animals with and without thyroparathyroidectomy.

roparathyroidectomized dogs with chronic renal insufficiency challenged with 500 mg phosphorus orally exhibit the same blunted phosphate excretion as non-thyroparathyroidectomized equally uremic but hyperparathyroid dogs (Fig. 4) (10). Finally, the hypothesis does not explain the inverse relationship that must exist in chronic renal disease between serum phosphorus and serum calcium, a relationship that is not always present in fasting patients early in the course of chronic renal disease (13). These observations indicate that phosphorus retention, although important in the genesis of hyperparathyroidism, is not the sole and only an indirect factor since phosphorus has no direct effect on parathyroid gland secretion (30). Rather than being directed at phosphorus homeostasis, the hyperparathyroidism of renal insufficiency may be a compensatory mechanism directed at calcium homeostasis whereby development of dangerous hypocalcemia after a phosphorus load is prevented. Indeed, in the absence of PTH, administration of phosphorus leads to severe hypocalcemia, tetany and death (15).

The evidence that altered vitamin D metabolism contributes to abnormal calcium metabolism in chronic renal disease is considerable. Patients with advanced renal failure have little or no production of $1,25(OH)_2D_3$, an important metabolite for intestinal calcium absorption and for a normal skeletal response to PTH. In the absence of adequate production of $1,25(OH)_2D_3$, a lowered intestinal calcium absorption and skeletal resistance to the calcemic action of PTH would reduce ionized calcium in blood, thereby stimulating the secretion of PTH and leading to secondary hyperparathyroidism.

Since hyperphosphatemia or phosphorus retention inhibits $1,25(OH)_2D_3$ formation in the kidney, a variant of the phosphorus retention hypothesis has been proposed in which changes in $1,25(OH)_2D_3$ would mediate the effects of phosphorus on serum ionized calcium (20). As renal mass is reduced, there may be a slight decrease in the renal generation of $1,25(OH)_2D_3$ leading to a fall in serum calcium and a rise in the secretion of PTH. The latter, in turn would stimulate the renal production of $1,25(OH)_2D_3$ leading to normal levels of the sterol in blood and return of intestinal calcium absorption to normal. This tendency to normalization is maintained only at the expense of a sustained elevation in serum iPTH level and would continue as long as the surviving nephrons of the diseased kidney are capable of increasing their production of $1,25(OH)_2D_3$. Phosphate retention may be the signal to the impaired generation of $1,25(OH)_2D_3$. Preliminary results in patients with early renal failure show that dietary phosphorus restriction may lead to an increase in $1,25(OH)_2D_3$ production, return of blood PTH levels to normal, improvement in the calcemic response to PTH and intestinal calcium absorption and healing of bone disease (14).

Infusion of PTH is normally attended by an increase in serum calcium. In comparison with normal subjects or animals, the same dose of PTH results in a markedly blunted calcemic response in patients or dogs with renal insufficiency (21,31) (Fig. 5). This skeletal resistance to PTH is independent of serum phosphorus and is not reversed by hemodialysis (31). It occurs after two days of acute uremia and is seen in patients with GFR's above 50 ml/min (31-33). Pretreatment with $1,25(OH)_2D_3$ improves the response in anephric and in remnant animals (32,34) (Fig. 4) while $1,25(OH)_2D_3$ alone in acutely uremic dogs with an intact renal mass (33) and $1,25(OH)_2D_3$ plus $24,25(OH)_2D_3$ in anephric animals completely normalize the skeletal response (35). The effects of the metabolites com-

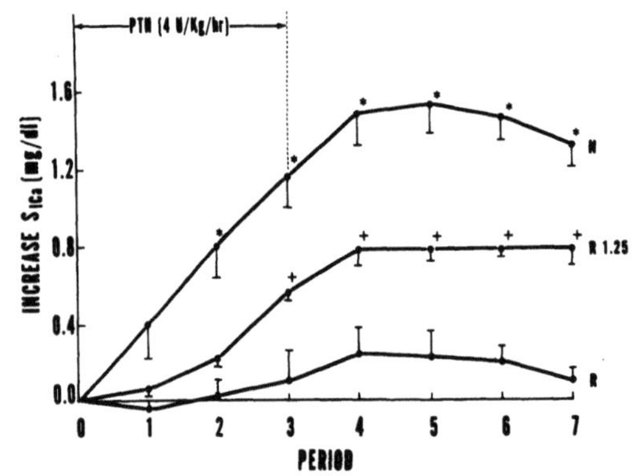

FIG. 5. Changes in serum ionized calcium in five normal (N) dogs (GFR 71 ± 4 ml/min) and in ten dogs with a remnant (R) kidney and chronic renal insufficiency (GFR 11 ± 2 ml/min) during and after intravenous infusion of a standard dose of purified bovine parathyroid hormone (Inolex Corp.). Half of the remnant dogs were tested after pretreatment for 3 days with 400 µg $1,25(OH)_2D_3$ (Data from 34).
*Indicates greater calcemic response in normal (N) dogs than in each remnant group ($P < 0.05$).
+Indicates greater calcemic response in $1,25(OH)_2D_3$ treated (R 1,25) than in untreated remnant (R) dogs.

bined need to be evaluated in chronic uremia. The pathogenesis of the skeletal resistance to PTH, thus, may relate to an impaired vitamin D metabolism. Uremia per se, however, has been implicated (33,36) and, in vitro, an increased phosphate medium concentration has been shown to decrease the release of calcium from bone in response to PTH (36,37).

This skeletal resistance has been viewed as a major factor in the genesis of secondary hyperparathyroidism (17,21). Although bone resistance to PTH may contribute to hyperparathyroidism, the blunted calcemic response to PTH in renal insufficiency does not appear to be a predominant factor in the pathogenesis of hyperparathyroidism since the chronically uremic dog treated with reduction of phosphorus intake, which prevents phosphorus retention and maintains a normal iPTH level, also demonstrates this abnormality (34).

In addition to phosphorus retention, alterations in vitamin D metabolism and skeletal resistance to PTH, other mechanisms contributing to hyperparathyroidism in renal insufficiency include an abnormal PTH metabolism, a decreased sensitivity of the parathyroid glands to calcium inhibition and possibly a lack of suppression of PTH secretion by vitamin D metabolites.

Although under conditions of hypercalcemia fragments of PTH may be released by the parathyroid glands, PTH is usually secreted as the intact molecule (9,38) and undergoes metabolism in the liver and the kidney (39). The fragments containing the amino end of the molecule are extracted by bone and by the kidney through peritubular capillary uptake and glomerular filtration while those fragments containing the carboxyl end are catabolized in the kidney where they only undergo glomerular filtration. Thus, as GFR decreases, the clearance of the C-terminal fragments also decreases, resulting in retention and increasing circulating levels of immunoreactive PTH (40,41). This metabolism of PTH explains why immunoassays directed at different portions of the PTH molecule provide different results. Thus, in chronic renal insufficiency, the levels of iPTH are increased not only because of increased production and secretion by the parathyroid glands but also because of impaired elimination. The biologic activity of the C-terminal fragments accumulating in uremia is unknown.

An altered negative calcium feedback on parathyroid gland secretion adds another reason for the sustained hyperparathyroidism of chronic renal insufficiency. A loss of the negative feedback mechanism of calcium on PTH secretion is evident in patients with end stage renal disease who progressively become hypercalcemic and develop "tertiary hyperparathyroidism". Abnormalities in the calcium ion regulation of PTH secretion, however, has also been observed in eucalcemic patients with chronic renal failure (9). In vitro, an increased affinity for magnesium, a decreased sensitivity for calcium and an abnormal cyclic nucleotides metabolism have been described in hyperplastic parathyroid glands from chronically uremic subjects (42).

Finally, although conflicting data exist, observations suggest that some metabolites of vitamin D may affect PTH secretion via a direct action on the parathyroid glands independent of changes in serum ionized calcium (43-48). If one of the vitamin D metabolites has a direct inhibitory effect on PTH release, its deficiency in advanced renal insufficiency would remove one of the negative feedback mechanisms of PTH secretion.

Vitamin D Deficiency

The metabolism of vitamin D, though a very important subject, will only be briefly commented upon. Vitamin D is generated by ultraviolet light in the skin. It is also present in food. Its absorption is intact in chronic renal disease. In the liver, vitamin D is hydroxylated to 25(OH) cholecalciferol. This metabolite undergoes further hydroxylation in the kidney to form $1,25(OH)_2D_3$ or $24,25(OH)_2D_3$ which are under strong regulatory influences. Formation of $1,25(OH)_2D_3$ is stimulated by PTH but inhibited by phosphorus. Conversely, in the absence of PTH or when serum phosphorus is normal, there is preferential hydroxylation in the 24 rather than in the 1 position and formation of $24,25(OH)_2D_3$. $1,25(OH)_2D_3$ is exquisitely active in stimulating active intestinal calcium absorption possibly through a calcium-binding protein. In addition, $1,25(OH)_2D_3$ acts on bone (49-51).

Until recently it was believed that only $1,25(OH)_2D_3$ had biologic activity. Indeed, on a molar basis $1,25(OH)_2D_3$ is the most potent metabolite of vitamin D. However, $1,25(OH)_2D_3$ circulates in blood in very small amounts of about 20-40 pg/ml. Other vitamin D metabolites which circulate in much higher concentrations (about 50-100 fold larger for $24,25(OH)_2D_3$ and 1000-fold for $25(OH)_2D_3$) have also been shown to possess biologic activity on gut and on bone.

In chronic renal failure, the levels of $25(OH)_2D_3$ are usually normal. On the other hand, preliminary data indicate that $1,25(OH)_2D_3$ levels are low in advanced renal failure and may be undetectable in anephric patients (15,52-54). Thus, chronic renal failure is a vitamin D deficient state. However, early in the course of renal disease, the levels of the di-hydroxy metabolites of vitamin D are normal and an absolute deficiency of $1,25(OH)_2D_3$ or $24,25(OH)_2D_3$ has not been demonstrated (14,15). Nevertheless a state of relative deficiency has been postulated by investigators who noted improvement of osteodystrophy with $1,25(OH)_2D_3$ treatment at an early stage of renal insufficiency (14,20).

The impaired intestinal calcium absorption was well recognized forty years ago when patients with chronic renal failure were shown to absorb only 7 percent of dietary calcium as opposed to 28 percent for normal subjects given the same calcium diet (55). The defect in calcium absorption may be apparent in patients with GFR's of 75 ml/min and is corrected by $1,25(OH)_2D_3$ (14,56). Normalization of calcium absorption also occurs with administration of 25(OH) D_3 in pharmacological doses or with 24,25$(OH)_2D_3$ (57). Other consequences of vitamin D deficiency include defective mineralization of bone and osteomalacia, myopathy and possibly impaired suppression of PTH (see above).

It is interesting to compare the biologic actions of 1,25 and 24,25$(OH)_2D_3$ in the context of renal osteodystrophy. 1,25$(OH)_2D_3$ increases intestinal calcium absorption. It also increases serum calcium and urinary calcium excretion and has variable effects on calcium balance. It has only late effects on serum alkaline phosphatase and decreases iPTH indirectly by increasing serum calcium (20,49-51). Although 24,25$(OH)_2D_3$ also increases intestinal calcium absorption, it does not increase serum calcium or urinary calcium excretion (20,45,57,58). Nevertheless it leads to a positive calcium balance presumably with deposition of calcium in bone. Thus, 24,25$(OH)_2D_3$ may have an anabolic effect on bone which is often not apparent for 1,25$(OH)_2D_3$. 24,25$(OH)_2D_3$ also decreases circulating iPTH as a result of a direct effect on the gland (43, 44). However this effect has not been observed consistently (57).

As discussed earlier it is presently unclear whether the decreased production of 1,25$(OH)_2D_3$ in renal failure is due to loss in renal mass or to phosphorus retention. Other factors contributing to a decreased production of renal metabolites of vitamin D include the lack of precursor formation in the skin due to seasonal variation in sunlight exposure, accelerated metabolism of 25(OH) D_3 in the liver by drugs (barbiturates, dilantin) or excessive urinary losses of 25(OH) D_3 in the nephrotic syndrome (20,59).

Treatment

Because of the evolving state of the art of the vitamin D field, a complete therapeutic regimen cannot be proposed presently. Nevertheless the pathogenic mechanisms discussed above allow the development of a rational approach of prevention and treatment of renal osteodystrophy (Table 3). Efforts must be directed at controlling serum phosphorus and the hyperparathyroidism, while correcting the vitamin D deficiencies and providing enough calcium for patients to maintain a positive calcium balance without hypercalcemia.

Evidence reviewed earlier clearly indicates that hyperparathyroidism can be minimized by decreasing dietary phosphorus intake. Although not practical on a long term basis, administration of a phosphate restricted diet is effective in lowering serum phosphorus. The use of phosphate binding antacids (aluminum hydroxide) seeks to achieve the same goal and is a more practical and now common, although unpalatable, means to decrease serum phosphorus. These antacids bind phosphorus in the intestinal lumen preventing its ab-

Table 3. Treatment of Renal Osteodystrophy

1.	Phosphorus:	- diet	
		- $Al(OH)_3$	
2.	Calcium:	- diet	
		- dialysate	
3.	Vitamin D:	- $25(OH)\ D_3$	
		- $1,25(OH)_2D_3$	
		- other preparations	
4.	Parathyroidectomy:		
		- surgical	
		- "mediçal":	- calcium
			- propranolol
			- $24,25(OH)_2D_3$
			- cimetidine

sorption across the gut. As a consequence, postprandial hyperphosphatemia and hypocalcemia are blunted and the stimulation of PTH after each meal is attenuated (60). Enough antacids should be given to lower and maintain a serum phosphorus level of about 4 to 5 mg/dl without inducing hypophosphatemia (61-63).

Passive intestinal absorption of calcium can be increased by providing enough calcium in the diet to avoid development of a negative calcium balance (64). When necessary, calcium supplementation should be given to provide a daily intake of 1.5 g calcium. To increase active intestinal absorption of calcium, a vitamin D preparation is necessary. Vitamin D therapy is beneficial not only for improving enteric calcium absorption but also to provide the hormone to other target organs (bone, kidney, parathyroid gland, muscle).

Which specific preparation should be used remains uncertain. The literature abounds with conflicting data on the effects of specific vitamin D metabolites in apparently similar disease entities. Only a few metabolites have been tested and a number of others have been described with undetermined biologic activity. It is quite possible, if not probable, that some of these may prove more specific than currently available preparations for certain pathophysiologic conditions. One must remember that the generic term of renal osteodystrophy masks heterogeneous disease entities of different pathogenesis (20). Hopefully, these uncertainties will resolve as stable preparations of different metabolites of vitamin D become available for experimental and clinical use together with reliable assays of vitamin D metabolites in blood. The use of a precursor, such as 25(OH) D_3, may be more beneficial than a renal metabolite when kidney function is normal to allow renal production of the metabolite or metabolites that may be most useful for the disabled body. When kidney function fails a precursor may be an ineffective substitute for a specific metabolite formed in the kidney.

The only metabolite of vitamin D presently available on the market is 1,25$(OH)_2D_3$. Although some report beneficial effects with the use of 1,25$(OH)_2D_3$ in renal osteodystrophy, this experience is not universal (2,3,65-67). The high potency of the drug requires careful monitoring. Indications for its use in renal disease include symptomatic uremic bone or muscle disease. Asymptomatic bone disease with roentgenographic evidence of bone resorption, increased alkaline phosphatase, increased iPTH, and histologic evidence of osteitis fibrosa is another indication. However, prophylactic use cannot be systematically recommended at this time in asymptomatic patients. It is less effective when osteomalacia predominates (20). 24,25$(OH)_2D_3$ may then be more useful whether renal disease is present (68-68a) or absent (69). Whenever 1,25$(OH)_2D_3$ is used, serum concentration of calcium and GFR must be carefully monitored (20,70-72). Other indications for 1,25$(OH)_2D_3$ may include hypocalcemia associated with the nephrotic syndrome or renal tubular acidosis. It is possible that renal osteodystrophy results from an imbalance between 1,25 and 24,25$(OH)_2D_3$ rather than from a single metabolite deficiency. Future therapeutic regimens may very well include both metabolites.

When all measures fail and hyperparathyroidism persists with progressive bone disease or hypercalcemia develops, parathyroidectomy is necessary (73). Subtotal parathyroidectomy is performed or total parathyroidectomy with implantation of parathyroid fragments in a site easily accessible in the event of later recurrence of hyperparathyroidism (74-76). A recent census in the Miami area indicates that 50 percent of patients undergoing chronic hemodialysis for four years needed parathyroidectomy while 100 percent of patients treated for eight years or more had been subjected to parathyroid surgery (W. Anderson, personal communication).

An alternative to surgical parathyroidectomy may be pharmacologic inhibition of PTH secretion. The most physiologic way to inhibit PTH secretion is with calcium ions. Calcium administration is obviously contraindicated in hypercalcemic patients and dangerous in hyperphosphatemic subjects. However, oral pharmacologic agents, propranolol, a beta-adrenergic antagonist, 24,25$(OH)_2D_3$, a vitamin D metabolite, and cimetidine, an H_2 histamine receptor antagonist, have been shown to decrease iPTH in patients or animals with chronic renal failure, presumably by acting directly on the parathyroid glands. Although the data available are scanty, they introduce the concept of "medical parathyroidectomy" as a possible future means of treatment of uremic hyperparathyroidism and renal osteodystrophy.

iPTH, alkaline phosphatase and radiologic bone lesions of lesser magnitude have been observed in chronic hemodialysis patients receiving propranolol for 4-22 months than in a comparable population not receiving the beta blocker (77). Propranolol has also been shown to decrease iPTH following intravenous administration (78). In primary hyperparathyroid patients propranolol normalized circulating iPTH in 5 of 8 patients but convincingly decreased serum calcium only in 3 patients (79). iPTH in hyperparathyroid chronically uremic dogs given 2 μg $24,25(OH)_2D_3$ daily p.o. decreased by 50 percent after 3 weeks of treatment (45). Finally, cimetidine administered prospectively to chronically hemodialyzed patients at a dose of 600-900 mg daily p.o. decreased circulating iPTH from 419 to 107 μlEq/ml (normal values: less than 75 μlEq/ml) after 10 weeks of treatment (80). Similar observations with cimetidine have been made in dogs with chronic renal insufficiency (26). Interestingly, with each drug, the inhibition of iPTH occurred without an increase in serum ionized calcium and was reversible upon withdrawal of the drug but none inhibited iPTH completely. For all three agents these preliminary data are experimental and need confirmation. Although for all three drugs the PTH inhibition is supported by physiologic data (81-87), the effectiveness of these agents in the long term treatment of renal osteodystrophy remains an open question. Nevertheless, they could prove useful in individual patients to correct the hypercalcemia of tertiary hyperparathyroidism when contraindication to surgical parathyroidectomy exists (88).

REFERENCES

1. Kumar, B.: Renal osteodystrophy: A complex disorder. J. Lab. Clin. Med. 93: 995-897, 1979.

2. Coburn, J.W., Kurokawa, K. and Llach, F.: Altered divalent ion metabolism in renal disease and renal osteodystrophy. In: Maxwell, M.H. and Kleeman, C.R. (eds.): Clinical Disorders of Fluid and Electrolyte Metabolism. New York: McGraw Hill, 1980, pp. 1153-1251.

3. Kurokawa, K., Klein, K. and Hartenbower, D.L.: Disorders of calcium and phosphate homeostasis. In: Gonick, C. (ed.): Current Nephrology. New York: Houghton Mifflin, 1979, Vol. 3, pp. 135-197.

4. Avioli, L.V.: Renal osteodystrophy. In: Avioli, L.V. and Krane, S.M. (eds.): Metabolic Bone Disease. New York: Academic Press, 1978, Vol. 1, pp. 142-218.

5. de Graaf, P., Schicht, I.M., Pauwels, E.K.J. et al.: Bone scintigraphy in renal osteodystrophy. J. Nucl. Med. 19: 1289-1296, 1978.

6. Malluche, H.H., Ritz, H., Lange, H.P. et al.: Bone histology in incipient and advanced renal failure. Kidney Int. 9: 355-372, 1976.

7. Dent, C.E. and Stamp, T.C.B.: Vitamin D, rickets and osteomalacia. In: Avioli, L.V. and Krane, S.M. (eds.): Metabolic Bone Disease. New York: Academic Press, 1978, Vol. 1, pp. 237-302.

8. Bordier, P., Rasmussen, H., Marie, P. et al.: Vitamin D metabolites and bone mineralization in man. J. Clin. Endocrinol. Metab. 46: 284-294, 1978.

9. Habener, J.F. and Potts, J.T., Jr.: Parathyroid physiology and primary hyperparathyroidism. In: Avioli, L.V. and Krane, S.M. (eds.): Metabolic Bone Disease. New York: Academic Press, 1978, Vol. 1, pp. 1-149.

10. Kaplan, M.A., Canterbury, J.M., Gavallas, G. et al.: Interrelations between phosphorus, calcium, parathyroid hormone, and renal phosphate excretion in response to an oral phosphorus load in normal and uremic dogs. Kidney Int. 14: 207-214, 1978.

11. Reiss, E., Canterbury, J. and Kanter, A.: Circulating parathyroid hormone concentration in chronic renal insufficiency. Arch. Int. Med. 124: 417-422, 1969.

12. Slatopolsky, E., Rutherford, W.E., Hruska, K. et al.: How important is phosphate in the pathogenesis of renal osteodystrophy? Arch. Int. Med. 138: 848-852, 1978.

13. Massry, S.G. The pathogenesis of secondary hyperparathyroidism of renal failure. Is there a controversy? Arch. Int. Med. 138: 848-852, 1978.

14. Massry, S.G. Pathogenesis of secondary hyperparathyroidism in early renal failure: a multifactorial system including phosphate retention, skeletal resistance to PTH, and altered vitamin D metabolism. In: Norman, A.W. et al. (eds.): Vitamin D. Basic Research and its Clinical Application. New York: W. de Gruyter, 1979, pp. 1203-1208.

15. Slatopolsky, E., Gray, R., Adams, N.D. et al.: The pathogenesis of secondary hyperparathyroidism in early renal failure. In: Norman, A.W. et al. (eds.): Vitamin D. Basic Research and its Clinical Application. New York: W. de Gruyter, 1979, pp. 1209-1216.

16. Ritz, E., Malluche, H.H., Krempien, B. et al.: Pathogenesis of renal osteodystrophy: Roles of phosphate and skeletal resistance to PTH. In Advances in Experimental Medicine 103: 423-437, 1978.

17. Massry, S.G., Ritz, E. and Verberckmoes, R.: Role of phosphate in the genesis of secondary hyperparathyroidism of renal failure. Nephron 18: 77-81, 1977.

18. Bricker, N.S., Slatopolsky, E., Reiss, E. et al.: Calcium, phosphorus and bone in renal disease and transplantation. Arch. Int. Med. 123: 543-554, 1969.

19. Slatopolsky, E., Caglar, S., Pennell, J.P. et al.: On the pathogenesis of hyperparathyroidism in chronic experimental renal insufficiency in the dog. J. Clin. Invest. 50: 492-500, 1971.

20. Levine, B.S. and Coburn, J.W.: Physiology of the vitamin D endocrine system and disorders of altered vitamin D metabolism. In: Brenner, B.M. and Stein, J.H. (eds.): Contemporary Issues in Nephrology, Vol. 4. Hormonal Function and the Kidney. New York: Churchill Livingstone, 1979, pp. 215-251.

21. Llach, F., Massry, S.G., Singer, F.R. et al.: Skeletal resistance to endogenous parathyroid hormone in patients with early renal failure. A possible cause for secondary hyperparathyroidism. J. Clin. Endocr. Metab. 41: 339-345, 1975.

22. Reiss, E., Canterbury, J.M., Bercovitz, M.A. et al.: The role of phosphate in the secretion of parathyroid hormone in man. J. Clin. Invest. 49: 2146-2149, 1970.

23. Rutherford, W.E., Bordier, P., Marie, P. et al.: Phosphate control and 25-hydroxycholecalciferol administration in preventing experimental renal osteodystrophy in the dog. J. Clin. Invest. 60: 332-341, 1977.

24. Kaplan, M., Canterbury, J., Bourgoignie, J. et al.: Reversal of hyperparathyroidism in response to dietary phosphorus restriction in uremic dog. Kidney Int. 15: 43-48, 1979.

25. Slatopolsky, E. and Bricker, N.S. The role of phosphorus restriction in the prevention of secondary hyperparathyroidism in chronic renal disease. Kidney Int. 4: 141-146, 1973.

26. Jacob, A.I., Canterbury, J.M., Gavellas, G. et al.: Effect of cimetidine on calcium and phosphate homeostasis in normal and uremic dogs. Clin. Res. 28, 450A, 1980.

27. Swenson, R.S., Weisinger, J.R., Ruggeri, J.L. et al.: Evidence that parathyroid hormone is not required for phosphate homeostasis in renal failure. Metab. Clin. End. 24: 199-204, 1975.

28. Tröhler, U., Bonjour, J.P. and Fleisch, H. Inorganic phosphate homeostasis. Renal adaptation to the dietary intake in intact and thyroparathyroidectomized rats. J. Clin. Invest. 57: 264-273, 1976.

29. Steele, T.H. and DeLuca, F. Influence of dietary phosphorus on renal phosphate reabsorption in the parathyroidectomized rat. J. Clin. Invest. 57: 867-874, 1976.

30. Sherwood, L.M., Mayer, G.P., Ramberg, C.F., Jr. et al.: Regulation of parathyroid hormone secretion: proportional control by calcium, lack of effect of phosphate. Endocr. 83: 1043-1052, 1969.

31. Massry, S.G., Coburn, J.W., Lee, D.B. et al.: Skeletal resistance to parathyroid hormone in renal failure. Studies in 105 human subjects. Ann. Int. Med. 78: 357-364, 1973.

32. Massry, S.G., Stein, R., Garty, G. et al.: Skeletal resistance to the calcemic action of parathyroid hormone in uremia: role of $1,25(OH)_2D_3$. Kidney Int. 9: 467-474, 1976.

33. Massry, S.G., Dua, S., Garty, J. et al.: Role of uremia in the skeletal resistance to the calcemic action of parathyroid hormone. Min. Electrolyte Metab. 1: 172-180, 1978.

34. Kaplan, M.A., Canterbury, J.M., Gavellas, G. et al.: The calcemic and phosphaturic effects of parathyroid hormone in the normal and uremic dog. Metab. 27: 1785-1792, 1978.

35. Massry, S.G., Tumas, S., Dua, S. and Goldstein, D.A.: Reversal of skeletal resistance to parathormone in uremia by vitamin D metabolites. J. Lab. Clin. Med. 94: 152-158, 1979.

36. Wills, M.R. and Jenkins, M.V.: The effect of uremic metabolites on parathyroid extract - induced bone resorption in vitro. Clin. Chim. Acta 73: 121-125, 1976.

37. Raisz, L.G. and Niemann, I.: Effect of phosphate, calcium and magnesium on bone resorption and hormonal responses in tissue culture. Endocr. 85: 446-453, 1969.

38. Habener, J.F. and Potts, J.T.: Biosynthesis of parathyroid hormone. N. Engl. J. Med. 299: 580-585 and 635-644, 1978.

39. Hruska, K.A., Kapelman, R., Rutherford, W.E. et al.: Metabolism of immunoreactive parathyroid hormone in the dog. J. Clin. Invest. 56: 39-48, 1975.

40. Freitag, J.J., Martin, K., Hruska, K.A. et al.: Impaired parathyroid hormone metabolism in patients with chronic renal failure. N. Engl. J. Med. 298: 29-32, 1978.

41. Martin, K., Hruska, K.A., Freitag, J.J. et al.: The peripheral metabolism of parathyroid hormone. N. Engl. J. Med. 301: 1092-1098, 1979.

42. Bellorin-Font, Martin, K.J., Freitag, J.J. et al.: Altered adenylate cyclase kinetics in hyperfunctioning human glands. Comparison with normal human and bovine parathyroid tissue. J. Clin. Invest. In press.

43. Canterbury, J.M., Lerman, S., Claflin, A.J. et al.: Inhibition of parathyroid hormone secretion by 25-hydroxycholecalciferol and 24,25 dihydroxycholecalciferol in the dog. J. Clin. Invest. 51: 1375-1383, 1978.

44. Canterbury, J.M., Gavellas, G., Bourgoignie, J. et al.: In-vivo suppression of parathyroid hormone secretion by 24,25 dihydroxycholecalciferol in hyperparathyroid dogs. In: Norman, A.W. et al. (eds.): Vitamin D. Basic Research and its Clinical Application. New York: W. de Gruyter, 1979, pp. 297-305.

45. Canterbury, J., Gavellas, G., Bourgoignie, J. et al.: Metabolic consequences of oral administration of $24,25(OH)_2D_3$ to uremic dog. J. Clin. Invest. 65: 571-576, 1980.

46. Care, A.D., Pickard, D.W., Papapoulos, S.E. et al.: Inhibitory effect of 25,26-dihydroxycholecalciferol on the rate of secretion of parathyroid hormone in goats. J. Endocr. 78: 303-304, 1978.

47. Golden, P., Mazey, R., Greenwalt, A. et al.: Vitamin D: A direct effect on the parathyroid gland? Min. Electrolyte Metab. 2: 1-6, 1979.

48. Tanaka, Y., DeLuca, H.F., Ghazarian, J.G. et al.: Effect of vitamin D and its metabolites on serum parathyroid hormone levels in the rat. Min. Electrolyte Metab. 2: 20-25, 1979.

49. DeLuca, H.F.: Vitamin D and calcium transport. Annals N.Y. Acad. Sci. 356-376, 1978.

51. Haussler, M.R. and McCain, T.: Basic and medical concepts related to vitamin D metabolism and action. N. Engl. J. Med. 297: 974-983 and 1041-1050, 1977.

52. Taylor, C.M.: 24,25-dihydroxyvitamin D in human serum. In: Norman, A.W. et al. (eds.): Vitamin D. Basic Research and its Clinical Application. New York: W. de Gruyter, 1979, pp. 197-204.

52a. Russell, R.G.G., Kanis, J.A., Smith, R. et al.: Physiological and pharmacological aspects of 24,25-dihydroxycholecalciferol in man. In: Advances in Experimental Medicine 103: 487-504, 1978.

53. Horst, R.L., Shepard, R.M., Jorgensen, N.A. et al.: Assays of vitamin D and its metabolites. In: Norman, A.W. et al. (eds.): Vitamin D. Basic Research and its Clinical Application. New York: W. de Gruyter, 1979, pp. 213-220.

54. Lund, B., Clausen, E., Friedberg, M. et al.: Serum 1,25-dihydroxycholecalciferol in anephric, haemodialyzed and kidney transplanted patients. Effect of vitamin D_3 supplement. Nephron 25-33, 1980.

55. Liu, S.H. and Chu, H.I.: Studies of calcium and phosphorus metabolism with special reference to pathogenesis and effect of dihydrotachysterol (AT10) and iron. Medicine (Baltimore) 22: 103-162, 1943.

56. Malluche, H.H., Werner, E. and Ritz, E.: Intestinal absorption of calcium and wholebody calcium retention in incipient and advanced renal failure. Min. Electrolyte Metab. 1: 263-270, 1978.

57. Kanis, J.A., Keyner, G., Russell, R.G.G. et al.: Biological effects of 24,25-dihydroxycholecalciferol in man. In: Norman, A.W. et al. (eds.): Vitamin D. Biochemical, chemical and clinical aspects related to calcium metabolism. New York: W. de Gruyter, 1977, pp. 793-796.

58. Llach, F., Brickman, A.S., Singer, F.R. et al.: 24,25-dihydroxycholecalciferol, a vitamin D sterol with qualitatively unique effects in uremic man. Metab. Bone Dis. and Rel. Res. 2: 11-15, 1979.

59. Malluche, H.H., Goldstein, D.A. and Massry, S.G. Osteomalacia and hyperparathyroid bone disease in patients with nephrotic syndrome. J. Clin. Invest. 73: 494-500, 1979.

60. Slatopolsky, E., Rutherford, W.E., Rosenbaum, R. et al.: Hyperphosphatemia. Clin. Nephrol. 7: 138-146, 1977.

61. Goldsmith, R., Furszyfer, J., Johnson, W.J. et al.: Control of secondary hyperparathyroidism during long-term hemodialysis. Am. J. Med. 50: 692-699, 1971.

62. Bouillon, R., Verberckmoes, R. and DeMoor, P.: Influence of dialysate calcium concentration and vitamin D on serum parathyroid hormone during repetitive dialysis. Kidney Int. 7: 422-432, 1975.

63. Goldsmith, R.S. and Johnson, W.J. Role of phosphate depletion and high dialysate calcium in controlling dialytic renal osteodystrophy. Kidney Int. 4: 154-161, 1973.

64. Clarkson, E.M., Eastwood, J.B., Koutsaimanis, K.G. et al.: Net intestinal absorption of calcium in patients with chronic renal failure. Kidney Int. 3: 258-263, 1973.

65. Goldstein, D.A., Malluche, H.H. and Massry, S.G. Management of renal osteodystrophy with $1,25(OH)_2D_3$. I. Effects on clinical, radiographic, and biochemical parameters. Min. Electrolyte Metab. 2: 35-47, 1979.

66. Malluche, H.H., Goldstein, D.A. and Massry, S. Management of renal osteodystrophy with $1,25(OH)_2D_3$. II. Effects on histopathology of bone: evidence for healing osteomalacia. Min. Electrolyte Metab. 2: 48-55, 1979.

67. Fournier, A., Bordier, P , Gueris, J. et al.: Comparison of 1α-hydroxycholecalciferol and 25-hydroxycholecalciferol in the treatment of renal osteodystrophy - greater effects of 25-hydroxycholecalciferol on bone mineralization. Kidney Int. 15: 196-204, 1979.

68. Hodsman, A.B., Sherrard, D.J., Wong, E.G.C. et al.: Vitamin D resistant osteomalacia without secondary hyperparathyroidism in dialysis patients. Clin. Res. 28: 560A, 1980.

68a. Coburn, J.W., Wong, E.G.C., Sherrard, D.J. et al.: Use of 24, 25-dihydroxyvitamin D_3 in dialysis osteomalacia: preliminary results. Clin. Res. 28: 532A, 1980.

69. Eastwood, J.B., de Wardener, H.E., Gray, R.W. et al.: Normal plasma $1,25-(OH)_2$ - Vitamin-D concentrations in nutritional osteomalacia. Lancet 1: 1377-1378, 1979.

70. Bell, N.H. and Stern, P.H. Hypercalcemia and increases in serum hormone value during prolonged administration of 1,25-dihydroxyvitamin D. N. Engl. J. Med. 298: 1241-1243, 1978.

71. Christiansen, C., Redbro, P., Christensen, M.S. et al.: Deterioration of renal function during treatment of chronic renal failure with 1,25 dihydroxycholecalciferol. Lancet 2: 700-703, 1978.

72. Nielsen, H.E., Romer, F.K., Melsen, F. et al.: 1α-hydroxy vitamin D3 treatment of non-dialyzed patients with chronic renal failure. Effects on bone, mineral metabolism and kidney function. Clin. Nephrol. 13: 103-108, 1980.

73. Wilson, R.E., Hampers, C.L., Bernstein, D.S. et al.: Subtotal parathyroidectomy in chronic renal failure. A seven year experience in a dialysis and transplant program. Ann. Surgery 174: 640-652, 1971.

74. Wells, S.A., Gunnells, J.C., Shelburne, J.D. et al.: Transplantation of the parathyroid glands in man: clinical indications and results. Surgery 78: 34-43, 1975.

75. Schneider, A.B., Wells, S.A., Gunnells, J.C. et al.: Regulation of function of transplanted parathyroid glands. Am. J. Med. 63: 710-718, 1977.

76. Cordell, L.J., Maxwell, J.G. and Warden, G.D. Parathyroidectomy in chronic renal failure. Am. J. Surgery 138: 951-956, 1979.

77. Caro, J.F., Besarab, A., Burke, J.F. et al.: A possible role for propranolol in the treatment of renal osteodystrophy. Lancet 2: 451-454, 1978.

78. Coevoet, B., Andrejak, M., Desplan, C. et al.: Acute effects of propranolol and metoprolol on plasma concentrations of parathyroid hormone and calcitonin in uremic patients. In: Thurm, R.H. (ed.): Essential Hypertension. Chicago: Yearbook Medical Publ., 1979, pp. 219-229.

79. Caro, J.F., Castro, J.H. and Glennon, J.A.: Effect of long-term propranolol administration on parathyroid hormone and calcium concentration in primary hyperparathyroidism. Ann. Int. Med. 91: 740-741, 1979.

80. Jacob, A.I., Lanier, D., Jr., Canterbury, J.M. et al. Reduction of serum parathyroid hormone levels in uremic patients. N. Engl. J. Med. 302: 671-674, 1980.

81. Kukreja, S.C., Williams, G.A., Hargis, G.K. et al.: Dual control of suppressibility of parathyroid hormone by calcium and by beta-adrenergic blockade. Min. Electrolyte Metab. 2: 316-322, 1979.

82. Brown, E.M., Gardner, D., Windeck, R.A. et al.: B. Adrenergically stimulated 3', 5' monophosphate accumulation in and parathyroid hormone release from dispersed human parathyroid cells. J. Clin. Endocr. Metab. 48: 618-626, 1976.

83. Kukreja, S.C., Johnson, P.A., Ayala, G. et al.: Role of calcium and beta-adrenergic system in control of parathyroid hormone secretion. Proc. Soc. Exp. Biol. Med. 151: 326-328, 1976.

84. Longley, R.S., Hargis, G.K., Bowser, E.N. et al.: Parathyroid hormone and calcitonin secretion: role of histamine H_2 receptors. Clin. Res. 28: 398A, 1980.

85. Brown, E.M.: Histamine receptors in parathyroid adenomas. Clin. Res. 28: 388A, 1980.

86. Williams, G.A., Longley, R.S., Hargis, G.K. et al.: Effect of histamine on secretion of parathyroid hormone. Clin. Res. 27: 794A, 1979.

87. Fischer, J.A. and Blum, J.W.: Noncalcium control of parathyroid hormone secretion. Min. Electrolyte Metab. 3: 158-166, 1980.

88. Lanier, D., Favre, H., Jacob, A.I. et al.: Cimetidine therapy for severe hypercalcemia in two chronic hemodialysis patients. Ann. Int. Med. In press.

HYPERTENSION OF RENAL ORIGIN IN CHILDHOOD

Michel Broyer, M.D. and Jean-Louis Bacri, M.D.

Serv. Nephrol. Pediatr., Hôpital Necker Enfants-Malades
Paris, France

From 1960 to 1980, 280 children and adolescents were referred to the pediatric nephrology department of the hospital "des Enfants Malades" in Paris for hypertension (HT). This series was defined by a diastolic blood pressure (BP) > 90 mm Hg. Of these 280 patients, the hypertension in 86% (240) was of renal origin. This percentage is an overestimation of the frequency of renal causes of childhood HT since these patients were referred to a specialized service. However, the amount is in accordance with previous studies performed under the same conditions; Still and Cotton found renal causes in 70% (1), Gill et al. in 83% (2), Royer et al. in 90% (3), and Aderele and Siriki in 95% (4). In contrast, Londe et al. found renal causes in only 5% but here hypertension was defined by the 97.5th percentile (5).

Thus, the exact prevalence of HT of renal origin in childhood is not known; it depends upon the definition of HT and also on age: the younger the child, and the higher the BP, the more likely the HT is secondary and of renal origin. Consequently, and in spite of the increasing interest raised by essential hypertension in the pediatric age, renal causes warrant careful analysis, as is attempted in this paper.

SYMPTOMS AND BLOOD PRESSURE VALUES

The majority of cases of renal HT reported here were symptomatic. The most frequent signs/symptoms were headaches, dizziness, abdominal pain, vomiting, polyuria, polydipsia, weight loss, sight defect, seizures, facial nerve palsy, and mucosal or post surgical bleeding. Nevertheless, nearly half of these cases (10 of the last 22 cases) have been detected by incidental physical examination at times indicated by the discovery of proteinuria, but often without any reason.

Severe complications have been observed, including congestive heart failure, blindness, coma and hypertensive encephalopathy. Malignant hypertension as defined by accelerated renal failure with very high blood pressure and hemolytic anemia, which looks like hemolytic uremic syndrome, was rare; 4 such cases were observed in this series.

Blood pressure values at time of diagnosis generally were very high. In 27 children with small, scarred kidneys for whom there were at least 3 BP measurements before any treatment, the mean BP was 185/119 mm Hg. In 38 children with renovascular HT by the same criteria, the mean BP was 192/114 mm Hg. In contrast with these figures, 15 patients belonging to the same series and finally classified as essential hypertension, had a mean BP of 158/96 mm Hg.

ETIOLOGY (Table 1)

The main causes of these 240 cases of HT were: glomerular disease, 71 cases; hemolytic uremic syndrome, 15 cases; scarred small kidneys, 77 cases (of which 30 were histologically defined as segmental hypoplasia); vascular changes (renovascular HT), 48 cases; obstructive uropathies, 18 cases; and various, 11 cases (Wilm's tumor 4, trauma 3, polycystic kidneys 3, sequellae of renal ischemia 1).

Glomerular Nephropathies (GN)

Only patients with persistent HT beyond the first weeks of the onset of the disease have been selected here. Acute GN, which represents a major cause of HT in childhood but generally is transient, is not included in this list. Rapidly progressive or crescentic GN frequently was associated with HT (15/22), as was periarteritis nodosa (12/14), and lupus GN (10/25); in contrast, membranoproliferative GN rarely was complicated by HT (2/106), neither was membranous GN (3/60) nor idiopathic steroid unresponsive nephrotic syndrome (4/136). Henoch Schönlein GN had an intermediate position (10/100). Berger's disease, frequently associated with HT in adult patients, was not in children (3/100). Whatever type of GN, there was generally a correlation between microscopic arterial lesions and the development of HT.

Hemolytic Uremic Syndrome

Severe HT may develop and persist beyond the acute phase of the disease. The frequency of this complication was nevertheless

Table 1. Etiology of 240 Cases of Renal Hypertension in Children

Cause	Cases	%
Glomerular disease	71	29.4
Hemolytic uremic syndrome	15	6.3
Scarred small kidneys	77	32.3
histologically defined	(30)	
without histology	(47)	
Renovascular	48	19.7
Obstructive uropathy	18	7.5
Various	11	4.6
Wilm's and other tumors	(4)	
post traumatic	(3)	
polycystic kidneys	(3)	
sequelae of renal ischemia	(1)	

different according to the age of the patient. It was rare in children under 2-3 years of age (5 of 60 cases), and frequent in those above 3 years (10 of 15 cases). Here again, important vascular lesions were found upon microscopic examination of the kidney. This form of renal HT sometimes was extremely severe, especially in older children; bilateral nephrectomy was required in 10 cases.

Small Scarred Kidneys

Considerable controversy remains about this group of patients, one of the most important in all series of renal hypertension in children under different eponyms (Ask-Upmark kidney, pyelonephritis, segmental hypoplasia, etc.). Calling it "segmental hypoplasia", Habib et al. (6) can be credited with giving the precise description of this histological lesion and drawing attention to the fact that this kind of renal alteration is often observed without any antecedent infectious episode and proposing an alternative to the general opinion that pyelonephritis is its usual cause.

Segmental hypoplasia is well defined anatomically and histologically (7). At macroscopic examination, the kidney appears reduced in volume. The atrophy involves both cortex and medulla with dilatation of corresponding calices. At microscopic examination, the main characteristic is the sharp demarkation of the scarred zone from the apparently normal zone. In the cortex the major alterations involve tubules and vessels. Tubules are either totally collapsed or dilated and their lumen is filled with colloid casts. Arcuate and interlobar arteries are severely altered with sclero-elastic endarteritis and complete obstruction of their lumen. The medulla is reduced to a thin layer of fibrous mesenchymatous tissue with occasional collecting ducts. These changes are not accompanied by an inflammatory infiltration of the interstitial tissue. In this series, using these histological criteria, 30 cases of HT were found fitting the definition of segmental hypoplasia. Age at diagnosis was 5-14 years. There was a predominance of female patients (22/30). The diagnosis was suspected after IV pyelography (IVP) which showed abnormalities affecting one or both kidneys, reduced size or abnormalities of the renal contour and of the calices. These lesions often were found at the upper pole with blunting or clubbing of calices and parenchymal amputation. Voiding cystourethrography (VCU) showed vesico ureteral reflux in 2/3 cases, usually marked and bilateral. Of 30 cases, only 8 had unilateral lesion with compensatory hypertrophy on the other side, suggesting that the lesion was unilateral.

HT was completely cured by nephrectomy in unilateral cases when this operation was performed before the development of contralateral lesions of nephroangiosclerosis. In cases of bilateral lesions, treatment was purely symptomatic and evolution toward terminal renal failure (TRF) was observed in the most severe forms and when HT was not easily under control.

Physiopathology of HT is linked to renin secretion in the scarred zone of the kdiney; this was shown by PRA assay from renal vein in unilateral cases, or by finding granules of renin in the pathologic arteries. The cause of scars remains a subject of discussion. Three hypotheses which have been proposed are: defect of renal development, reflux nephropathy during fetal life or the first months after birth, or late sequelae of early infection of renal parenchyma.

Vascular Changes
(Renovascular Hypertension)

This group of 48 cases is defined by HT associated with alterations of the main renal vessel and its first branches (1). HT was generally severe. Arterial stenosis was suspected in 7 patients after finding an abdominal bruit; in 4 others, clinical symptoms of neurofibromatosis oriented the diagnosis toward a renovascular cause.

IVP generally drew attention to the kidney, but was noninformative in 13 of the 48 cases. Kidney size usually was reduced, and the contrast material appeared more opaque in the renal pelvis on the side of ischemia. After IV furosemide administration, this last finding was observed in 75% of the cases with unilateral lesions. The diagnosis in all cases was confirmed by arteriography. Two main subgroups may be described.

Localized alteration of renal arteries occurred in 22 cases. Of these, 5 were cases of *renal artery stenosis*; only one was clearly related to a precise cause - radiotherapy done 13 years before for neuroblastoma. *Renal artery thrombosis* was suspected on clinical grounds in 3 infants who underwent umbilical artery catheterization after birth and had cardiac failure. Two were nephrectomized; the HT of the third one was successfully treated but he was left with a small kidney. One girl whose first symptom was lumbar pain, rapidly developed severe HT which was cured only by nephrectomy; renal artery thrombosis was discovered upon histological examination. She had an important and persistent increase of factors V and VIII. A diagnosis of lupus was confirmed 3 years later based on biological criteria. Three other cases of renal artery thrombosis remained idiopathic. There were 4 cases of *renal artery aneurysm*. This diagnosis was based on arteriography in 3. In the fourth, the right kidney was not visualized and arteriography did not show a right renal artery; the diagnosis of massively thrombosed aneurysm was made at laparotomy. No systemic disease was found in these patients. Several types of *fibromuscular dysplasia* have been described in adult patients but the four cases in this series were unusual. Two were characterized by an anarchic proliferation of muscle fiber in the media, the rarest type; in another case, this abnormality was limited to a segment of the vessel. Two cases of *endarteritis* remained without an explanation.

Alteration of renal artery as part of a generalized vascular disease occurred in 20 cases. *Neurofibromatosis of Von Recklinghausen* is the most frequent cause of generalized angiodysplasia. Out of the seven cases in this series, five had unilateral and two, bilateral lesions. The diagnosis was suspected because of "cafe au lait" spots or familial antecedents in 5 of the 7 cases. Arteriography showed a banal stenosis in 4 cases, and multiple vascular abnormalities in the others. In two cases the diagnosis was made after microscopic examination of the renal artery which showed the specific lesion characterized by irregular proliferation of fusiform cells in the tunica intima, breaching of the lamina elastica interna and, here and there, disappearance of the tunica media. *Pseudoxanthoma elasticum* (2 cases), a rare hereditary disease, is clinically characterized by skin lesions (yellow papuli), specific abnormalities of the eyegrounds (angioid streaks), gastrointestinal bleeding and progressive obstruction of arteries. HT is rare in children. Diagnosis was ascertained on familial antecedents, microscopic examination of arteries, and ultrastructural abnormalities of skin elastic fibers. Multiple thrombosis and fusiform aneurysms of branches of renal, iliac and mesenteric arteries were noted in our cases, giving a characteristic feature to the arteriography. *Ehlers-Danlos syndrome* (type IV of Sack) was found in one case, a boy of 14 years who had an aneurysm of the aorta with an irregularly dilated left renal artery; he had recurring pyeloureteral stenosis after surgery and an abnormal skin.

Takayasu's disease or coarctation of abdominal aorta occurred in 5 children ages 2-14 years (3 from north Africa). Three had no or feeble peripheral pulses. Arteriography revealed extended stenosis of the abdominal aorta and ostial stenosis of renal arteries. Histological examination in two cases confirmed the diagnosis of nonspecific aortitis with predominant lesions in the adventitia. The pathogenesis of this disease remains obscure. A congential malformation may be considered in very young children. An infectious process has been proposed. Tuberculosis was found frequently in some areas. Two out of these 5 patients had strongly positive tuberculin skin tests. An autoimmune inflammatory process has also been advocated. *William and Beuren syndrome* was observed in one case. This child had the characteristic "elf" facies. He became hypertensive at age 13. Arteriography showed stenosis of one renal artery and of the aorta. *Idiopathic arteritis with calcification of the media* was found in 2 cases with severe HT, ages 3 and 12 years with diffuse microscopic calcification of arteries including renal, without coronary involvement. The relationship between these 2 cases and the classical idiopathic infantile arterial calcification is not clear. *Unclassified abnormalities* were found in 2 cases.

Miscellaneous causes of renovascular HT included renal vein thrombosis followed by HT in 2 cases and external compression of the renal artery by hematoma or a tumor in 4 cases.

Treatment of renovascular HT. This type of HT is of great interest because there is the possibility of surgical cure. In the past, nephrectomy often was thought to be the only way to avoid the problems stemming from renal ischemia. Now, efforts are as conservative as possible, to try to repair vascular lesions by eventually using *ex vivo* surgery or autotransplantation. Each case raises a particular problem which can be solved only after complete investigation which includes renal vein plasma renin assay (PRA).

In the last 3 years, 8 patients with renovascular HT underwent vena cava and renal vein sampling for PRA. Six of them had unilateral arterial lesions and a ratio R/RC between 1.5 and 10; all have been cured by surgery. Two patients had asymetrical bilateral vascular disease and had a ratio R/RC > 1.5; they also had a ratio RC/VC > 2 which gave evidence of a persistent renin secretion on the better side. They were treated medically.

Overall results of the present series are difficult to interpret because of the long period of time during which the cases were collected. Out of 27 cases of unilateral lesions, 25 have been operated. Thirteen nephrectomies have been performed as first operation with 12 definitive cures. Ten surgical reconstructions of renal arteries have been undertaken, and if 3 subsequent nephrectomies are included, 7 of these patients are completely cured of their HT. The case with renal artery stenosis secondary to irradiation underwent autotransplantation with improvement of HT. Another case healed after evacuation of a hematoma. Of the 19 children with bilateral lesions, 10 underwent surgery but only 3 with Takayasu disease could be satisfactorily recontructed with complete cure of HT.

Obstructive Uropathies

Eighteen cases of HT were recorded under this title but only 6 of them really may be considered as such. In these 6 cases HT was cured or improved after correction of the urinary obstruction. In the other cases the result of surgery was less clear and the kidneys gnerally were altered. These patients might be classified with the group defined as "small scarred kidneys".

OTHER CAUSES

Hypertension Associated with Renal Tumor

Wilm's tumor classically may be complicated by severe HT as was the case for 2 children of the present series. There was also one case of hamartoma of the kidney and one case of compressive sympathoblastoma.

Hemangiopericytome or renin secreting tumor is lacking in this series. This cause has to be carefully looked for in children with high renin HT without obvious etiology. Arteriography usually detects the tumor but this investigation may be negative and the tumor is then only suspected after segmental renal vein sampling for PRA.

Post Traumatic Hypertension

Three cases of mild HT developed after renal trauma, without apparent involvement of the main renal artery, but with a reduction of renal size.

Polycystic Disease and Hypertension

Of a total of 12 cases followed with polycystic disease, 3 exhibited HT during the first 2-3 years of life.

Sequelae of Renal Ischemia - Unclassified Case

One case difficult to classify deserves to be reported. N.J., a boy 11 years old, became suddenly and severely hypertensive; IVP showed a right kidney smaller than the left but without any abnormality of calices. Arteriography did not show any alteration of the renal arteries, but scintigraphy and ultrasonography revealed a slight abnormality in the right kidney structure. As PRA was higher on this side (R/RC = 1.8), a biopsy and a right nephrectomy were successively performed and hypertension disappeared. Histological examination revealed a limited zone of ischemic lesions without any vascular alteration. Antecedents of prematurity and neonatal difficulties were the only explanation that could be suggested.

In conclusion a number of renal causes may be involved in childhood and adolescent hypertension. These causes should be carefully looked for in these age groups because of surgical possibilities for correction. From a practical point of view, it must be recalled that renal hypertension usually is severe. We propose limiting complete investigation to patients who have blood pressure consistently at least 10 mm of Hg above the 97.5th percentile of normal distribution, or in the case of symptomatic or complicated HT.

SUMMARY

Two hundred and eighty cases of hypertension in children and adolescents were collected over a twenty year period (1959-1980). Definition of hypertension was a diastolic BP > 90 mm Hg. Two hundred and forty cases were of renal origin. Seventy-one cases (29.5%) were related to glomerulonephritis, the majority of which were rapidly progressive GN, periarteritis nodosa and lupus nephritis. Fifteen (6.03%) cases occurred after hemolytic uremic syndrome, especially in children older than 3 years. Seventy-seven cases (32.3%) had small scarred kidneys of which 30, after histological examination, were classified as "segmental hypoplasia". Forty-eight cases (19.7%) had abnormalities of renal arteries or branches, 22 had localized alterations of the renal artery, 20 were part of a general vascular disease (7 neurofibromatosis, 5 Takayasu's disease, 2 renal vein thrombosis, and 4 external compression by tumor). There also were 19 cases (7.5%) of obstructive uropathy and 11 (4.6%) miscellaneous causes.

The mean blood pressure before treatment was 185/119 in patients with small scarred kidneys and 192/114 in renovascular HT. It is proposed in childhood hypertension to limit complete renal investigation to those cases where BP is consistently at least 10 mm Hg above the 97.5 percentile.

REFERENCES

1. Still, J.L. and Cotton, D.: Severe Hypertension in Childhood. Arch. Dis. Child. 42: 34, 1967.

2. Gill, D.G., Mendes da Costa, B., Cameron, J.S., et al.: Analysis of 100 children with severe and persistent hypertension. Arch. Dis. Child. 51: 951, 1976.

3. Royer, P., Habib, R., Mathieu, H. et al.: Nephrol. Pediatr. Flammarion Medecine, 2 eme edition, p. 333, 1975.

4. Aderele, W.I. and Seriki, O.: Hypertension in Nigerian children. Arch. Dis. Child. 49: 313, 1974.

5. Londe, S., Bourgoignie, J.J., Robson, A.M. and Goldring, D.: Hypertension in apparently normal children. J. Pediatr. 78: 569, 1971.

6. Habib, R., Courtecuisse, V., Ehrensperger, J. et al.: Hypoplasie segmentaire du rein avec hypertension arterielle chez l'enfant. Ann. Pediatr. 12: 262, 1965.

7. Olivier, C., Broyer, M. and Habib, R. In XXIV Congres de l'Association des Pediatres de Langue Francaise, Paris. l'Expansion Scientifique, vol. 1, p. 43, 1975.

USAGE OF ANTIBIOTICS IN CHILDREN WITH RENAL INSUFFICIENCY

Alan B. Gruskin, M.D., H. Jorge Baluarte, M.D., Martin A. Polinsky, M.D., James W. Prebis, M.D. and Abdelaziz Y. Elzouk, M.D.

Sect. Nephrol, St. Christopher's Hosp. for Child., Dept. Pediatr., Temple Univ. Sch. Med., Philadelphia, Pa. 19133 USA

The control of infection remains an important aspect of treatment in patients with renal insufficiency. A large fraction of deaths associated with acute renal failure as well as the three phases of end stage renal disease, the period of chronic uremia, dialysis and transplantation, are due to infection. A large fraction of patients with renal disease need antibiotics for treating bacterial infections exclusive of urinary tract infection. Little data is available in children with renal failure on the incidence of infection or its treatment with anti-infectious agents. In a recent survey of our transplantation experience involving 107 transplants at St. Christopher's Hospital for Children, positive blood cultures were obtained in 10 patients in the initial 21 days following the transplant (1). Moreover, antibiotics have been administered for a variety of infectious problems to virtually all of our patients with end stage renal disease. In one report of 497 children undergoing maintenance dialysis, infection was responsible for death in 13 percent (2). Thus, the need to understand how best to administer antibiotics to uremic children is obvious.

We are aware of three publications dealing with the subject of the pharmacokinetics of usage in children with renal failure. Two deal with the use of gentamycin (3,4). The third is a study performed by us. We have recently completed a study which to the best

Supported in part by General Clinical Research Center Grant RR-75, the Smith Kline and French Corporation, and Hoechst-Roussel Pharmaceuticals.

of our knowledge is the first to evaluate the pharmacokinetics of antibiotic elimination following the administration of a single dose of antibiotic to stable uremic children and to evaluate the relationship between drug removal and progressive renal insufficiency as well as maintenance hemodialysis in children.

The purpose of this presentation is four-fold:

1. To review a few pharmacokinetic principles involved in clinically evaluating antibiotic usage.
2. To illustrate these principles using our experience with Cefazolin in children with chronic renal failure.
3. To consider the use of antibiotics in children undergoing maintenance dialysis based on our experience with Cefazolin.
4. To provide on the basis of our experience with Cefazolin some suggested guidelines for using other antibiotics in children with renal insufficiency.

PHARMACOKINETIC GENERALITIES

Studies of the pharmacokinetics of antibiotics have been performed in two clinical settings (6,7). The first involves the study of drug elimination after administering a single dose of antibiotics to a stable, non-infected patient with normal and reduced renal function. The second approach involves administering a minimum of three doses of antibiotic at appropriate intervals to an infected patient and then evaluating drug kinetics. The former permits the study of drug elimination in a stable patient under controlled conditions while the latter approach often necessitates study in patients whose renal function may be changing. The latter approach, however, may be somewhat more representative of what actually happens in an ill patient who is receiving multiple doses of drugs and has had time for maximal distribution and binding of the drug to occur.

The goal of antibiotic therapy is to administer sufficient drug so that the concentration of drug within the plasma and in cells will exceed the minimum inhibitory concentration necessary to obtain antibacterial activity. Simultaneously, toxic levels must be avoided. In general, a loading dose of antibiotic is initially given. Subsequently, maintenance doses are administered. The frequency of drug administration must be at intervals which permit adequate drug levels to be achieved for periods long enough to destroy infectious agents, yet avoid toxic levels. In general, the frequency of antibiotic administration used in clinical medicine is to administer the antibiotic at intervals equal to 2 to 4 times the half-life of the drug. Drugs will accumulate in the body if they are administered more often than intervals less than

1.4 times the half-life. Theoretically after 1,2,3 and 4 half-lifes the concentration of drug remaining is 50,25,12.5 and 6.25 percent of the original peak concentration. Depending on the drug involved, the maintenance dose given at times corresponding to 1,2 or 3 half-lifes would be 50,75 and 87.5 percent of the loading dose. The administration of drugs at such intervals permits the serum level of drug to fall to a level which is sufficiently low so that the next dose will not raise drug levels to toxic levels. Practical considerations, however, require that the frequency of administration of antibiotics be greater so as to prevent toxic accumulations.

Exclusive of the effect of dialysis on drug removal, the sum of the contribution of other factors can be estimated by ascertaining the serum half-life, i.e. biologic half-life, of the antibiotic. It should be remembered that the half-life of an antibiotic is quite variable and may change daily in a given patient for a number of reasons. The biologic half-lifes of antibiotic are determined by administering the antibiotic either orally, intramuscularly, or intravenously, waiting 30-60 minutes for mixing to occur within the body and then obtaining blood samples at periodic intervals over a number of hours, usually 1-12 (5,6,7). The formula used is: $C = C_0 \cdot e^{-kt}$ where C = drug concentration at time t, C_0 = drug concentration at time zero, e^{-kt} = natural logarithm of two raised to the power kt where k represents the elimination rate constant and t equals time. The elimination rate constant (k) is usually determined by plotting the log of the concentration of the drug against time and the slope of this line or k determined by a least squares regression line. Once k has been determined, the half-life, $t\frac{1}{2}$, is easily calculated. Half-life can be shown to be equal to $-0.693/k$ equals $t\frac{1}{2}$. C or the peak concentration of the drug and the volume of distribution of drug can also be determined by extending the slope of the line back to time zero. Peak levels should not exceed toxic levels.

A number of parameters influence the removal of antibiotics from the body (7,9). They include the renal elimination rate, i.e. the level of renal function, the non-renal excretion rate, the level of function of organ systems involved in the non-renal excretion of drugs, the rate of biotransformation of antibiotics, the volume of distribution of antibiotic, and the influence on the rate of removal of antibiotic by dialysis. Alterations in any one of these parameters by altering the $t\frac{1}{2}$ of an antibiotic will either increase its toxicity or render the drug less effective. In addition to the above, a number of other factors are known to influence drug metabolism in uremic individuals. These factors include the effects of uremia on drug biotransformation (9), protein binding sites (10,11), gastrointestinal function, altered volumes of distribution of drug, i.e. increased extracellular volume, and reduced quantities of albumin. In order to simplify matters, the discussion to follow will assume that all factors other than renal function have remained constant.

ANTIBIOTIC USAGE IN PROGRESSIVE RENAL FAILURE

With the above as a background, we can now proceed to illustrate how alterations in renal function in children influence the drug elimination. As already mentioned, this will be done using our experience with Cefazolin (5) and comparing our results to studies on Cefazolin pharmacokinetics in adults with renal insufficiency (12,13,14,15). Cefazolin is a cephalosporin with a broad spectrum of antimicrobial activity. It is highly bound to serum proteins, but not tightly bound, and readily dissociates from serum proteins when the free level of drug decreases. The principal mode of excretion of Cefazolin is through the kidney by means of glomerular filtration. We have studied its pharmacokinetics in two groups of children with renal insufficiency. The first group included 11 children with varying levels of renal function. We found that the $t_{1/2}$ of Cefazolin increased as the GFR fell. As the GFR fell from 60 to 1.0 ml/min/1.73 m^2 the $t_{1/2}$ of cefazolin increased from 3.8 hours to 115 hours. In evaluating how best to express GFR so that children of varying age and body size could be considered together, we found that the classical hyperbolic relationship between GFR and drug half-life was best demonstrated when the GFR was corrected for surface area. When this was done, the $t_{1/2}$ for Cefazolin in relation to creatinine clearance was similar to values previously reported in adults. When the GFR was not corrected for surface area the anticipated relationship was not as apparent. When the creatinine clearance was estimated, using the formula GFR in ml/min/1.73 m^2 equals $\frac{.55 \text{ Ht in cm}}{\text{serum creatinine mg/dl}}$ (16), close agreement between the estimated clearances were obtained.

On the basis of our studies, our current practice in using antibiotics in children over 1 year of age with renal failure is as follows. First, obtain a serum creatinine and estimate the GFR per 1.73 m^2. Secondly, if pharmacokinetic data are available in children with renal failure modify the dose according to specifically available pediatric data. The specific recommendations which have been developed for the use of Gentamycin and Cefazolin in children with renal failure are tabulated in Table 1. When such data is unavailable - the usual case - we make the assumption that the antibiotic will be handled in uremic children over age one in a manner analogous to that in adults and modify the dose and/or interval according to the recommendations based on pharmacokinetic data developed in adults (17-20). For example, if a child age 7 with a height of 47 inches or 120 cm had a serum creatinine of 2.4 mg/dl, we would assume his clearance to be 27.5 ml/min/1.73 m^2 and would follow the recommendations made for adults whose renal function is 25-30 percent of normal assuming a normal creatinine clearance of 100-120 ml/min/1.73 m^2, or use the recommendation for adult individuals with a GFR of 24-40 ml/min (Table 2). Unfortunately the level of renal function in the majority of pharmacokinetic studies in

Table 1. Dose Recommendations for the Use of Cefazolin and Gentamicin in Children with Renal Failure

		Range $t_{1/2}$ hrs	Interval between doses (hrs)
Gentamicin[a]			
> 50	1 mg/kg	1-6[a]	6-9
25-50	1 mg/kg	22-12[a]	9-21
10-25	1 mg/kg	4-27	21-48
> 10	1 mg/kg	9.5->100	48-72
Cefazolin[b]			
> 50	7 mg/kg	1.8-2.2 (adults)[b]	6
25-50	7 mg/kg	3.8-4.8[c]	12
10-25	7 mg/kg	19-20[c]	24-36
> 10	7 mg/kg	29->100[c]	48-72

[a]Reference 3 (95% confidence limit).
[b]Reference 13.
[c]Reference 5.

adults report clearances simply as ml/min and do not take into account the body size of the individual. The current recommendations for the use of antibiotics as derived for adults with renal insufficiency are summarized in Table 2 (17-20). The variable intervals are due to differences in the biologic half-life which in turn reflect the influence of those factors previously mentioned as influencing drug metabolism. The recommendations are based on giving the usual dose at prolonged intervals rather than a lower dose at the usual interval. We are unaware of any clinical data supporting the superiority of either approach.

ANTIBIOTIC USAGE IN DIALYSIS PATIENTS

The second aspect of our studies with Cefazolin focused on the rate of removal of Cefazolin during five hours of hemodialysis. We found that the $t\frac{1}{2}$ for Cefazolin varied with the efficiency of a particular dialysis as evaluated by the percentage drop in either BUN and/or creatinine occurring during the dialysis. In these children the $t\frac{1}{2}$ for Cefalozin ranged from 8-29½ hours. The parameters which are known to influence antibiotic removal during dialysis are modified by the mechanics involved in the dialysis procedure itself. The more important factors (18,19) are: the molecular weight of the drug, the degree of protein binding, the rate of ultrafiltration and its accompanying solute drag, the rate of blood flow through the coil, ongoing biotransformation of drug, the intrinsic characteristics of the dialysis membrane, including surface area and size of pores, and the extra-renal excretion of drug. The reasons for the large individual variation in the change in drug concentration observed in our studies are multiple. We individualize each dialysis treatment and often vary both the rate of ultrafiltration and the rate of blood flow throughout a dialysis. Both will affect drug removal, especially those drugs which are highly and/or tightly bound to serum proteins. The smaller the transcoil drop in drug concentration the longer the $t\frac{1}{2}$ of the drug, as only a small quantity of drug is removed during each passage through a dialysis coil. The transcoil difference in the concentration of Cefazolin by virtue of its being highly protein bound is small. Rates of removal of antibiotics occurring during peritoneal dialysis may be different from those occurring during hemodialysis, for the overall efficiency of a single peritoneal dialysis as evaluated by changes in BUN and creatinine is not as great as in hemodialysis. Moreover, the type of peritoneal dialysis being performed, i.e. continuous hourly exchanges, continuous ambulatory, or chronic intermittent will influence the rate of removal of antibiotic. Solute removal of small molecular weight compounds is slower during peritoneal dialysis, yet the peritoneal membrane permits the removal of as much larger molecular weight compounds as does hemodialysis. This occurs because the peritoneal membrane is more permeable to large molecular weight compounds, that is, the artificial membranes used

Table 2. Recommendations for modification of anti-infectious agents in adults with renal insufficiency and following dialysis. (Information obtained from references 17,18,19,20)

	Maintenance Dose (Intervals in Hours) GFR ml/min				Modification for Dialysis	
	>100	>50	50-10	<10	Hemodialysis	Peritoneal
Amikacin	8-12	12-18	24-36	36-48	Yes	Yes
Aminosalicylic Acid	8	8	12	Avoid	Yes	
Amoxicillin	8	8	12	16	Yes	-
Amphotericin B	24	24	24	36	No	No+
Ampicillin	6	6	9	12-15	Yes	No
Carbenicillin	4	4	6-12	12-16	Yes	No
Cefamandole	4-6	6	6-9	9	No	No
Cefazolin	8	8	12	24-48	Yes	No
Cephalexin	6	6	6	6-12	Yes	Yes
Cepholothin	6	6	6	8-12	Yes	Yes
Cephapirin	6	6	6	12	Yes	
Cephradine	6	100*	50*	25*	Yes	Yes
Chloramphenicol	6	NC	NC	NC	Yes	No
Chloroquine	24	NC	NC	50	No	-
Clindamycin	6-8	NC	NC	NC	No	No
Cloxacillin	6	NC	NC	NC	No	No+
Colistimethate	12	75	50	25	No	Yes
Dicloxacillin	6	NC	NC	NC	No	No+
Doxycycline	12	NC	NC	NC	No	No
Erythromycin	6	NC	NC	NC	No	No
Ethambutol	24	24	24-36	48	Yes	Yes
Five-Fluorocytocine	6	6	12-24	24-48	Yes	Yes

Table 2 Cont.

Gentamycin	8	8-12	12-24	24-48	Yes	Yes
Isoniazid	8	NC	NC	8-12	Yes	Yes
Kanamycin	8	24	24-72	72-96	Yes	Yes
Lincomycin	6	6	12	24	No	No
Methenamine Mandelate	6	NC	NC	Avoid	?	No
Methicillin	4	4	4	8-12	No	No
Metronidazole	8	8	12	24	Yes	?
Minocycline	12	12	18-24	24-36	No	No +
Nafcillin	6	NC	NC	NC	No	No
Nalidixic Acid	6	NC	NC	Avoid	?	?
Neomycin	6	6	12-18	18-24	Yes	?
Nitrofurantoin	8	Unch.	Avoid	Avoid	Yes	-
Oxacillin	6	NC	NC	NC	No	No
Penicillin G	8	8	8	8-12	Yes	No
Pentamidine	24	24	24-36	48	?	?
Pyrimethamine	24	NC	NC	NC	?	?
Quinine	8	8	8-12	24	Yes	No
Rifampin	24	NC	NC	NC	?	?
Streptomycin	12	24	24-72	72-96	Yes	Yes+
Sulfamethoxazole Trimethoprim	12	12	18	24	Yes	No
Sulfisoxazole	6	6	8-12	12-24	Yes	Yes
Tetracycline	6	8-12	12-24	24	No	No
Ticarcillin	4-6	4	8	12	Yes	Yes
Tobramycin						Yes
Vancomycin	24	24-72	72-240	240	No	No

(-) Unable to find information.

NC No change.

(+) Although in vivo data are not yet available, it has been suggested that when such data become available these agents will be classified as indicated.

(*) Available data reported as a percentage of the usual dose.

in hemodialysis. The ability of peritoneal dialysis to remove antibiotics is also summarized in Table 2. We are aware of only one study which deals with the pharmacokinetics of an antibiotic, Gentamycin, during peritoneal dialysis in children (4). Following an intravenous injection of 1 mg/kg of Gentamycin the half-life ranged from 9-37 hours (mean 21 hours). The large range of half-life may have reflected in part the varying length of dwell time of dialysate. It was felt that the peritoneal clearance of Gentamycin of 4 ± 2.6 ml/min/m^2 in the five children ages 8-15 years was similar to values reported in adults. On the basis of the large variation in half life it was suggested that therapy should be individualized and if possible, drug levels measured.

Insofar as the amounts of dialysate in relation to body size and dwell times are similar to those in adults, rates of removal of antibiotic in children undergoing peritoneal dialysis should be similar assuming that the peritoneal surface area and permeability are also similar. This state probably applies to older children and adolescents, but not to neonates and infants. We have recently demonstrated in the experimental animal that the peritoneal membrane of the young is relatively larger than that of the adult and that it is also more permeable (21). On the basis of the available data and the need to know more about peritoneal dialysis kinetics in infants, we feel that additional information is needed prior to developing more specific guidelines for using antibiotics in children undergoing peritoneal dialysis.

It is apparent that antibiotic dosimetry must be modified twice in patients undergoing dialytic therapy in order to insure that the maximum therapeutic benefit is attained. First, the dose must be appropriately modified for the interdialytic period according to the level of renal function. Second, the dose must be again modified in accordance with the amount of drug removed during dialysis.

A summary of the dialyzability of antibiotics is provided in Table 2. As indicated, a number of antibiotics are dialyzable to an extent that requires that their use be modified. By establishing the relation between the overall efficacy of dialysis and the $t\frac{1}{2}$ for antibiotic removal during dialysis, the concentration of antibiotic remaining in the blood at the end of the dialysis can be estimated and a post dialysis dose calculated to again raise the serum level to a therapeutic level. We have utilized this approach in our studies with Cefazolin. For example, if the drug level at the start of dialysis was assumed to be ½ of its peak level because dialysis was started a number of hours after administering the drug, and the drug level was estimated by the change in serum creatinine or urea to fall by 50% during dialysis, the assumed drug concentration would be 25% of its peak level at the end of dialysis and a dose equal to 3/4 of a maintenance dose could be given to again achieve a therapeutic concentration of antibiotic.

Bear in mind that the relationship between dialysis efficiency and drug remaining in the body, i.e. drug removal, would vary for different antibiotics. Some antibiotics are so highly diffusable that the concentration of drug remaining in the body after hemodialysis approaches zero. When this happens, a full sustaining dose of antibiotic should be given at the end of dialysis.

SUMMARY

In conclusion, much still remains to be learned in children with renal insufficiency about the metabolism and pharmacokinetics of antibiotics. More meaningful data about the pharmacokinetics of antibiotics in neonates and infants as well as the influence of uremia per se on antibiotic metabolism in developing children are needed. Meanwhile, the development of knowledge about the pharmacokinetics of antibiotics in uremic children has begun. We feel that we have contributed toward establishing a clinical basis upon which rational decisions concerning antibiotic dosimetry in uremic children can be based. It should be remembered that the actual measurement of serum levels of drug remains the best method of monitoring treatment and avoiding toxicity. The complexity of drug measurements as well as their availability continues to limit the practical use of measuring drug levels and requires that we continue to use doses of drugs and intervals of administration of drugs based on carefully performed pharmacokinetic studies of antibiotics.

REFERENCES

1. Fisher, M.L., Baluarte, H.J., Cote, M.L. et al.: Bacteroides fragilis infection in renal allograft recipients. Abstract. 19th Interscience Conference on Antimicrobial Agents & Chemotherapy, October, 1979.

2. Scharer, K., Brunner, F.P., Dehn, H. et al.: Combined report on regular dialysis and transplantation of children in Europe, 1972. Proc. Eur. Dial. Transplant. Assoc. 10: LVIII, 1973.

3. Yoshioka, H., Takimoto, M., Matsuda, I. et al.: Dosage schedule of gentamycin for chronic renal insufficiency in children. Arch. Dis. Child. 53: 334, 1978.

4. Jusko, W.J., Baliah, T., Kim, K.H. et al.: Pharmacokinetics of gentamycin during peritoneal dialysis in children. Kidney Int. 9: 430, 1976.

5. Hiner, L.B., Baluarte, H.J., Polinsky, M.S. et al.: Cefazolin in children with renal insufficiency. J. Pediatr. 96: 335, 1980.

6. Cutler, R.E. and Christopher, T.E.: Drug therapy during renal insufficiency and dialytic treatment. In: Massry, S.E., Sellers, A.L. (eds.). Clinical Aspects of Uremia and Dialysis. Springfield, Ill.: Charles C. Thomas, 1976, p. 427.

7. Gambertoglio, J.G.: Pharmacokinetic principles and renal disease. Dial. & Transplant. 8: 8, 1979.

8. Jusko, W.J.: Pharmacokinetic principles in pediatric pharmacology. Pediatr. Clin. N. Am. 19: 81, 1972.

9. Reidenberg, M.M.: The biotransformation of drugs in renal failure. Am. J. Med. 62: 482, 1977.

10. Greene, D.S. and Tice, A.D.: Effect of hemodialysis on cefazolin protein binding. J. Pharmacol. Sci. 66: 1508, 1977.

11. Gulyassy, P.F. and Depner, T.A.: Abnormal drug binding in uremia. Dial. Transplant. 8: 19, 1979.

12. Craig, W.A., Welling, P.G., Jackson, T.C. et al.: Pharmacology of cefazolin and other cephalosporins in patients with renal insufficiency. J. Infect. Dis. 128 (Suppl.): S347, 1973.

13. Levison, M.E., Levison, S.P., Ries, K. et al.: Pharmacology of cefazolin in patients with normal and abnormal renal function. J. Infect. Dis. 128 (Suppl.): S354, October, 1973.

14. McCloskey, R.V., Forland, M.F., Sweeney, M.J. et al.: Hemodialysis of cefazolin. J. Infect. Dis. 128 (Suppl.): S358, October, 1973.

15. Kirby, W.M.M. and Regamey, C.: Pharmacokinetics of cefazolin compared with four other cephalosporins. J. Infect. Dis. 128 (Suppl.): S341, 1973.

16. Schwartz, G.J., Hyacock, G.B., Edelmann, C.M. Jr. et al.: A simple estimate of glomerular filtration rate in children derived from body length and plasma creatinine. Pediatrics 58: 259, 1976.

17. Bennett, W.M., Singer, I., Golper, T. et al.: Guidelines for drug therapy in renal failure. Ann. Intern. Med. 86: 754, 1977.

18. Gibson, T.P.: Dialyzability of common therapeutic agents. Dial. & Transplant. 8: 24, 1979.

19. Golper, T.A.: Drugs and peritoneal dialysis. Dial. & Transplant. 8: 41, 1979.

20. Anderson, R.J., Gambertoglio, J.G. and Schrier, R.W.: The clinical use of drugs in renal failure. Springfield, Ill.: Charles C. Thomas, 1976.

21. Elzouki, A., Gruskin, A.B., Baluarte, H.J. et al.: Age related changes in peritoneal dialysis kinetics. Abst., Society Pediatr. Res. 14: 618, 1980.

PANEL DISCUSSION

Moderator: José Strauss, M.D.

Div. Pediatr. Nephrol., Dept. Pediatr., Univ. Miami
Sch. Med., Miami, Fla. 33152 USA

QUESTION: What are the hematological aspects of the hemolytic uremic syndrome?

RESPONSE: I don't know what the exact nature of the hemolytic uremic syndrome is. I happen to believe that it occurs following GI or other types of infection. It is a disease characterized by intravascular coagulopathy and microangiopathic hemolytic anemia leading to the renal problem. That is, the vascular problem is the primary one and the renal disease is secondary. I believe it is a variant of thrombotic thrombocytopenic purpura and that virtually there are no differences between the two entities. There has been a significant breakthrough in management of thrombotic thrombocytopenic purpura (TTP) which I believe would apply to the hemolytic uremic syndrome.

Some of you may be familiar with it. Based on observation that exchange transfusion is effective in some patients with TTP, a fellow by the name of John Byrnes in the Department of Medicine of the University of Miami, tried an infusion of plasma in patients with TTP. Now there are some 20 patients who were treated with the infusion of plasma in various amounts who had complete remission in the majority of cases. Furthermore, lately an important aggregating factor has been found in the plasma of these patients; normal plasma, on the other hand, contains an inhibitor of this aggregating factor. So by infusing plasma you are providing the inhibitor which apparently causes the complete remission. However, I should point out that the nature of this factor or factors is currently under study. I would urge pediatricians who see patients with the hemolytic uremic syndrome to administer plasma to them. As a matter of fact, I know a pediatrician who already has applied this treatment to two patients and obtained very interesting results.

COMMENT: There is a group who has done some work along these lines and they have hypothethesized that maybe a deficiency of prostacycline production is responsible for the development of the vascular lesions. I don't know whether you would care to comment on that or whether there have been measurements of prostacycline metabolism. The argument is that there is a deficiency in a serum factor which is responsible for prostacycline generation.

COMMENT: This is an interesting possibility. I am sure that it has to be studied. I think that it obviously is an acquired problem. What happens when it recurs, for example, sometimes after years of remission, has to be studied.

QUESTION: The normal creatinine clearance in children reported per surface unit is not the same as in adults or children older than one. It starts around 40 and goes up to around 100, reaching 100 quite late. I wondered if it wouldn't be more exact to take as a coordinate the proportion of glomerular filtration of an individual patient to the normal for age.

RESPONSE: Of course there is a problem of dealing with the changes of GFR. (We are not talking about all children, only about those less than 1 year of age). When you look at creatinine clearances, there are two aspects. One, I agree that there may be a small increase over age but in a practical setting your GFR's for most children over two, at least my understanding of it, is a number that's greater than 80 or 90 to 100 ml/min/1.73 m^2. From a practical point of view the recommendations based on broad ranges of GFR appear to work. Obviously, if you have a child who has a GFR of 60 you can look at and interpret it in two different ways. You could say 60 ml-this will correspond to some recommendation between this level and that level. You could also say percent of 100% and then decide what you wanted for your 100% value, whether you wanted 100, 90, or 120 ml of GFR, and it would work out in a very similar way.

COMMENT: I would like to comment on the problem of shortcutting, using a Schwartz formula on a creatinine clearance. There is a group of patients in whom it is totally inapplicable. That's your patients who are paraplegic and patients with muscle disease. We always seem to forget where creatinine comes from. I take care of a large number of paraplegic patients and I have lost two when they entered other hospitals where it was not recognized that 1.5 mg/dl is much too high a creatinine level for a teenager who has no muscle below a T 10 or a C 7 level. I really think we ought to encourage people to use creatinine or glomerular filtration rate particularly when aminoglycosides are used.

These patients, of course, have frequent urinary tract infections and an undue number of them are being done in because we don't recognize the fact that their creatinine levels really have different norms.

COMMENT: You are obviously right. We run into the problem with a number of our cases. We must remember that there are two components. Obviously you are always better off measuring clearance. If you can't get a clearance, what do you then do? I think that Schwartz's formula is an approach dealing with the problem when you can't get a clearance. Probably, the most reasonable and practical thing to do would be to get a serum creatinine and one respectable measurement of clearance; if you have an acute problem, monitor drug changes on the basis of what that individual serum creatinine is in comparison to the clearance and the rate of change of serum creatinine. By the way, I don't think you need a 24 hr urine collection to get a respectable, usable creatinine clearance for this purpose. I know of very few places that can consistently collect respectable 24 hr urines in children. You probably are better off using one hour or two hour timed urines.

MODERATOR: We are going to review some of these subjects (such as treatment modalities) in other sessions; but since we may overlook this particular one later on we can talk a little bit about treatment of systemic disorders with the hypertensive syndromes that were presented. In particular, I am referring to something that we have been interested in: the use of cyclophosphamide in polyarteritis and other situations. I wonder whether the panel would like to address that subject. I'm sure that the subject will come back again, when we discuss the treatment of rapidly progressive nephritis. Would you have any comments on that? We've had a patient with Takayasu arteritis that our group published recently and we have some very exciting results with the use of immune suppression and aggressive anti-hypertensive medication. We have in the audience a nurse who is the mother of one of our prize patients in this regard-a patient who, according to a consensus evaluation at one of the Seminars should not have survived and who is now, for all intents and purposes, with normal kidney function, doing very well, though still receiving antihypertensive medication. Do you have any comments?

COMMENT: Of course, polyarteritis nodosa is a cause of severe hypertension which could be modified by immunosuppressive treatment. We have several cases with good evolution under long term treatment associating prednisone and cyclophosphamide. But the results on hypertension were never rapid and medical treatment, symptomatic treatment of hypertension, was always necessary for at least some months. I think that I haven't seen good persistent control with improvement of the vascular damage in polyarteritis nodosa, though it may happen. But at the beginning of the disease, it is necessary to use in addition, symptomatic treatment of hypertension. About Takayasu's disease, I have no experience with immunosuppressive treatment, but when you have a severe narrowing of the aorta, I doubt that you can change the histological lesions and return the aorta to its normal size with immunosuppressive treatment.

MODERATOR: We have not repeated those studies, but the patient with Takayasu, by some coincidence also the daughter of a nurse, was expected to die. She had documented progression of her disease and had severe symptomatic expression of her disease. She was put on triple therapy (cyclophosphamide, azathioprine and prednisone). The pathologist got fooled because he was expecting the autopsy but it has not arrived because the patient is alive and fairly well; it has been about three years or so now. We have not repeated the studies. That's another question, how to document progression of the diseases or lack of progression by either repeating the biopsy or other means in cases as complicated as those two. Do you have any suggestions about that?

RESPONSE: We have operated on three of five cases of stenosis of the aorta. I don't know if all these cases are the same disease. It may be the same; there are several processes described under this pathology. I don't know whether in some countries where Takayasu's disease is frequent, if there is some experience with immunosuppressive treatment. For example, in Southwest Asia and in Korea they reported patients with a kind of aortitis, probably related to tuberculosis. I wonder about the results of immunosuppressive drugs with such an infection.

MODERATOR: Obviously, we had absolutely not even the slightest suggestion of tuberculous infection and the patient had a negative tuberculin test. That is basic and should be always ruled out before starting such treatment.

COMMENT: On this problem in a general way, it is very difficult to draw conclusions about the value of treatment in rare diseases. You can either go on the body of previous limited experience and show cases who, as in your patient, have done remarkably better and take that as some indication that the therapy is of value--nothing more; or you can try and set up a controlled trial which is difficult to do in rare diseases even if you are involved in many centers because the standards and uniformity of management and diagnosis and all the rest of it are very difficult to achieve. You need a uniformity of management and diagnosis in order to get a proper trial. It's inherent in the design. The second approach is difficult and all that remains is to hope that there are some good ways of monitoring effective treatment. The point is to have some kind of parameter or variable to be measured and shown immediately to be altered by the kind of intervention that you carry out. That in itself can't prove that the treatment works, but it adds to the body of knowledge. Difficulties in evaluating treatment regimens in rare diseases are almost insuperable. We've been with this problem in nephrology now since the early controlled trials in the 1960's, and we are not much farther along. It does make life very difficult. In response to your point about hypertension in polyarteritis, for example, it's almost inevitably the case. You are dealing with a large vessel disease in the kidney, medium sized vessel disease. One advantage to that is that one can see an ischemic segment afterwards. But, of course, it's conceivable that this will go away or become no longer responsible for producing renin. You can imagine the opportunities for variation in the natural history. It's a mess. So, I think that if you have a case that has done well, you have a case that's done well and that's about all you can say about it--until we have accumulated a substantial body of information and everybody agrees that things have changed dramatically since a certain treatment was introduced.

MODERATOR: We contacted the people with most experience in the world (in Mexico and in Japan). Corticosteroids were most frequently used with Takayasu arteritis and their results, like ours, were just anecdotal statements.

COMMENT: We doctors very often are inclined to draw conclusions from some successful treatments that we have had. For instance, I had a case of periarteritis nodosa which I treated with aspirin with very good results. But it does not mean that aspirin would be good for any kind, any type of periarteritis nodosa. This particular child had received aspirin for one month; then the disease disappeared and the child was completely well until one year later when he had a relapse. Then, as we were aware of the severity of the disease, we did not want to give aspirin; we gave prednisone and the disease subsided. If we had had at the very beginning the idea of giving the triple therapy, then it would have been the cause of this success. Now, talking about the Takayasu's disease, the unspecific arteritis, we have several cases in Mexico of renal artery hypertension. We haven't been able to demonstrate very well the relationship with tuberculosis. But the first case we had subjected to surgical treatment, was a unilateral renal artery stenosis in whom a segment of the artery was removed; by histopathology it was unspecific arteritis. The hypertension was corrected but remained with normal growth ratio for about three months. After this time, hypertension came back again. We repeated the arteriogram and we saw exactly the same feature. Then we didn't want to repeat the surgical operation.

We tried with the prednisone for about two months, 60 mg/m^2 daily dosage. The blood pressure went down and remained so even though the new arteriogram showed that the stenosis was still there through the two or three years that we were able to follow this patient. Since that time, many other patients have been receiving similar treatment with generally good results. There was not complete disappearance of the hypertension but at least there was improvement in the majority of the cases.

MODERATOR: Regarding the patient that improved with aspirin which was documented by biopsy, would you say that it was a severe disease?

RESPONSE: Yes. As a matter of fact we didn't know that it was a periarteritis nodosa until we presented the case to another pathologist and she made the diagnosis. But the child was already in a good state from receiving only the aspirin.

MODERATOR: I want to emphasize the fact that we have not concluded anything about treating these patients nor recommend that all patients that look alike be treated similarly. We are asking questions, not presenting gospels or magical solutions. Recently there have been some reports, one in particular, in the New England Journal of Medicine, proposing that cyclophosphamide made a significant difference in polyarteritis nodosa. The problem is that it was an uncontrolled study. It was not a single blind or double blind design. But the proposal has been made, and it's in the literature. It's a question that needs to be resolved. We need to talk about the theoretical possibilities of that type of medication being desirable or being justified in its use. Do you have any comments about that? Also, what about the logic behind the combination of cyclophosphamide with azathioprine and prednisone?

RESPONSE: There are two questions. Do I share the views which many people hold that cyclophosphamide has a place to play in the management of severe generalized arteritis? I certainly do. I think there is a body of information which is not controlled but which is persuasive that cyclophosphamide has a positive effect. I don't have any doubt in those patients who've got a syndrome of generalized vasculitis with something that amounts to Wegener's Granulomatosis. There's really very little doubt in my mind, based on our own quite substantial experience--more than twenty or so patients with Wegener's Granulomatosis--and the group at NIH, that this drug produces a dramatic and immediate improvement in aspects of this disease including the granulomata and vasculitic lesions. The natural history of the development of ideas is that somebody tries a treatment that works and is very obvious, and controlled trials are not generally regarded as a major necessity. It's only when the effect of treatment is more marginal or that someone can claim that it doesn't work that a controlled trial starts to become much more compelling.

To come back to vasculitis, at one end of the spectrum I also think that it's of value in patients with systemic vasculitis without clearly defined Wegener's Granulomatosis. There the data are slightly less convincing, I think. I just don't know how it's to be evaluated. My guess is that there are enough patients around for that kind of thing to be subjected to a controlled study. The difficulty is what kind of placebo-what kind of control group you have when someone's got a fulminating, rapidly progressive disease which is likely to lead to death shortly, the type of patient which will be left untreated by most physicians under those circumstances. So, that's on one question.

You also asked me what are the grounds for triple therapy. There are very few rational grounds for combining azathioprine and cyclophosphamide. I could produce arguments that would have some kind of scientific basis. The two drugs do seem to have different effects on the immune system. But since in man we don't know what we are aiming at when we treat patients with these severe vasculitic diseases, it's hard to go from what is known in experimental animals about taking azathioprine and cyclophosphamide to man. To summarize some of the more major differences, it does seem as if azathioprine has slightly different effects on the immune system, slightly more depressive effects on the T arm of immunity whereas cyclophosphamide seems, under some circumstances, to have different effects along the B side of immunity. Also, under experimental circumstances and possibly in man, cyclophosphamide may induce the formation of specific suppressor cells which actually switch off the immune response under some circumstances. So, there are differences. All I can say is, if there were to be empirical experience suggesting that cyclophosphamide and azathioprine together were better than either alone, I wouldn't be that surprised. But I think that what's going to happen is that empiricism is going to rule, that we are not going to find a treatment that works better, and that it will be a long time before this is analyzed in scientific basic terms. Of course, a major part which again is to unravel, it may well be that these drugs, corticosteroids, cyclophosphamide and azathioprine, certainly in the short term, have very little immunosuppressive properties as we are currently using them, and that the effects are almost entirely anti-inflammatory. I doubt if that will turn out to be a complete explanation. I have grounds for saying this. For example, in patients undergoing plasma exchange, you compare the rate of rebound of IgG levels after it's been removed from the circulation and patients who have been recently started on cyclophosphamide, azathioprine and steroids, against people not receiving that triple combination of drugs and you find a highly significant inflammatory properties are more likely to be important. I'm afraid that we have to go by empirical clinical results and then have people start to unravel the components of the system that has been effected by the treatment.

MODERATOR: Several times in past Seminars, we have quoted experimental work which suggested that the combination of the three drugs was better than prednisone and cyclophosphamide, as I recall.

RESPONSE: In doses that were comparable to those used in man? I think not. This is one of the great problems. The doses of drugs that are effective as immunosuppressive agents in mice are enormously greater than what we normally use under usual circumstances.

QUESTION: I would like to ask if anybody has had any experience with treatment of vasculitis with hypertension using pulses of methyl prednisolone? We treated a number of children who have had different types of vasculitides with pulse therapy along with the subsequent switch to more conventional triple therapy. It seems to have been effective.

MODERATOR: Anybody want to comment?

RESPONSE: I am not sure that pulse therapy has much to offer in the treatment of vasculitis. I also think that it is pretty dangerous as well. There was a report from a London group on the effects on circulating immune complex, for example, which has not been confirmed, not even by them. My own impression in studying mainly adult nephrology patients, is that there are many more complications associated with pulse therapy, severe infections, for example, than we see in patients who don't use it. I'm not at all convinced that it does anything that a non-methyl prednisone won't do. I don't know how my colleague here feels. He must have many patients with this problem.

COMMENT: Yes. I fear the complications of pulse therapy. We experienced a burst of severe hypertension during pulse therapy used for transplant rejection and some deaths were reported in this country. I am not completely certain that it is useful therapy for vasculitis. I am reserving this treatment for transplanted children because it seems to be less toxic than very high doses of every day prednisone.

MODERATOR: Not in patients with vasculitis, but in patients with systemic lupus erythymatosus, we are using pulse therapy. Again, in an uncontrolled fashion, we feel that we are getting acceptably good results. Would you comment on that?

RESPONSE: Yes. You may be interested to know that I recently reviewed a paper on corticosteroid treatment in lupus. I think nephrologists would agree that high dose steroids are indicated in patients with severe lupus nephritis. That's based upon work of nearly twenty years ago. If that data are analyzed properly-by proper statistical methods, mainly life-table analysis, the differences between the treated and the non-treated groups will not be found to be significant. Now, it's very interesting. So far as I know that is the only study which compares in any reasonably formal way, although again historical cases were probably used, high dose versus normal doses of corticosteroids in lupus.

Now you asked me to comment on pulse (high intravenous) doses of therapy under these circumstances. You can see that we really are in the jungle of ignorance. If you want my own bias, I see a lot of patients with lupus. My own feeling is that high dosages of corticosteroids administered as pulse therapy are very rarely indicated for systemic lupus. Most patients I see for lupus have been controlled with conventional doses of steroids and when they are not being controlled with conventional doses of steroids, it is usually because other clinical aspects have been ignored. For example, the problem of undiagnosed or inadequately treated infection is a major factor. The only type of lupus where I am sometimes tempted to use pulse therapy is in cerebral lupus which can be extremely difficult to manage. I'm not sure at all that pulse therapy is of value in those people. I'm quite sure of one thing-that if more people with lupus would be "calmed" by pulse therapy then they would be better off. That I have seen. You know, I work in a major tertiary referral center where patients are referred from other hospitals-I get lots of patients referred with lupus. Should we carry out a plasma exchange on them because they are not responding to treatment? In the majority of them, you don't have to do it. All they need is the proper care, proper general medical therapy. I'm not suggesting that that is the state of affairs here but certainly it is a major problem where I come from.

MODERATOR: We have had the experience of patients who have progressed to end stage renal disease. We have an adolescent girl right now undergoing hemodialysis. In cases like that where we see that the conventional, even high doses of continued oral corticosteroid therapy do not induce any change, we are trying either pulse therapy or triple therapy. In one case which came to us last year about this time, we were again at a loss. This adolescent girl with systemic lupus had a progressive down hill course. She had reached end stage renal disease levels, pulse therapy was applied and she was readied for hemodialysis. She did not require even one dialysis as I recall. She is doing well now.

COMMENT: I think the problem that has to be addressed in something like severe lupus is: now that dialysis and transplantation are, relatively speaking, an effective form of treatment, is it safer to give patients sufficient doses of steroids just to control their sort of systemic features of the disease and let the renal disease take its course, if it's already moderately severely advanced? Or, is it better to go all out with the dangerous combination of treatments that are available (plasma exchange is one of these)? Is it better to go all out to save glomeruli at all costs? I think that this is a judgement which will have to vary from patient to patient, depending upon social, economic, other factors. But I strongly suspect that many patients with severe renal lupus are in fact overall being damaged more by agressive treatment than they would be if they were given just enough steroids to keep them systemically controlled and allowed to go into renal failure and then take their chances by getting treatment for renal failure. Again, I would like to hear what my colleague has to say about this. I know you've had lots of experience with problems like these.

RESPONSE: I would agree with you at this point that the treatment could be the cause of death of the patient. We have had some patients in the past who died, for example, from viral infection and probably would not have died without this kind of treatment. So, your remarks are quite pertinent. I feel that in the absence of renal involvement, the aggressive treatments are questionable.

MODERATOR: I guess it's a philosophical problem which is very difficult to resolve. In practical terms also it is difficult in our hands to decide when to treat those patients with what, whether to follow the renal disease or the systemic disease. We attempt to follow both, but, again, who has the answer?

QUESTION: On a different topic, in discussing the evaluation of the efficacy of the reticuloendothelial system, you mentioned that clearances of antibody coated red cells and heat damaged red cells were improved by plasmapheresis. I was wondering if you thought that the plasmapheresis itself could in any way mechanically damage these red cells to further enhance their clearance.

RESPONSE: No, I don't think that's a possible explanation. To enlarge on this for a moment, the reason that this project developed was the observation in some patients that after one or two plasma exchanges or after a series of small volume plasmapheresis, there was sometimes protracted clinical improvement. In patients who had certain of the immune complexes, they disappeared promptly and they stayed away for periods of sometimes three, four, or five weeks-much longer than could have been accounted for on the basis of the simple, physical removal from the circulation of what was there at the time.

There are several explanations one could have drawn under these circumstances. One is that the generation of immune complexes returned very, very slowly and that they gradually accumulated over a period of three or four weeks; this just didn't seem inherently likely. The other explanation is that plasmapheresis was doing more than simply removing something. It was allowing physiological mechanisms for clearances to be restored to normal. Now, based on that problem, the question was, how is it possible to study what the RES is doing? It is extremely difficult, and all that is really useful and technically possible in man at the moment is to take heat damaged red cells or antibody for red cells which are cleared by the spleen. Then, one assumes that the cleared red cells are a reflection of splenic macrophage function although there are other things that could be happening such as changes in blood viscosity, blood flow, arterial disease in the spleen, lots of other things which affect delivery of these cells to sites where they are going to be removed from the circulation. So, that is how that came about. It is inconceivable that there could be any changes in red cells induced by plasma exchange which would be reflected two or three weeks later. I don't see how that kind of process could possibly have happened as a result of the plasmapheresis procedure due to the spinning in the bowl.

The real trouble is, how do I know that this test is a good test of RES function? We don't really know. It's all we have at the moment. The evidence that we are measuring something which is relevant is that in patients who got immune complexes, and became infected, there is a correlation between the level of complexes and performance of their spleens. If their spleens are good, the complexes are not present. If the spleens go bad, the complexes tend to reappear.

MODERATOR: I would like to go to another subject now from an earlier presentation. I may have missed the point about the indication for Vitamin D administration. Let's not get into the clinical part yet; I believe that it has been found experimentally, that administration of Vitamin D when GFR starts decreasing, may prevent or decrease some of the changes that accompany osteodystrophy or increased PTH production. Is that correct? What are your thoughts on that? Have you done work on it?

RESPONSE: No. We have not studied that directly. There are studies in rats that were made uremic and then followed. One group was fed a normal diet; the other group was fed a low phosphate diet. The result was, I think, that after five months the animals fed the normal diet all died while the group fed the low phosphate diet, all survived. These studies have been amplified. Until now there are some strange observations that have been made. For example, these animals become nephrotic, with time. If you do a parathyroidectomy, in time the nephrotic syndrome disappears which may have some implications in terms of the pathogenesis of the nephrotic syndrome and the relationship between PTH and GFR. This is a very active area of research at the present time.

In uremic dogs that we have followed on a long term basis, some animals were studied, for instance, with either a low phosphate diet or administration specifically of 24,25 or cymetidine which decreased in these animals also. The normal course in these animals is that the GFR drifts slowly down in time; in the animals in which PTH was prevented from increasing, the GFR went down more slowly. This is very preliminary but it is very exciting, obviously.

MODERATOR: At Pediatric Grand Rounds, the State of the Art was presented two or three years ago. At that time, the speaker described some experiments that I believe were done by him where the vitamin D administration seemed to have prevented changes in the animals. He was reluctant to extend those benefits to the clinical situation. You are not aware of those studies?

RESPONSE: No, I am not.

COMMENT: Aren't there some data that the use of 1,25 DHC may result in a more rapid loss of GFR because of problems related to hypercalcemia?

RESPONSE: Yes. Indeed, if you give 1,25 (the most active vitamin D metabolite), the danger is to induce hypercalcemia. Usually you don't see hypercalcemia when you start treatment. At the time when alkaline phosphatase goes down, suddenly calcium goes up. If the patient has osteomalacia, then he will become hypercalcemic immediately. Indeed, the effect of calcium per se on the kidney is to enhance progression of the disease.

QUESTION: We've had some problems with the interval extension method for adjusting aminoglycoside dosages because a single dose may cause acutely toxic levels. I was wondering if you have run into the problem and if, for that reason, you use smaller doses more frequently or how do you handle this?

RESPONSE: No. We use aminoglycosides with a prolonged interval regimen rather than a lower dose. Clinically, our documented infections seem to have responded to that treatment regimen. I think the available data would suggest, from a practical point in terms of the therapy of infection, that we can do it either way and still get effective eradication of bacteria. Are you saying that you had problems with the treatment of the infectious process?

RESPONSE: No. Just toxicity.

COMMENT: The toxicity issue becomes one, of course, of how much you give in relation to what the GFR is. There is one paper describing the use of gentamycin given intramuscularly, looking at recommended doses, but their range mean $\pm$ 2 standard deviations for any level of GFR was quite wide. If you pick a number that's a little higher, you will have more toxicity. If you pick a number that's a little lower, you may not have enough antibiotic. The classical conflict.

MODERATOR: Thank you. We must adjourn now.

PRINCIPLES OF DIURETIC THERAPY IN EDEMATOUS CONDITIONS

George A. Richard, M.D., Eduardo H. Garin, M.D., Abdollah Iravani, M.D., Robert S. Fennell, III, M.D. and John K. Orak, M.D.

Div. Pediatr. Nephrol., Dept. Pediatr., Col. Med. Univ. Fla., Gainesville, Fla. 32610, USA

The clinical use of diuretics should be based on a good understanding of the pathophysiology of edema and the disease being treated, the pharmacology of the diuretics and their reported side effects. This knowledge allows one the best opportunity to effectively and safely match the mechanism of action of the diuretic to the altered physiology caused by the disease. The major clinical conditions for which diuretics have been used in the treatment of edema are shown in Table 1. It is generally agreed that, whatever the pathophysiology of the primary disease, the retention of sodium by the kidney ultimately determines the magnitude of the fluid overload and consequent edema formation. Thus, an understanding of normal salt and water handling by the kidney is essential.

SALT AND WATER HANDLING BY THE KIDNEY

Regulators of Salt and Water Handling (1-4)

The amount of sodium excreted into the urine is equal to the filtered load at the level of the glomerulus minus the sodium reabsorbed as the filtrate passes down the tubule. At least *three factors* are known to regulate sodium balance within the kidney. *Glomerular filtration rate (first factor)* has been most extensively studied and therefore the best understood. However, the overall roles of *aldosterone (second factor)* and the *third factor(s)* remain controversial. The mean *glomerular filtration rate (GFR)* in man is 125 milliliters per minute per 1.73 meters squared. Each day, the kidneys produce approximately 180 liters of glomerular filtrate containing about 25,000 mEqs of sodium. Ninety-nine point 5 percent of the filtered sodium load is reabsorbed along

Table 1. Clinical Conditions Associated with Edema

Renal Failure, acute and chronic
Nephrotic Syndrome
Congestive Heart Failure
Hepatic Failure and Cirrhosis
Protein Losing Enteropathy

the nephron, yielding an average of 125 mEqs excreted in the urine. The amount of sodium filtered is directly proportional to the GFR, and if only GFR were involved, a 1% change in the GFR would result in changes of as much as 250 mEqs of sodium excreted in the urine. These large changes in the amount of filtered sodium are modified by a corresponding decrease or increase in tubular reabsorption of sodium. This cooperative working relationship between GFR (first factor) and tubular reabsorption is called glomerulotubular balance.

Aldosterone (second factor) is the most potent of the mineralocorticoids in sodium reabsorption. The principal site of action is in the collecting duct where sodium is reabsorbed in association with but not directly dependent upon the secretion of potassium and hydrogen ions. Since only one percent of the filtered sodium load reaches the collecting duct, aldosterone would have a relatively small effect on sodium excretion. Aldosterone requires 30-60 minutes to induce the intracellular or membrane-bound proteins which allow for potassium secretion and subsequent sodium reabsorption, and thus could not participate in minute to minute control of sodium reabsorption. Chronic administration of mineralocorticoids causes only a transient salt retention after which sodium balance is restored. This phenomenon called "DOCA release" mitigates against aldosterone's relative importance as a regulator of sodium balance.

Because of such circumstantial evidence, factors other than GFR and aldosterone have been hypothesized to explain minute to minute control of the concentration and volume of the extracellular fluid. Direct evidence for the existence of additional factor(s) was first established by de Wardener (5). While maintaining GFR and aldosterone concentration constant, he was able to demonstrate in the dog a brisk diuresis and natriuresis in response to an intravenous saline infusion. Because neither the first nor second factor could account for the diuresis, he postulated the existence of a natriuretic or *third factor(s)*. In two decades since de Wardener's original work, several hypotheses have been proposed to explain the mechanism(s) by which third factor(s) participates in glomerulotubular balance. A circulating substance of *hormonal* nature (6,7), changes in the peritubular *physical forces* (8), and changes in the distribution of *intrarenal blood flow* (9) are the three most accepted mechanisms for third factor activity. Several animal and clinical studies appear to demonstrate the existence of a circulating hormone possessing natriuretic properties. This natriuretic or salt losing hormone inhibits proximal tubular transport of sodium under conditions of volume expansion. However, the search to isolate and identify this factor has been unsuccessful.

Since the majority of the filtered sodium is isosmotically reabsorbed in the proximal convoluted tubule, examination of factors influencing sodium reabsorption in this area would seem appropriate. Brenner and colleagues postulate a second mechanism for third factor activity (8). In their experiments on volume-expanded states, diuresis and natriuresis depended largely on changes in the peritubular *physical forces*. These changes include a decrease in plasma colloid oncotic pressure resulting from dilution of plasma proteins and the increase in capillary hydrostatic pressure which act in concert to inhibit the outflow of reabsorbate from the tubular lumen and to increase the rate of back-flux. The reversal of these mechanisms during contraction of the extra-cellular volume would result in an increase in proximal tubular reabsorption of salt and water.

Changes in *intrarenal blood flow* have been proported to contribute to third factor activity. During volume expansion, there is a redistribution of *intrarenal blood flow* from the inner juxtamedullary nephrons (salt-retaining, long loop) to the outer cortical nephrons (salt-losing, short loop). This would result in a decrease in the fraction of sodium reabsorbed with a consequent natriuresis and diuresis. With contraction of extracellular volume, redistribution of the blood flow to the juxtamedullary nephrons results in salt and water retention. Recent studies have cast some doubt on this hypothesis, suggesting that changes in the distribution of intrarenal blood flow may not be as significant as previously indicated (10). Earley has proposed a somewhat different theory which states that the increase in medullary blood flow, occurring with volume expansion, inhibits sodium reabsorption in the ascending limb of Henle by a wash-out of the medullary interstitium (11).

Finally, the renal *prostaglandin, PGE,* may have a direct natriuretic action on the tubule. Preliminary studies in normal man show increased levels of urine PGE following a saline load. However, the prostaglandin antagonist, indomethacin, does not inhibit the natriuresis. Thus a direct role for prostaglandin on sodium balance in normal man remains unproven, but it may play an indirect role on sodium balance through the effects of prostaglandins on renal blood during renal ischemia (12).

Major Sites of Tubular Reabsorption

There are four major sites for the tubular reabsorption of salt and water. The *proximal tubule (Site 1)* accounts for 50-70% of the salt and water reabsorbed along the nephron (1). The process involves the energy dependent active extrusion of sodium from the tubular epithelial cell into the intercellular spaces and peritubular interstitium of the cortex. Chloride follows sodium passively and water is isosmotically reabsorbed. The high rate of cortical blood flow rapidly removes the salt and water deposited in the peritubular interstitium. As the remaining fluid passes down the straight proximal tubule and the descending thin limb of Henle, sodium passively diffuses into the tubular lumen from the area of high concentration within the surrounding interstitium. The highly concentrated tubular fluid enters the *ascending loop of Henle (Site 2)* where chloride is actively extruded into the interstitium and sodium follows passively. This segment of the tubule is impermeable to water; thus, the solute reabsorption leads to a hypotonic tubular fluid and a hypertonic medullary interstitium. At each level an osmolar gradient develops between the ascending loop and medullary interstitium. This process is called countercurrent multiplication of the concentration. The osmotic gradient increases from the cortex to the deep medulla from 300 milliosmols to 1200 milliosmols per kilogram of water, respectively. Urea and sodium are the major solutes which contribute to the osmolality. Approximately 20-25% of the sodium is reabsorbed in the ascending loop of Henle (Site 2). The *distal convoluted tubule (Site 3)*, lies between the juxtaglomerular connection (macula densa) and the confluence with other distal tubules which marks the beginning of the cortical collecting tubule. At this site sodium is actively reabsorbed and chloride transport is passive. Water is isosmotically reabsorbed in the presence of ADH, but if the level of circulating ADH is low as with water diuresis, the epithelium of the distal tubule and collecting duct is impermeable to water and a very dilute urine results. Site 3 accounts for approximately 10% of the reabsorbed salt and water. The remaining one percent of the salt and water is reabsorbed in the *collecting ducts (Site 4)*. Aldosterone influences sodium reabsorption and potassium secretion at this site; but, the sodium concentration and volume of the collecting duct fluid are the major factors which affect the final reabsorption of sodium and secretion of potassium and hydrogen ions.

The Pathophysiolosy of Edema (1,2)

Edema is a condition in which there is an increase in the amount of fluid within the extracellular space of the body, particularly the interstitial space. Clinically, edema becomes apparent when either the extracellular fluid volume has increased by approximately 50% or the body weight by 7 to 10%. It is produced by an imbalance between the intravascular hydrostatic pressure generated by the pumping action of the heart and the plasma colloid oncotic pressure produced by serum proteins, principally albumin. Starling showed that these forces normally are in balance with each other such that hydrostatic pressure is higher than colloid oncotic pressure at the arteriolar end of the capillary beds (13), allowing fluid to leak into the interstitial spaces. At the venular ends, the colloid oncotic pressure is higher than the hydrostatic pressure allowing the fluid to be absorbed into the intravascular compartment of the circulation. The small amount of fluid remaining returns to circulation via the lymphatic system. Edema occurs when a disruption in this normal balance allows fluid to accumulate within the interstitial space at a rate greater than it can be returned by the lymphatic system (13).

Sodium and water are so important to the survival of the organism that a complex system has evolved to maintain their balance. This integrated system includes the heart and blood vessels, Starling's Law of tissue perfusion, salt and water handling by the kidneys, the pituitary-adrenal axis and protein metabolism by the liver. The entire process is dependent upon normal renal physiology. Other than the syndrome of inappropriate release of the antidiuretic hormone, generalized edema is due to sodium retention by the tubular system of the kidney or a decrease in GFR. In either situation, it is the retained sodium rather than the water which determines the extracellular fluid volume and the degree of edema (2).

In the various edematous conditions listed in Figure 1, several intrarenal mechanisms are activated to play an essential role in producing and maintaining the excess salt and water. The initial signal for the kidney to retain salt and water is a decrease in plasma volume and particularly effective arterial volume (14). This decrease in plasma volume may result from loss of plasma colloid oncotic pressure as seen with the nephrotic syndrome or cirrhosis of the liver. It may also occur in congestive heart failure where the decreased cardiac output causes a decrease in effective arterial volume. The kidney compensates for the deficit by retaining salt and water. Both renal blood flow and glomerular filtration rate are reduced to decrease the amount of salt and water presented to the nephron for excretion. The renin-angiotensin-aldosterone system is activated, allowing for an increased recovery of sodium in the collecting duct. Other forces which contribute to increase salt and water retention include the previously discussed redistribution of intrarenal blood flow, peritubular physical forces, suppression of the postulated natriuretic hormone and possibly a suppression of PGE.

Table 2. Pharmacology of Commonly Used Diuretics

Diuretics	Mercurials (Thiomorin)	Osmotic (Mannitol)	Carbonic Anhydrase Inhibitor (Acetazolamide)	Thiazides (Chlorothiazide)
Dose	0.1-0.2 ml Titrate dose	Test dose: 200 mg/kg over 3 min. Diuresis: 1-2 g/kg over 30-60 min.	5 mg/kg/qd	10-15 mg/kg
Route of Administr.	I.M.	I.V.	P.O.	P.O., b.i.d.
Major Sites of Action	ascend. loop & cortical dil. seg.	prox. tub. & ascend. loop	proximal tubule	cortical diluting seg. distal convoluted tubule
Onset of Maximum Action	8 hours	minutes	2 hours	3-4 hours
Duration of Action	18 hours	1 hour	24 hours	8-10 hours

Mean Diuretic Potency	> 15%	< 5% do not use at low GFR	>5%	5-10% ineffective at GFR < 20 ml/min
Effect on GFR & RBF	none	none	little	mild decrease
Effect on Potassium Excretion	mild ↑	mild ↑	moderate ↑	moderate ↑
Effect on Acid Excretion	↑ H+	little effect H+, but ↑ HCO3-	↓ H+ ↑ HCO3-	little effect
Effect on Uric Acid Excretion	inhibits	none	inhibits	inhibits
Major Side Effects	metab. alk. nephrotox.	vascular overload	metab. acidosis	hypokalemia, metab. alk.

Table 2. Pharmacology of Commonly Used Diuretics Cont'd.

Diuretics	Metolazone*	Ethacrynic Acid & Furosemide	Potassium Retaining Diuretics Spironolactone (SP) Triamterene (TRIAM)
Dose	2-5 mg/1.73 m^2 per day	Ethacrynic Acid: P.O.: 2-3 mg/kg/day I.V.: 0.5-2 mg/kg/dose (titrate) Furosemide: P.O.: 1-2 mg/kg q6h I.V.: 0.5-1.0 mg/kg q2h	SP: 0.5-1 mg/kg q8h TRIAM: 4 mg/kg/day divided b.i.d. Max. of 300 mg q.d.
Route of Administr.	P.O.		P.O.
Major Sites of Action	cortical diluting seg. distal convoluted tubule	ascend. loop & cortical diluting segment	collecting duct
Onset of Maximum Action	3-4 hours	P.O. - 2 hours I.V. - minutes	SP: several days TRIAM: 2-4 hours
Duration of Action	18-24 hours	P.O. - 6 hours I.V. - 2 hours	SP: 12-24 hours TRIAM: 7-9 hours

Mean Diuretic Potency	5-10% effective at GFR < 20 ml/min	> 15% effective at GFR < 20 ml/min	< 5% do not use at low GFR
Effect on GFR & RBF	mild decrease	Redistrib. RBF Large doses may increase GFR	Triamterene may decrease GFR
Effect on Potassium Excretion	moderate ↑	mild ↑	moderate ↓
Effect on Acid Excretion	little effect	↑ H+ with less Furos. than E.A.	SP: ↓ H+ TRIAM: ↓ H+
Effect on Uric Acid Excretion	inhibits	inhibits	SP: none TRIAM: variable
Major Side Effects	hypokalemia, metab. alk.	hypokalemia hyponatremia hypovolemia ototoxicity	K+ retained ↓ GFR

*FDA approved for adults only.

PHARMACOLOGY AND SITES OF ACTION OF DIURETICS (TABLE 2)(15-17)

Several decades ago, sodium reabsorption was considered to be a single bulk operation performed by the renal tubules. However, through the study of the modes of action of the various diuretics, we have come to realize that there are at least four sites for sodium reabsorption within the tubular system affected by different hormonal and hemodynamic signals. It is apparent that these same mechanisms are also operative along the renal tubule to produce the edema seen in the nephrotic syndrome, heart failure, cirrhosis of the liver and in renal failure. Having previously reviewed the tubular reabsorption of salt and water by the kidney, we will now review the pharmacology and sites of action of the various diuretics. Knowledge of the site of action of these drugs permits the appropriate choice of therapy to reverse or counterbalance the pathophysiologic processes causing the edematous state. Table 2 outlines the pharmacology of the various diuretics.

Water Diuresis

In patients with normal heart and kidney function, the ingestion of water allows for the production of dilute urine and a marked diuresis (1). Water is the ideal diuretic to irrigate the lower urinary tract in infections, and to prevent deposits of insoluble urinary substances as in prophylaxis for urinary calculi. Of course, it can not be utilized as a diuretic in edematous states.

Osmotic Diuretics

The osmotic diuretics, mannitol and urea, increase the urine volume by their osmotic attraction of fluid into the lumen of the tubule. This has been the basis for the use of mannitol in the prevention or early treatment of acute tubular necrosis. Research with mannitol diuresis has demonstrated clearly that although the reduction in fractional reabsorption of sodium and water in the proximal tubule was only 5% and 10% respectively, excretion into the urine amounted to as much as 30% of the filtered water and sodium. Micropuncture studies demonstrated a continued effect of mannitol diuresis within the ascending thick loop of Henle. In essence, this confirmed the suspicion that any drug exerting its primary action on the proximal tubule will have its overall potency as a diuretic affected by transport processes at more distal tubular sites. In a similar way, the tubular reabsorption of sodium chloride and water in the ascending loop of Henle (15) will be affected by the mechanisms that control reabsorption in the distal convoluted tubule and collecting duct. For example, in clinical conditions complicated by secondary hyperaldosteronism, considerable salt and water will be reabsorbed in the collecting duct in exchange for potassium and hydrogen. This will decrease the effect of diuretics acting at more proximal tubular sites. It is also very possible that various intrarenal and extrarenal hemodynamic and transport processes may increase proximal tubular reabsorption of sodium to compensate for losses secondary to these induced distal losses. These mechanisms are essential to the homeostasis of the patient and they may vary with the disease process, potency of the diuretic and duration of its use. These concepts must be strongly considered in the use of any diuretic and may be an indication for combination therapy.

Xanthines Diuretics

The *xanthines* (caffeine, theophylline and theobromine) are weak diuretics and have no role in the treatment of edema. They have been shown to cause a slight increase in both glomerular filtration rate and medullary renal blood flow.

Carbonic Anhydrase Inhibitors

The *carbonic anhydrase inhibitor,* acetazolamide (Diamox), produces a decrease in the fractional reabsorption of sodium and bicarbonate in the proximal tubule. Although these diuretic agents are excellent inhibitors of salt and water reabsorption in the proximal tubule, their net effect is nullified by an almost complete recovery of the sodium and water within the ascending loop of Henle, For this reason they are weak diuretics and have no place in the treatment of edematous patients. The carbonic anhydrase inhibitors work well in the presence of a metabolic alkalosis; but with their continued use, the loss of bicarbonate and potassium within the proximal convoluted tubule produces a metabolic acidosis and hypokalemia.

Organomercurials

The *organomercurials* are potent diuretics which inhibit the tubular reabsorption of sodium chloride in the ascending loop of Henle and the distal convoluted tubule. They inhibit 15% of the fractional reabsorption of sodium. Their use is limited, because they must be given parentally, they are potentially nephrotoxic, and they depend on a state of hyperchloremic metabolic acidosis for effectiveness. They interfere with both diluting capacity (free water clearance) and concentrating capacity (negative free water clearance). With the advent of less toxic and equally effective oral diuretics, the organomercurials are no longer used in the treatment of patients with edema.

The remaining discussion will be limited to examples of the most commonly used diuretics. These include the *thiazides,* (chlorothiazide), metolazone, the *loop blockers* (furosemide and ethacrynic acid) and the *potassium sparing compounds* (spironolactone, triamterene and amiloride). As organic acids, they are protein bound, limiting their filtration by the glomerulus. There is evidence to suggest that these drugs and acetazolamide are taken up from the peritubular capillaries and secreted into the luminal fluid of the proximal straight tubule in a manner similar to paraminohippurate (PAH). The advantage of these drugs being secreted by the tubule is that even at low plasma concentrations, relatively high concentrations may be obtained at the site of drug action of the luminal surface of the tubular epithelial cell (16). Recent evidence suggests that these diuretics can be blocked by drugs that inhibit this organic secretory pathway.

Thiazides

The *thiazides,* particularly chlorothiazide, remain the diuretics of choice in clinical practice. Although they inhibit proximal tubular carbonic anhydrase, this is of little clinical significance since the ascending thick loop of Henle compensates to reabsorb the extra salt and water. The major effect of the thiazides is to interfere with the tubular reabsorption of sodium in the distal convoluted tubule. This results in a decrease in diluting capacity (decreased free water clearance) but there is no effect on concentrating capacity (negative free water clearance). The thiazides are not influenced by acid-base balance. They may decrease renal blood flow and glomerular filtration rate. The thiazides are not effective at glomerular filtration rates below 20 ml/min since they are very much dependent upon an adequate load of filtered sodium. The thiazides are able to increase the fractional excretion of sodium and water by approximately 5%. The many types of thiazides, some more powerful than others by weight, offer no advantage of increased potency or margin of safety over chlorothiazide when utilized at the maximum recommended dose. There have been some claims that certain of these agents have lesser degrees of kaliuresis, hyperchloremia or hyperuricemia, but this has not been proven. Thiazide diuretics have been commonly used in the prevention of renal calculi in patients with hypercalciuria. Thiazides enhance distal tubular reabsorption of calcium through a mechanism probably separate from the inhibition of sodium reabsorption. The increased reabsorption of calcium appears to be a direct tubular effect rather than through parathormone (17).

Metolazone

One of the newer compounds which deserve special mention is quinazolinone, metolazone (18). This has been approved for use in adults and is currently being investigated in children. This is a safe and effective diuretic with moderate potency. The major site of action is in the cortical diluting site of the distal convoluted tubule. It differs from the thiazides in that the proximal site of action does not seem to be related to carbonic anhydrase. Metolazone offers at least two advantages. First, its duration of action allows it to be given once each day. Second, when glomerular filtration rate falls to less than 20 ml/min, metolazone maintains diuretic potency.

Loop Blockers

Furosemide and *ethacrynic acid* are the most potent diuretics in clinical use today. These two compounds are chemically different, although very similar in their pharmacologic behavior. They also share many properties in common with chlorothiazide. These agents work at the level of the thick ascending limb of Henle's loop. The mechanism by which they inhibit the active tubular reabsorption of chloride at this site remains unknown. Maximal doses of these agents are able to completely abolish urinary concentrating action at both the medullary and cortical portions of the ascending thick limb. Furosemide and ethacrynic acid increase the fractional secretion of sodium to as much as 30%. This can be increased considerably by prior saline infusion inhibiting proximal tubular reabsorption of sodium and thus increasing the amount of sodium presented to the loop of Henle. These studies support the concept that for a diuretic to be maximally potent, it must not only inhibit sodium chloride transport in the loop of Henle, but have an additional inhibitory effect in the proximal tubule enhancing sodium delivery to the loop of Henle. Furthermore, those factors which reduce the concentration of sodium in the proximal tubule, such as reduced glomerular filtration rate and volume depletion, must also reduce the effectiveness of all diuretics.

Potassium-Retaining Natriuretic Agents

There are two types of diuretic agents which act on the collecting duct to induce potassium retention while at the same time causing a natriuresis. The first, spironolactone, is a true competitive inhibitor, blocking cell receptor sites of aldosterone. This agent is most effective in conditions associated with secondary hyperaldosteronism such as cirrhosis of the liver and the nephrotic syndrome. Examples of the second type are triamterene and ameloride. They act independently of aldosterone. Triamterene inhibits the tubular reabsorption of sodium in the collecting duct while at the same time causing potassium retention. Ameloride acts both on the distal convoluted tubule and the collecting duct. Although both triamterene and ameloride are more rapidly acting, spironolactone has been shown to be safer. Both of these non-steroidal inhibitors block hydrogen ion secretion and cause a metabolic acidosis. They also produce a reversible decrease in glomerular filtration rate with a consequent azotemia. Although these drugs are not potent diuretics, they are very helpful in preventing potassium loss and may produce a significant diuresis in conditions that are caused by secondary hyperaldosteronism. Ameloride has yet to be approved by the Food and Drug Administration for pediatric use.

REPORTED COMPLICATIONS OF DIURETIC THERAPY (19)

All drugs have potentially harmful side-effects, diuretics being no exception. They rarely cause serious toxic and allergic complications. Patients with a prior history of either sulfonamide sensitivity or photosensitive skin eruptions should not receive thiazides or furosemide. The metabolic disorders produced by the chronic use of diuretics have been reported frequently. These include: hyponatremia, hypokalemic alkalosis, other acid-base disturbances, hyperuricemia, and hyperglycemia. Additional complications which may occur and need to be considered as one monitors a patient on diuretics include severe decreases in extracellular fluid volume, decreased glomerular filtration rate and renal blood flow, and rarely vasculitis, pancreatitis, cholecystitis, and occasional hematologic disorders. *Hypokalemia* and *metabolic alkalosis* usually occur together. They may be seen following the use of either the loop blockers or the thiazides. The increase in sodium presented to the collecting duct is exchanged with either hydrogen or potassium ions. The loss of hydrochloric acid and potassium chloride produces the metabolic alkalosis and potassium deficiency. The degree of alkalosis is further augmented by the contraction of the extracellular fluid volume which stimulates increased bicarbonate reabsorption in the proximal tubules. The severity of the hypokalemia and metabolic alkalosis will depend on the potency of the diuretic and the quantity of sodium which reaches the collecting duct. It may also be affected by the co-existence of hyperaldosteronism which would aggravate the hypokalemia. The common complications of potassium depletion include weakness, neuromuscular disorders, ileus, and an increased susceptibility to digitalis glycoside toxicity. Recognizing that the chloride depletion is the common denominator of the hypokalemia and the alkalosis, the treatment of choice is potassium chloride. Supplementing the diet with potassium or using potassium-retaining diuretics such as spironolactone or triamterene may help to minimize the incidence of alkalosis and hypokalemia. The potassium-retaining diuretics should not be utilized in patients with azotemia. Treatment should be limited to patients on diuretics with serum potassium concentration of less than 3.0 mEq/liter, and used prophylactically in patients receiving cardiac glycosides or prednisone. Although diuretics frequently cause *hyperuricemia*, gouty attacks are rare, particularly in children. Two mechanisms have been proposed for the hyperuricemia. First, both uric acid and diuretics compete for secretion in the proximal straight tubule. Second, there may be an enhanced tubular reabsorption of uric acid caused by the diuretic induced plasma volume contraction. This reduction in blood volume acts to augment the proximal reabsorption of uric acid and may possibly inhibit the distal secretion due to the increases of angiotensin II. Hyperuricemia may be treated with allopurinol, an inhibitor of uric acid production. *Hyponatremia* occurs when the diuretic has caused severe contraction of the extracellular fluid volume. This will result in increased ADH levels with retention of water in excess of sodium, as well as a decrease in glomerular filtration rate. The decrease in urine volume occurs in the face of a continued intake of hypotonic fluids either orally or parentally. The treatment of choice is to restrict hypotonic fluids and carefully re-expand the extracellular fluid volume with isotonic fluids. Diuretics, particularly the thiazides, are known to produce *hyperglycemia*. Some investigators have attributed the carbohydrate intolerance to potassium depletion. The importance of this diabetogenic effect of diuretics need not be exaggerated. In non-diabetic patients, the administration of diuretics rarely has been associated with diabetes. In the prediabetic patient diuretics may induce definite diabetes but this also occurs infrequently. The complications of a decreased extracellular fluid volume, decreased *vascular volume* and *azotemia* are preventable by closely monitoring the patient's clinical condition. The more potent diuretics, such as furosemide, may acutely produce a marked diuresis to decrease extracellular and vascular volumes to levels which cause a decrease in renal blood flow and glomerular filtration rate. The chronic use of thiazides may also cause a reversible decrease in renal function. On the other hand, the non-steroidal diuretics, triamterene and ameloride may decrease GFR independent of changes in vascular volume. These complications are reversible with expansion of vascular volume and reducing drug dosages. Gynecomastia is a reported complication of spironolactone therapy. Table 2 outlines some of the side effects of the various diuretics.

PATHOPHYSIOLOGY AND TREATMENT OF EDEMATOUS STATES (20-24)

Congestive Heart Failure (20)

Congestive heart failure results in an increase in hydrostatic pressure at the venous end of the capillary circulation, due to the increased fluid and pressure within the venous system. The inability of the lymphatic system to handle the increased load of interstitial fluid causes generalized edema beginning in the feet and legs. Both the decrease in cardiac output and the loss of fluid into the interstitium contribute to decrease the effective arterial volume. There are several responses within the kidney which result from the decrease in effective arterial volume. First, total renal blood flow decreases and redistributes to the juxtamedullary, salt retaining, long loop nephrons at the expense of blood flow to the cortical, salt losing, short loop nephrons. Efferent arteriolar constriction, possibly due to angiotensin II or norepinephrine, increases the filtration fraction to maintain GFR despite the decrease in renal blood flow. Changes in peritubular physical forces, particularly decreased hydrostatic pressure and increased plasma colloid oncotic pressure, produce an increase in proximal tubular reabsorption of salt and water. The decrease in effective arterial volume is also a stimulus for the release of renin by the kidney to activate the renin-angiotensin-aldosterone system. Aldosterone increases salt reabsorption and potassium secretion within the collecting ducts. The overall effect of the kidney through the altered intrarenal hemodynamics is to increase salt and water reabsorption, and thereby produce an increase in the effective arterial volume. This is accomplished in the face of a further accumulation of edema.

Because decreased renal perfusion is a major factor in the disturbed salt and water retention of congestive heart failure, therapeutic management must begin with improvement of renal blood flow. This can be best accomplished by the use of an inotropic agent such as digitalis which acts on the myocardial muscle to decrease the left ventricular end diastolic pressure and increase cardiac output. Once good cardiac function has been re-established, dietary salt restriction and diuretic therapy will help further to improve the patient's clinical condition. The proximal tubular acting diuretics have not been efficacious in treating the edema of congestive heart failure. On the other hand, the loop diuretics, furosemide and ethacrynic acid, have been shown to be very effective. As previously mentioned, patients treated with the loop blockers must be monitored closely since serious extracellular fluid volume and electrolyte problems might develop in these patients who are receiving digitalis therapy. The loop diuretics are particularly effective since they have a rapid onset of action, especially when given intravenously. The thiazides are excellent drugs in the long term management of patients with mild to moderate congestive heart failure. However, they are not as effective in patients with severe congestive heart failure, particularly those with glomerular filtration rates of less than 20 ml/min. An exception to this would be metolazone which seems to maintain its diuretic potency at lower glomerular filtration rates. Metolazone has yet to be approved by the Food and Drug Administration for use in children. A potassium sparing diuretic should not be used as a single agent in congestive heart failure. However, spironolactone is indicated in combination with other diuretics because of its effectiveness in treating the secondary hyperaldosteronism of congestive heart failure. When prescribed, supplemental potassium chloride should be discontinued in order to reduce the risk of hyperkalemia. In summary, the approach to the treatment of congestive heart failure must be to improve cardiac output so that renal blood flow and glomerular filtration rate might return to normal. Following this, dietary salt restriction and diuretic therapy can be effective. The success of therapy depends on the cooperation of the patient and commitment of the physician to closely monitor treatment.

Cirrhosis of the Liver

The initial effect of cirrhosis of the liver is to increase the portacaval venous pressure and to increase flow through the lymphatics. These hemodynamic changes result in the development of an extensive portacaval venous collateral network. This increase in the volume of the venous system causes a relative decrease in the effective arterial volume. The decreased effective arterial volume stimulates various renal compensatory mechanisms; however, renal blood flow and GFR remain normal. Acites becomes evident as more salt and water are retained. The mechanism by which the kidney continues to reabsorb salt and water is unknown. As the cirrhotic process progresses, albumin synthesis by the liver decreases to further compromise the plasma albumin concentration and the plasma colloid oncotic pressure. The increased hydrostatic pressure, decreased plasma colloid oncotic pressure and obstruction of the lymphatics combine to further aggravate the acites and generalized edema. The first steps in the treatment of edema of cirrhosis of the liver should be to limit the amount of salt and water through careful dietary management. When these conservative measures are no longer effective, diuretic therapy should be considered. Satisfactory therapy usually includes a combination of furosemide and spironolactone. In some refractory patients one may also add chlorothiazide, keeping in mind that the maximum response from spironolactone will take several days. During therapy the patient must be monitored closely for weight loss, clinical changes and alterations in serum electrolytes. One must be careful that the aggressive use of potent diuretics does not cause vascular collapse and decreased renal blood flow. This is especially true for the patient with severe hypoproteinemia. The patient should participate actively in the therapeutic regimen by closely monitoring his salt and water intake, as well as daily weight.

Nephrotic Syndrome and Protein Losing Enteropathies (22,23)

The edema of the nephrotic syndrome is secondary to an increased permeability of the glomerular basement membrane which allows for loss of plasma proteins, principally albumin into the urine. A similar gastrointestinal loss of plasma proteins occurs with the protein losing enteropathies. Thus, the subsequent pathophysiology of these conditions is quite similar. The decrease of plasma albumin to less than 2.5 grams percent results in a significant decrease in plasma colloid oncotic pressure. The decrease in plasma colloid oncotic pressure at the venular end of the capillary beds reduces the amount of fluid returning to the intravascular compartment and increases the load of fluid which must be returned via the lymphatics. The residual fluid produces interstitial edema. The decrease in plasma volume and the effective arterial volume causes a decrease in renal blood flow. However, glomerular filtration rate is maintained by a compensatory increase in the filtration fraction. The latter is due to an increase in efferent arteriolar resistance. The increased filtration fraction produces a slight increase in the concentration of plasma proteins within the peritubular capillaries; however, this probably does not affect salt and water retention as would occur with normal concentrations of plasma proteins. The increased efferent arteriolar resistance also produces a decrease in hydrostatic pressure within the peritubular capillaries. These changes in the peritubular capillary physical forces, do not completely explain the retention of salt and water seen in the nephrotic syndrome. The decrease in effective arterial volume also stimulates the renin-angiotensin-aldosterone axis to increase sodium reabsorption in the collecting duct. However, this effect is too small to explain the edema. The intrarenal hemodynamic and physiologic processes which produce the edema of the nephrotic syndrome require further research.

Prednisone is the treatment of choice for minimal change nephrotic syndrome of childhood. Diuretics should not be used in the nephrotic syndrome unless the patient is clinically resistant to prednisone therapy and has biopsy findings compatible with a steroid resistance process. Because these patients are hypovolemic, treatment with diuretics, particularly those with significant potency, could result in hypovolemic shock and vascular thrombosis. However, in those children with severe edema, particularly when there is respiratory embarrassment, diuretics can be helpful. Initial therapy should utilize a thiazide or metolazone, perhaps in combination with spironolactone. This may often permit the gradual loss of edema fluid, as well as protect the patient from developing severe hypokalemia. In those patients with generalized acites resistant to therapy, more potent diuretics such as the loop blockers can be used. Recently, Garin reported good success in the treatment of refractory edema of the nephrotic syndrome in children using a combination of furosemide and metolazone (25). Patients with severe refractory edema may need to be admitted to the hospital for parenteral therapy with a combination of salt-poor albumin in a dose of 1 gm/kg body weight, administered over 2-4 hours in combination with an intravenous dose of a loop blocker. In this way, generalized edema can be often successfully managed without the necessity of abdominal paracentesis or peritoneal dialysis.

Acute and Chronic Renal Failure

The pathophysiology of renal failure in producing edema is even more complex. In both acute and chronic renal failure there is a severe compromise of glomerular filtration rate, usually in the face of a normal plasma colloid oncotic pressure. Consequently, these conditions are most often associated with hypervolemia, increased hydrostatic pressure, and generalized edema. The increase in hydrostatic pressure in the face of a normal plasma colloid oncotic pressure results in a loss of plasma water at the arteriolar end of the capillary beds which is in excess of what can be returned to the circulation at the venular end of the capillary beds and via the lymphatics. This type of generalized edema may become complicated by congestive heart failure, pulmonary edema and cerebral edema. Effective treatment must incorporate an understanding of this basic pathophysiology.

The edema of the acute and chronic renal failure requires that limitations be placed on the patient's salt and water intake. This ceiling should equal urine output plus insensible water loss minus the volume of water which one can safely remove each day, usually through dialysis. One must take every effort to determine whether or not there is a way that renal function might be improved. The causes of reversible renal failure which should be considered are hyponatremia, hypovolemia, congestive heart failure, pericardial effusion, sepsis, severe anemia, hypertension, and surgically correctable obstructive processes of the urinary collecting systems. Often, acute renal failure of either glomerular or tubular origin is reversible, but may take several weeks to resolve. As soon as every measure to improve glomerular filtration rate has been exhausted, one should consider diuretic therapy. By definition, these patients have a severe decrease in glomerular filtration rate. For this reason, the diuretics available are limited, including only the loop blockers and sometimes metolazone. In general, furosemide is the drug of choice. It is potent and may slightly increase glomerular filtration rate in patients with lower levels of kidney function.

SUMMARY

In summary, the proper use of diuretics in clinical medicine requires that the physician becomes knowledgeable in understanding their mechanism of action on the kidney, particularly in various edematous and non-edematous states. In order to accomplish this, he must first understand the normal salt and water handling by the kidney, as well as the pathophysiology of various edematous conditions.

Two decades ago our understanding of diuretic action on the kidneys was limited to the overall effect on tubular readsorption of sodium. Today, we have a variety of agents which are well understood with respect to their sites of action and usefulness in various edematous conditions. The clinician will continue to have the excitement and challenge of new and more potent diuretics to utilize in his treatment of edema. It is essential that he maintain a basic knowledge of renal physiology and pathophysiology.

REFERENCES

1. Pitts, R.E.: Physiology of the Kidney and Body Fluids. Chicago, Ill: Year Book Medical Publishers, Inc., 1974.

2. Stein, J.H. and Reineck, H.J.: Regulation of Sodium Balance in Normal and Edematous States. In Contr. Nephrol., Basel: Karger, 1978, vol. 14, p. 25.

3. Kinne, R.: Current Choices of Renal Proximal Tubular Function. In Contr. Nephrol., Basel: Karger, 1978, vol. 14, p. 14.

4. Richard, G.A., Garin, E.H., Fennell, R.S. et al.: A Pathophysiologic Basis for the Diagnosis and Treatment of the Renal Hypertensions. In Advances in Pediatrics. Chicago, Ill.: Year Book Medical Publishers, Inc., 1977, vol. 24, p. 339.

5. de Wardener, H.E., Mills, I.H., Clapham, W.F. et al.: Studies on the Efferent Mechanism of the Sodium Diuresis Which Follows the Administration of Intravenous Saline in the Dog. Clin. Sci. 21: 249, 1961.

6. Buckalen, V.M. and Nelson, D.B.: Natriuretic and Sodium Transport Inhibitory Activity in Plasma of Volume Expanded Dogs. Kidney Int. 5: 12, 1974.

7. Levinsky, N.G.: Non-Aldosterone Influences on Renal Sodium Transport. Ann. N.Y. Acad. Sci. 139: 295, 1966.

8. Brenner, R.M., Troy, J.L. and Daugharty, T.M.: Quantitative Importance of Changes in Postglomerular Colloid Osmotic Pressure in Medicating Glomerular Tubular Balance in The Rat. J. Clin. Invest. 52: 190, 1973.

9. Barger, A.C.: Renal Hemodynamic Factors in Congestive Heart Failure. Ann. N.Y. Acad. Sci. 139: 276, 1966.

10. Lamere, N.H., Lifschitz, M.D. and Stein, J.H.: Heterogeneity of Nephron Function. Ann. Rev. Physiol. 39: 159, 1977.

11. Earley, L.E. and Friedler, R.M.: Observations on the Mechanism of Decreased Tubular Reabsorption of Sodium and Water During Saline Loading. J. Clin. Invest. 43: 1928, 1964.

12. Horton, R. and Zipser, R.: Prostaglandins: Renin Release and Renal Function. In Contr. Nephrol. Basel: Karger, 1978, vol. 14, p. 87.

13. Starling, E.H.: Physiologic Factors Involved in the Causation of Dropsy. Lancet 2: 1405, 1896.

14. Cannon, P.J.: The Kidney in Heart Failure. N. Engl. J. Med. 296: 26, 1977.

15. Seely, J.F. and Dirks, J.H.: Site of Action of Diuretic Drugs. Kidney Int. 2: 1, 1977.

16. Burg, B.: Mechanisms of Action of Diuretic Drugs. In Brenner, B.M., Rector, F.C. (eds.). The Kidney. Philadelphia: W.B. Saunders Co., 1976, vol. 1, p. 737.

17. Dirks, J.H.: Mechanism of Action and Clinical Uses of Diuretics. Hospital Practice, vol. 13, p. 99, 1979.

18. Belair, E., Kaiser, F. et al.: Pharmacology of SR 720-22. Arch. Int. Pharmacodyn. 177: 71, 1969.

19. Van Ypersele De Strihou, C.: Metabolic Complications in the Use of Diuretics. In Advances in Nephrology. Chicago: Year Book Medical Publishers, Inc., 1972, vol. 2, p. 241.

20. Porter, G.: The Role of Diuretics in the Treatment of Heart Failure. JAMA, vol. 244, 1980, p. 1614.

21. Sherlock, S.: Diuretics in Hepatic Disease in Modern Diuretic Therapy. In Lant, A.F. and Wilson, G.M. (eds.). Excerpta Medica, Amsterdam, 1973, p. 270.

22. Hollerman, Charles E.: Pediatric Nephrology. New York: Medical Examination Publishing Co., Inc., 1979, p. 305.

23. Lewy, J.E.: The Pathogenesis of Edema in Renal Disease and Other Disorders Affecting the Kidney. In Edelmann, C.M. (ed.). Pediatric Kidney Disease. Boston: Little, Brown and Co., 1978, vol. 1, p. 315.

24. Loggie, J.M., Kleinman, L.I. and Van Maanen, E.F.: Renal Function and Diuretic Therapy in Infants and Children. Part III. J. Pediatr. 86: 825, 1975.

25. Garin, E.G. and Richard, G.A.: Edema Resistant to Furosemide Therapy in Children with Nephrotic Syndrome: Treatment with Furosemide and Metolazone. J. Pediatr. Nephrol. and Urol. (In press).

PERITONEAL DIALYSIS KINETICS - A PEDIATRIC PERSPECTIVE

Alan B. Gruskin, M.D., Abdelaziz Y. Elzouki, M.D., H. Jorge Baluarte, M.D., James W. Prebis, M.D. and Martin S. Polinsky, M.D.

Dept. Pediatr., St. Christopher's Hosp. for Children and Temple Univ. Sch. Med., Philadelphia, Pa. 19133, USA

Although the technique of peritoneal dialysis is being used with increased frequency in children, relatively few studies dealing with dialysis kinetics, i.e. the movement of solute and water across the peritoneal membrane, have been performed in children and/or the developing animal. The purpose of this presentation is three-fold. Firstly, a few general principles of transperitoneal solute and water movement will be reviewed. Secondly, the available data describing peritoneal dialysis kinetics in children will be reviewed. Thirdly, certain aspects of studies which we have performed in order to increase our knowledge of peritoneal dialysis kinetics in the experimental animal as well as in children will be reviewed.

GENERAL PRINCIPLES OF PERITONEAL TRANSFER OF SOLUTE AND WATER

The peritoneal membrane functions as a passive semipermeable membrane through which solute diffusion occurs between the extracellular fluid compartment and the dialysate in the peritoneal cavity (1). The Fick equation for solute diffusion, $n = cAPt$, states that the number of particles of solute (n) crossing the diffusing membrane per unit time (t) is a function of the concentration gradient (c) across the membrane, the permeability (P) of the

---

Supported in part by the following grants; General Clinical Research Center RR-75, National Heart and Lung Institute Grant 1R01-HL23511-01, the University of Garyounis, Benghazi, Libya and Hoechst-Roussel Pharmaceuticals.

membrane for a given particle, and the functional area (A) of the membrane through which solute and water can move. Since the permeability of most solutes in physiologic solutions is inversely related to its radius, larger molecular weight solutes move across diffusing membranes slower than solutes having smaller molecular weights. The actual area as well as the size of the holes in the membrane which participates in the transperitoneal movement of solute and water is not known. As regards the peritoneum, there are differences between the anatomically measurable surface area of the peritoneum and the segment of the peritoneal membrane through which solute and water flow (2). The term, functional peritoneal surface area has been utilized to describe the latter.

It is not possible to determine the actual mass transfer coefficients for peritoneal membranes. The measurement of either peritoneal clearances and/or peritoneal dialysance are used in lieu of being able to measure mass transfer coefficients. Both clearances and dialysance measurements reflect the combined influence on transperitoneal transport of permeability and membrane area.

The more easily understood and widely utilized of the two measurements is peritoneal clearance (1): $Cl = \frac{DV}{Pt}$ where Cl = clearance in ml/min; D and P = the solute concentration in the drained dialysis fluid and plasma at the midpoint of the dialysis exchange; V = total volume in ml of the dialysis fluid drained; and t = the time in minutes from the start of the inflow of dialysis fluid at the beginning of an exchange to the end of the draining period. Peritoneal clearance is a direct measurement of what was actually accomplished; however it has certain limitations (3). No distinction can be made between the inflow, dwell and drain segments of a peritoneal exchange. During each of these segments different areas of the peritoneal membrane are utilized. Peritoneal clearance represents a mean clearance per exchange. It is highest during the initial moments of an exchange when the concentration gradient between blood and dialysate is greatest and diminishes throughout the exchange and becomes zero when the solute concentration in the dialysate equals that in the blood. Since the measurement of peritoneal clearance does not take into account the changing, decreasing gradient in solute concentration between blood and dialysate occurring with time during an exchange, there is no correction for the deteriorating gradient as the exchange progresses when peritoneal clearances are measured.

A more quantitative estimate of solute transfer can be obtained by measuring the peritoneal dialysance of a solute. The following formula which is used to determine peritoneal dialysance is especially helpful when the movement of molecules of varying weights, i.e. ratios of solute dialysance, is being evaluated (2,3).

$$D = \frac{\ln\left[1 - \frac{Sd\ (Vd+Vb)}{SbVb}\right]}{t} \times \frac{V_b V_d}{V_b + V_d}$$

D = peritoneal dialysance in ml/min
Sb = concentration of solute in blood or plasma at the midpoint of the dialysis exchange
Sd = concentration of solute in the dialysis fluid drained at t (time)
t = total time in minutes involved in a dialysis exchange including inflow, dwell and drainage
Vd = milliliters of dialysis fluid drained by the end of the exchange
Vb = the volume of distribution of solute within the body external to the peritoneal cavity

Peritoneal dialysance can be defined as the rate of solute movement across the peritoneal membrane per unit of concentration gradient. It also has been defined as the peritoneal clearance occurring at time zero of an exchange. In developing the concept of peritoneal dialysance, four assumptions were made: 1) that the volume of distribution of a solute within the body remains constant throughout an exchange, 2) that ultrafiltration resulting in solvent drag is not occurring, 3) that the exchange process is not limited by the rate of capillary blood flow within the peritoneum and 4) that exchanges are precisely performed as regards the duration of inflow, dwell and outflow periods of an exchange. Assumptions one and two are valid when peritoneal exchanges are performed with solutions isoosmotic to plasma. Assumption four permits comparative studies to be made as the error introduced by changes in the time permitted for inflow, dwell and outflow will be similar.

The dialysance of an individual solute is a function of both membrane area and permeability of the peritoneum. Changes which occur in dialysance indicate that a change in one or in both of these parameters has occurred (2,3). It has been demonstrated that changes in the dialysance of a low molecular weight solute such as urea (mol. wt. = 60), which has a comparatively high rate of diffusion, reflects alterations in either the membrane area or peritoneal capillary blood flow. Changes in the dialysance of a larger solute such as inulin (mol. wt. = 5200) have been shown to reflect changes in either the permeability of the peritoneal membrane and/or alterations in membrane area.

The ratio of the dialysance of inulin to urea, $\frac{DI}{DU}$, or the permeability index reflects the relative permeability of the dialyzing membrane. Since $\frac{DI}{DU}$ equals $\frac{\text{permeability/inulin}}{\text{permeability/urea}} \cdot \frac{\text{membrane area}}{\text{membrane area}}$, it is apparent that the membrane area for the simultaneously determined dialysances of multiple solutes is identical. When the dialysance ratio is calculated, the value corresponding to the size of the membrane area is cancelled. Because the DI/DU ratio provides a dimensionless index of permeability, changes occurring in this ratio, e.g. before and after the addition of vasodilators to dialysis fluid, reflect changes in permeability.

When comparing the technique of clearance versus dialysance certain similarities between the two measurements can be shown assuming that no ultrafiltration has occurred (1). It has been shown that clearance approximates dialysance only for large molecules when the surface area permeability product is low and the dwell time short. When the peritoneal surface area permeability product is large, when t is long and/or varied, and when small molecular weight compounds such as urea are being evaluated, significant differences between clearance and dialysance will occur.

The rate of ultrafiltration which is determined by the osmotic gradient between dialysis fluid and blood influences dialysis kinetics by increasing water movement across the membrane together with whatever solute may be trapped and moved across the diffusing membrane by solvent drag. The use of hyperosmotic dialysis fluid will increase peritoneal clearances and dialysance by virtue of increasing solute movement. It may also alter the SD/SB ratio and change the dialysance ratios of molecules of varying size. Thus, despite the obvious importance of ultrafiltration in the clinical care of patients, the process of ultrafiltration is best avoided when attempting to evaluate other aspects of dialysis kinetics such as the influence of peritoneal surface area, permeability, dialysate flow rate, and peritoneal blood flow, and the influence of growth, development and drugs on dialysis kinetics (4).

KINETICS OF PERITONEAL DIALYSIS IN THE YOUNG

When evaluating the kinetics of peritoneal dialysis in children the following factors need to be considered:

1) the actual size of the peritoneal membrane
2) the size of the membrane which participates in the exchange process
3) the permeability of the peritoneal membrane
4) the dialysate flow rate
5) the rate of delivery of water and solute to the peritoneal membrane, i.e. peritoneal blood flow
6) the manner in which studies of dialysis kinetics in infants, children and adults can be compared

Relatively few studies which deal with the question of the actual size of the peritoneal membrane are available (5,6,7). It has been suggested that the peritoneal membrane surface area approximates the surface area of the skin and is approximately 2.0 m^2 in area in the adult human (7). Two studies comparing the peritoneal surface area in children to that of adults are available (5,6)(Table 1). Both studies demonstrated as expected that the actual peritoneal surface area in children is smaller than in adults. When corrected for body weight, however, both studies indicate that the surface area of the peritoneum per unit of weight in infants is approximately twice as large as it is in adults.

The question arises as to what segment of the peritoneal membrane actually participates in the exchange process. The entire peritoneal membrane does not participate equally in the exchange process (1). It is probable that only the juxtacapillary peritoneal membrane participates in solute exchange. The visceral mesentery has been shown to be more permeable than the parietal peritoneum (8). A number of studies have shown that the capillaries involved in the exchange process can vasoconstrict and vasodilate in response to topically applied solutions such as hypertonic dialysate (3) and drugs (nitroprusside) (9). These agents are felt to act by altering the quantity of the peritoneal surface area participating in the exchange process.

If the functional peritoneal surface area is also twice as large in infants as it is in adults, similarly performed dialysance studies should yield a dialysance value per unit of body weight in infants twice that of the adults.

Table 1. Surface area of the peritoneal membrane measured by anatomical measurements. Data derived from references five and six.

Size	Surface area cm^2	Ratio of Surface Area to Weight cm^2/kg
Infant	1,512	522
Adult	20,281	284
Infant	2,743	383
Adult	10,379	177

The permeability of the peritoneal membrane may be examined by examining the relationship between the concentration of solute in the dialysate and blood (or plasma) after instilling dialysis fluid into the peritoneal cavity. It is difficult to decide how to compare individuals of differing sizes, realizing that the anatomic area of the peritoneum is relatively greater in infants than in adults. Because diffusion occurs across the peritoneal membrane according to concentration gradients and because the movement of water between various body compartments should remain constant throughout dialysis to maintain systemic hemodynamics, we decided to examine diffusion across the peritoneal membrane in children of different ages by performing diffusion curves after instilling an isoosmotic solution into the peritoneal cavity (9). Similar dialysis mechanics were utilized in all studies. Forty ml/kg of body weight of 5% dextrose in water was introduced into the peritoneal cavity over 5 minutes and allowed to remain in the peritoneal cavity for 60 minutes. Each 10 minutes a sample of dialysate was withdrawn and a sample of blood obtained.

Our initial studies suggested that the rate of movement of solute with time was similar in children below 2 years of age as well as in children greater than two years of age (9,10). The infants when compared to the older children had similar SD/SB ratios for urea, creatinine and uric acid suggesting that similar clearances and/or solute dialysance occurred in both groups. However, only two of the four children were less than 6 months of age and one had the hemolytic uremic syndrome which by virtue of its being a vascular disorder might also have affected peritoneal blood vessels and its transport characteristics. We have recently studied two premature infants requiring peritoneal dialysis for acute renal failure secondary to shock. A high dialysate to blood ratio for urea and creatinine and uric acid was found in both neonates when compared to the older children. This would suggest that peritoneal clearances and dialysance are higher in neonates than in older children.

Assuming that the dialysate flow rate relative to body weight remains constant, the finding of a high peritoneal fluid to blood ratio (SD/SB) of solute in young infants indicates that the young human has a higher peritoneal clearance than the adult and that if a dialysance were calculated on the basis of the above, the peritoneal dialysance in the young would also be greater than that of the adult. In order to critically evaluate this suggestion we have performed dialysance studies of urea C_{14} and inulin H_3 in a group of puppies less than 1 month of age and in a group of adult dogs (11,12). Because the dialysate to blood ratios of urea and inulin were higher in the puppies, the dialysance of both of these solutes were increased in the puppies. As already mentioned, if the SD/SB ratios were similar in both groups the dialysance would be similar. The results of these studies suggest that either the functional area and/or the permeability of the peritoneal membrane in infants is greater than in adults. The fact that the larger molecular weight species had a greater dialysance in infants than in adults suggests that not only is the surface area larger in infants, but that the permeability of the peritoneal membrane is also greater in infants than in adults.

The available studies reported by other investigations in infants and young animals suggest that the peritoneal membrane in the young permits a greater rate of transfer to solute than does the peritoneal membrane of adults. These studies also permit alternative explanations because the dwell time as well as the quantity of the dialysis fluid utilized had not been kept constant (6, 13). Inspection of either the clearance or dialysance formula demonstrates clearly that manipulation of either of these parameters can alter clearance or dialysance without any change in membrane permeability or functional area. Thus, exchange times and volumes of dialysate relative to body fluid compartments must be kept constant in order to obtain comparative data when large differences in body size exist. As regards the published studies dealing with peritoneal dialysis kinetics in young animals and children, data relative to dialysis volume and/or dwell time are often lacking. Also, dialysis volume and dwell times have not been maintained constant when individuals of different sizes have been dialyzed. The suggestion that peritoneal dialysis is more efficient in infants as compared to adults in these studies can be explained by the fact that volumes and dwell times were different. In retrospect these studies have not critically examined the issues of peritoneal permeability and functional surface area involved in the exchange process. We have performed clearance studies in children and dialysance studies in puppies and adult dogs using two different volumes of dialysate. As expected, clearances and/or dialysance varied with changes in dialysate flow rate. A doubling of dialysis volume did not double either clearance or dialysance. Consequently, if comparative studies are desired dialysate volume must remain constant in relation to body fluid compartments, otherwise any differences will be able to be explained in part by changes in dialysate volume.

There are no studies of peritoneal blood flow in infant and young animals. The available studies in adult animals suggest that the rate of peritoneal blood flow does not limit solute exchange in normal animals across the peritoneal membrane (14). However, in certain disorders such as diabetes, heat stroke and scleroderma the rate of blood flow through the peritoneum may limit solute exchange (15). Also, it has been demonstrated that vasodilatation of peritoneal capillaries increases the rate of movement of solute across the peritoneal membrane.

In summary, our various studies have addressed three of the four variables involved in the kinetics of peritoneal dialysis -

permeability, functional surface area, and dialysate volume. They demonstrate that the peritoneal permeability as well as the functional surface area of the peritoneum is greater in infants than in adults, and that changes in dialysate volume influences peritoneal clearance and probably dialysance. The practical implications of these studies on peritoneal dialysis kinetics in the young are that the rate of removal of solutes is quicker in the young than in the adult for a given set of dialysis mechanics. Also, the removal of larger molecular weight compounds, i.e. middle molecules, should be anticipated to be more efficiently dialyzed in the young because the peritoneal membrane in the young is more permeable to larger molecules.

REFERENCES

1. Henderson, L.W.: Peritoneal dialysis. In: Massry, S.G. and Sellers, A.L. (eds.): Clinical Aspects of Uremia and Dialysis. Springfield, Illinois: Charles C. Thomas, 1976, p. 555.

2. Henderson, L.W. and Kintzel, J.E.: Influence of antidiuretic hormone on peritoneal membrane area and permeability. J. Clin. Invest. 50: 2437, 1971.

3. Henderson, L.W. and Nolph, K.D.: Altered permeability of the peritoneal membrane after using hypertonic peritoneal dialysis fluid. J. Clin. Invest. 48: 992, 1969.

4. Henderson, L.W.: Peritoneal ultrafiltration dialysis: enhanced urea transfer using hypertonic peritoneal dialysis fluids. J. Clin. Invest. 45: 950, 1966.

5. Putiloff, P.V.: Materials for the study of the laws of growth of the human body in relation to the surface areas of different systems; the trail on Russian subjects of planigraphic anatomy as a means for exact anthropometry - one of the problems of anthropology. Report of Dr. P.V. Putiloff at the meeting of the Siberian Branch of the Russian Geographic Society. October 24, 1884, Omsk, 1886.

6. Esperance, M.J. and Collins, D.L.: Peritoneal dialysis efficiency in relation to body weight. J. Pediatr. Surg. 1: 162, 1966.

7. Dunea, G.: Peritoneal dialysis and hemodialysis. Med. Clin. N. Am. 55: 155, 1971.

8. Gosselin, R.E. and Berndt, W.G.: Diffusional transport of solutes through mesentery and peritoneum. J. Theor. Biol. 3: 487, 1962.

9. Gruskin, A.B. and Cote, M.L.: Kinetics of peritoneal dialysis in children. Abst. Soc. Ped. Res., 1970, p. 44.

10. Gruskin, A.B.: Peritoneal dialysis in acute renal failure: indications and technical considerations. Proc. Int. Congr. Pediatr., Nephrology Issue, Vienna, Aug.-Sept. 1971, p. 261.

11. Elzouki, A.Y., Gruskin, A.B., Polinsky, M.S. et al.: Age related changes in peritoneal dialysance. Abst. Ninth Ann. Clin. Dial. & Transplant Forum, Nat. Kid. Found., Nov. 16-19, 1979, p. 37.

12. Elzouki, A.Y., Gruskin, A.B., Baluarte, H.J. et al.: Age related changes in peritoneal dialysis kinetics. Abst. Soc. Ped. Res., April, 1980.

13. Feldman, W., Baliah, T. and Drummond, K.N.: Intermittent peritoneal dialysis in the management of chronic renal failure in children. Am. J. Dis. Child. 116: 30, 1968.

14. Aane, S.: Transperitoneal exchange: IV. The effect of transperitoneal fluid transport on the transfer of solutes. Scand. J. Gastroenterol. 5: 241, 1970.

15. Nolph, K.D., Stoltz, M.L. and Maher, J.F.: Altered peritoneal permeability in patients with systemic vasculitis. Ann. Intern. Med. 75: 753, 1971.

PANEL DISCUSSION

Moderator: José Strauss, M.D.

Div. Pediatr. Nephrol., Dept. Pediatr., Univ. Miami Sch. Med., Miami, Fla. 33152, USA

QUESTION: About Saralasin, do you think that has a future for therapeutic and various hypertension needs?

RESPONSE: Saralasin, I believe, is intravenous. As a blocking agent (with blocking activity), captopril (which is the generic name), Dr. Broyer was telling me during the coffee break that he has had a reasonable experience with it now using captopril to treat severe hypertension in 20-30 children; he thinks that it is the drug of the future. I would tend to agree. It is very difficult to get it in this country to study in children because of the questions which have been raised and bantered around because of the fact that it may produce proteinuria. I have a feeling that the proteinuria issue will get itself resolved and I think it is a drug that has tremendous potential as both a diagnostic and therapeutic agent. I foresee it being widely used if it doesn't have this problem of toxicity.

MODERATOR: We recently had a patient that had a nephritis of acute onset, went into acute renal failure with severe pulmonary distress. X-rays of the chest revealed a few infiltrates. We thought we had a sure case of Goodpasture. The mother described bloody striae in the sputum. The patient went home to recover completely after several peritoneal dialysis procedures. We obtained a kidney biopsy and the finding was endocapillary proliferation with typical electrodense and immunofluorescence of post-infectious glomerulonephritis. Since the initial clinical description of the so-called Goodpasture syndrome was renal and lung involvement, do you have any tips on how to differentiate those patients who look like one but are not from those that are the true Goodpasture syndrome?

RESPONSE: It's very important to get your terminology right. In the sort of patient you describe, measuring the hemoglobin is the way to distinguish pulmonary hemorrhage from pulmonary edema, if you have any doubt and there can be doubt sometimes. But, if somebody has got Goodpasture syndrome with a white out on chest x-ray and hemoglobin way down - 6 or 5 or 4 or 3 or sometimes even less - then, there is no doubt.

QUESTION: Just a mild decrease would not qualify?

RESPONSE: That's a clinical distinction to make in a few moments. Otherwise, Goodpasture syndrome, of course, is the clinical association of extensive pulmonary hemorrhage and nephritis. There are many patients who have lung hemorrhage from conditions such as polyarteritis, lupus, Wegener Granulomatosis, anti-TBM nephropathy, etc.

As I said yesterday, you can generally distinguish these if they have clearly a one system disease of some kind. It may not be the sort that you can diagnose specifically but you have a patient who is generally ill with weight loss, pyrexia, muscle aches, that type of thing while patients with anti-GBM disease are suffering from typical symptoms such as anemia, sometimes vomiting, a congested lung. The disease in the lung and the kidneys fares generally well.

MODERATOR: I should mention that Dr. Pardo did try for circulating anti-basement membrane antibodies and did not find them. So, we had the suspicion that the impression was not correct but we also thought that maybe his method was in error.

QUESTION: I would like to ask if you have any experience with the complement system in IgA nephropathy. Do you ever see decreased serum complement levels associated with this "disease"?

RESPONSE: The general pattern in IgA nephropathy is that the complement is normal. There is one very solitary patient described with a very curious system of complement activation with involvement of the alternate pathway of activation. At that time there was a great deal of uncertainty about the mechanism involved and this, as far as I know, has not been resolved. After that happened, people in my laboratory carried on an extensive search of serum properdin levels on patients with IgA nephropathy with no abnormalities found in the complement system. Some people at the Institute of Child Health in London have found IgA and IgE contained in immune complexes. Often these complexes in fact are not detected by C_{1q} binding but are detected by one of the other techniques.

QUESTION: The efficiency and safety of peritoneal dialysis in the case of post-operative period for pancreatic processes - could you comment?

RESPONSE: A number of people have used peritoneal dialysis following abdominal surgery for different types of procedures and have found that you can effectively use peritoneal dialysis after intra-abdominal surgery. We have used it in a couple of children who had abdominal surgery. I think if you are going to do that, though, you should use a smaller volume rather than larger volume so that you don't put too much stress on the inside, so to speak, of the suture. It certainly can be used without much difficulty. If you have a patient who has adhesions, for example, who has been on chronic peritoneal dialysis and has had some infection, then it makes sense to apply continuous peritoneal dialysis to such a patient so that one gets the mechanical factor - whatever that is - of preventing adhesions.

QUESTION: How long do you keep plasma exchange and immune suppression treatment in anti-GBM disease and which are the parameters of the treatment?

RESPONSE: That's a good question. Our practice has changed as we have gained experience. What we currently do is to carry out daily plasma exchanges until such time as the clinical evidence of disease activity ceases. By that I mean stabilization of serum creatinine, and a substantial clearing of the urinary red cells. That you can do in any routine laboratory. We also are fortunate in having anti-GBM assay available to us. What we now do is get daily assays of circulating antibody. When antibody is no longer detectable and has been undetectable for a period of two to three weeks, then we take the patient off of any special treatment. We stop plasma exchange when the disease becomes clinically quiescent. We stop immune suppressive treatment within two to three weeks. We start reducing anyway within two to three weeks of the antibody having been cleared from the circulation. Now, this applies particularly in the patient seen early and who suffers from moderately preserved renal function. The problem arises in what to do with a patient who presents anuric, whom you treat because of pulmonary hemorrhage and that resolves. You still are left with a patient with a high level of antibody in the circulation but with irreversible damage to the kidneys. How long should you continue with plasma exchange and treat the patient with drugs? I think the answer to that is a bit uncertain. The difficulty is that we've seen a number of patients in whom we've stopped treatment, who have been left with a high titer of antibody in the circulation and are apparently well, gone back to the referring physician and developed a respiratory infection. Some have died under those circumstances. So, that's a difficult judgement to make. I can't give you clear guidelines on it. It's still a course between the danger of continuing cyclophosphamide and steroids in an anuric patient who is on regular dialysis and that's a patient in considerable danger of infections and hemorrhage. But, in those patients, I think, probably you can start to reduce the cytotoxic drugs.

As I said yesterday, we've only very exceptionally continued cyclophosphamide anyway for more than 6-8 weeks.

QUESTION: I was going to ask if you might spend a minute or two just describing the mechanics of how you do your plasmapheresis - using shunts, grafts, single needle, double needle, etc.

RESPONSE: Well, it just depends upon what kind of problem you are dealing with. If you've got somebody who comes in with life threatening anti-GBM disease you can be pretty sure that you are going to need to do upwards of 14, 20 or even 30 daily plasma exchanges. Under these circumstances one needs top quality vascular access. I still think that under most circumstances you will be forced to have an arteriovenous shunt before that. I say that with some reluctance because I also told you that the infection of the shunt site causes trouble. For this reason, we tried other approaches such as femoral catheters, or more recently, subclavian catheters, after the experience of the group in Toronto, particularly, who have used it very extensively for hemodialysis. That does seem to be useful in an unfortunate patient who requires an intensive plasma exchange. I think that that is the easiest way you can get intermittent plasma exchange which may be of value and I'm referring now to patients with severe lupus where you may want a few plasma exchanges or some of these other immune complex diseases where the plasma exchange seems to tip the patient into a state of cardiac decompensation. Then, we would try, if possible, to use just a venous access. The trouble with that is that you get poor flow and the whole procedure drags on for three to four hours instead of the usual two hours. In a few patients with anti-GBM disease who, for example, look as though they are heading for renal failure and regular dialysis anyway, we have early fistulas put in. The problem is that you can't use them as soon as you would like to. In most circumstances where you want to do plasma exchange, you want to do it that night, not in two weeks.

QUESTION: I would like to ask you to give us a summary of your experience with chronic peritoneal dialysis.

RESPONSE: We have about fifteen patients dialyzed every other night. We have been able to compare about five patients that went into hemodialysis for a period of six months and then they decided or asked us to shift to peritoneal dialysis. We compared another period of six months. We were then able to see that we had had a good control of the hypertension. The patients who went to peritoneal dialysis, arrived with lower levels of urea, creatinine, and with normal levels of hemoglobin. So, I think we got very good results. Then, we thought that maybe these kids were stabilizing because of the previous periods of hemodialysis, but when we compared another number of patients who went from the very beginning to peritoneal dialysis, we got exactly the same results. So, I think it is an improvement.

On the other side we had two patients whom we put on chronic ambulatory peritoneal dialysis. It worked very well. We were able to keep these two patients for about six months in very good condition so I think that it also, is a good dialysis modality.

QUESTION: Did the infants grow on CAPD?

RESPONSE: No, I don't think so.

QUESTION: Regarding the individual variability in the amount of fluid needed to maintain balance, during intermittent peritoneal dialysis at times we must make adjustments in terms of the amount of fluid lost over and above that put in. Do you find that in chronic peritoneal dialysis?

RESPONSE: I am not aware of any studies looking at how much fluid you lose in children dialyzed with different glucose concentrations, different volumes, etc. I do know that there is some published data but I can't remember the numbers, as to how much fluid you remove in an average exchange with a certain concentration of glucose. In terms of acute dialysis, I agree with you. We see patients in whom the amount of water that has been removed is great; others in whom we can't get much out. We occasionally see some patients, when they first start, in whom we get almost nothing back in relation to what we put in for reasons which I am not sure about. Some of these children probably have had lots of stress, intermittent episodes of hyperglycemia with a gradient such that water will move into the patient. One of the things that we have done on a couple of occasions in children with post-operative open heart surgery and acute renal failure, who have had high blood sugars - even before we started - when the blood sugar even went further up to 400-500-600 mg/dl, we even had to administer intermittent insulin.

MODERATOR: By the way, your review of antihypertensive agents regarding hyperglycemia in peritoneal dialysis, using diazoxide when given under those conditions can really create havoc. We had that situation. We had not thought about it but the patient had crystals of glucose in his eyegrounds on fundoscopy. I wonder whether one of you could touch on the point of implantation of catheters in terms of surgical versus medical, whether you need to go into an operating suite, and whether it makes any difference whether the catheter is one that you buy for $40 or one that you make at home for $2-4?

RESPONSE: We've taken the easy way out. We have had the surgeons put our catheters in for practical reasons. We have used the Tenkoff catheters because they have been available. I do believe that there is a somewhat different catheter in Toronto that apparently has been helpful. There is some difference between the dacron sleeves at the two ends which if anybody is interested in getting the catheter I can provide names for them. The other thing we have done in acute patients, we have in the last few years used Tenkoff catheters rather than straight catheters with the idea that most of the children whom we dialyze, we don't dialyze but one or two days. Based on our past experience they will have dialysis for a week or ten days - a minimum of a week to ten days. So, having a catheter that you can use intermittently with less problems may be helpful.

MODERATOR: What do you do in those cases? Do you continuously dialyze those patients?

RESPONSE: When we put a Tenkoff in we need to do the dialysis every day for the first five days. Now it may not be 8 or 12 hours - it may be a few hours. It seems as though - and it's recommended by some people - that some exchange must be done daily for the first number of days. This allows trap formation to occur, inhibits the infection process, etc., and the catheter will work better. What we now do in anyone, either an acute or chronic patient who has a Tenkoff put in, we'll do some exchange daily for the first five or six days.

COMMENT: For chronic peritoneal dialysis we use the one made by our staff because it cuts down the cost from $40 to $4. We use either one of the implantation procedures according to the age of the patient. If it is a small infant we use the surgical procedure; in the older child, we do it by ourselves. We start using the peritoneal dialysis immediately daily for five or six days and then we start with the intermittent approach.

QUESTION: Could I ask a question from last night's workshop? I may not have understood exactly what you said, but I gather from what you said regarding treatment of apparent or presumed renal immunologic disease, based on your rationale, you use either one or two criteria: number one, documentation of the exact nature of the disease with definite, demonstrated evidence from scientific data that the therapy is going to work. Number two, I think you said that you must not treat such patients if there has not been previous experience with similar cases showing or indicating success. We had a case which we had never seen before and which had not been reported specifically in all its complexity which we happened to treat. Now, if we saw a similar case next year and treated her or him similarly and achieved the same good result, would you praise the treatment next year as opposed to condemning it this year?

RESPONSE: As you put it to me, basically, you either treat or try a treatment because you think you understand the nature of the disease - its rationale - and that, of course, happens fairly infrequently\ or you use drugs in an entirely uncritical way. Along those lines, who would have thought that the nephrotic syndrome associated with minimal change nephropathy, on the basis of the evidence that we have accumulated over the past 25-30 years, would have responded the way it has? Are there grounds for believing that there are mechanisms involved that steroids or cyclophosphamide are likely to influence? I don't think there are. But, the treatment works. When you come to a disease that you haven't seen before, that nobody else has seen before and don't know how to treat, then you are entitled to do almost anything within reason provided you don't - it's not a question of what you do, it's how you write it up. What I was objecting to last night was a mixture of empiricism and science.

QUESTION: I saw in one of your slides that you almost doubled the efficiency of your dialysis by increasing the dwell time to 60 minutes. I have been traditionally taught that when you increase the dwell time up to and beyond 60 minutes you are really going to decrease your efficiency. Have you carried out any studies to see what is the optimum dwell time?

RESPONSE: No, we haven't except that we have performed a number of diffusion curves, the data of which I did not show, as to changes of dialysate concentration with time. This has been done many times in adults. For example, urea with 30 minutes dwell time, you'll get maybe 40-50% of plasma level. If you leave it in for 60 minutes, you'll get 60 or 70% of plasma level; if you leave it in for three hours, you'll get 100% of plasma level. The calculation I showed you was a theoretical level calculation. That is, if you leave time as a factor, it would almost double. On the other hand, from a realistic point of view, if you leave the solution in there for a longer amount of time, the concentration builds up as well, but that's falling off with time. So when you have all of these variable things to field, you'll practically - most people, I believe, do exchanges that range from 30 to 40 minutes. Sixty minutes may be a tad too long. Some people have looked at several exchanges, one every 30 minutes versus one every 60 minutes versus one every two hours. I think it's decided that every 30-40 minutes probably you get the most solute removed.

QUESTION: Regarding the more efficient dialysis of infants versus the adult individuals, is there anything to do with peritoneal elasticity or surface area in relation to total body mass or weight?

RESPONSE: As far as the elasticity, I can't make any comments except to say that there are some data on the isolated perfused tubules studied suggesting that the endothelial membrane or basement membrane are more volume pliable in general. The question of surface area, I think there is no doubt that the surface area of the peritoneal membrane in relation to body size is larger in infants whereas it has been pointed out that it is not necessarily the entire surface area which participates in the exchange process. It is more likely to be the visceral peritoneum than the parietal peritoneum. There's also some data that suggest the length of capillaries may have something to do with the exchange process.

QUESTION: Do you find that peritoneal dialysis when peritonitis exists, is contraindicated?

RESPONSE: We have not looked at it. I am not aware of any data on that. But I'm not sure of any study supporting it.

QUESTION: I was wondering how the progression of the osteodystrophy in the peritoneally dialyzed children compared to those in hemodialysis.

RESPONSE: We haven't carefully looked at it. We get monthly calciums, phosphoruses, PTH's. Twice a year we get x-rays. I could not answer you whether the rate of progression is that much different or not.

MODERATOR: How solid are the data on increased ADH levels or production in patients with the nephrotic syndrome? You mentioned that that is evident.

RESPONSE: I can't answer that as far as how solid the data are. I guess I was assuming that because of the lowered effective arterial volume, that there would be a stimulus for ADH release.

MODERATOR: We are interested in this subject, as you know. We feel that the explanations that we have data for in terms of edema are insufficient and that probably ADH is increased; we are looking into that. It is obviously a logical assumption but it would be important to know how much of that has been documented.

RESPONSE: As you know, it is difficult to measure ADH levels. The accuracy or at least the availability is not the best. One thing I wanted to comment on is that in pediatrics my experience in the last 15 years, seeing a huge number of children with renal disease, I think Goodpasture below age 18 approaches about zero-zero. I would be interested to know what some of the others here have experienced with Goodpasture disease. We talked about plasma exchange. If I had had this procedure, over the last 15 years I would not have had any patients.

RESPONSE: I guess you would have been very fortunate, wouldn't you? I think the point that I was trying to make is not whether plasma exchange is or is not of value in this form of renal disease. I think that what we get from plasma exchange is an indication of how the treatment is to be brought about or which monitoring methods should be used. It's interesting that one rare disease, with this treatment, appears to be curable under some circumstances. As a proportion of patients in pediatric practice that's not very important. As an idea, as a concept of how diseases of this group may be treated, it's very important. I think that is really the point. In relation to immune complex disease it is much more important. As I say, I don't know how valuable plasma exchange is. Formal data of studies are not yet available. But, again, there are indications from plasma exchange of the sort of things one might wish to do. It's far less expensive, less dangerous, and less invasive than hemodialysis. Again, not what it does, it's the way it points. I run a clinical research department and my approach to renal disease has always been that existing forms of treatment are inadequate. Our knowledge is not adequate and what we have to do is fundamental research on methods of treatment and use those insofar as possible to try to help patients but to bear in mind constantly that empirical clinical observations may well turn out to be much more interesting in the long run.

MODERATOR: You also mentioned last night that there was an increase in the reported incidence or number of reported cases.

RESPONSE: I think that it's just in the diagnosing part. It's quite interesting. I remember going to a meeting in Paris in about 1971, I think it was, when an American immunologist came and spoke about pathogenic mechanisms in nephritis. It was a gathering of very distinguished French nephrologists. He talked about anti-GBM disease and described the mechanisms-a beautiful thing. He discussed immune complex disease in the most erudite manner. An elegant talk. Afterwards a French pathologist got up and showed his slides--an analysis of the past 400 cases of primary glomerulonephritis at his hospital--400 immune complex disease, zero anti-GBM disease. For a long time, the French nephrologists claimed that anti-GBM disease was exceedingly rare and even non-existent. It's very interesting how much the disease has increased in incidence recently. I have seen more reports coming through of anti-GBM and anti-TBM diseases than ever before. I think it's the usual thing. Once a form of treatment is apparently successful, these patients are identified. I used to see one case a year in a major internal medicine practice. Now we have two or three cases on the ward at the same time.

QUESTION: Changing the subject, did you have any problems in relation to body image with the Tenkoff catheter, particularly in adolescents? And, have you considered or used any of the reverse osmosis units?

RESPONSE: Our children have not, to the best of my knowledge, verbalized body image problems because of a catheter. I think they have sufficient body image problems without the catheter to begin with. They also have body image problems with access routes, etc. I would assume that they feel that it's a body image problem. On the other hand, you can conceal a Tenkoff or other catheter in terms of daily dress very easily. Reverse osmosis machines: the unit that I showed you, we opened approximately a year and a half ago. We do use reverse osmosis. So all of our hemodialysis patients now are hooked to water treated by reverse osmosis. The groups that have observed the epidemics of dialysis dementia (particulary I'm thinking of the Newcastle, England, group) make the statement that after they have switched from some other kind of water to reverse osmosis, the epidemic has disappeared-presumably from reducing the aluminum content in the dialysate water. So, in terms of hemodialysis, the use of reverse osmosis may have a significant impact in the future on the incidence of the whole problem of dialysis dementia-if you believe it's aluminum.

COMMENT: I have not been aware of the psychological impact of this procedure but I have to look at this particular aspect. I think that most of our patients are already depressed because of the disease or because of procedures they have had.

COMMENT: I would like to make one other point about the use of the Tenkoff catheter. At least in our experience, it always has been associated with going to home dialysis. I think these particular groups of children tending to themselves, because they have been at home, in more of a routine life style, in general have improved, so the trade off may be well worth the catheter.

MODERATOR: In terms of safety of plasmapheresis or plasma exchange, we hear some of the commercial companies say, "It's a very simple procedure; we can train the nurse in a couple of days and that's all you need". In our discussions, letters, etc. regarding the establishment of such a procedure in our hospital, it has been my assumption that we needed to approach this program very much like the establishment of a dialysis facility, with all the support personnel, monitoring and physician supervision. Could you give us your thoughts on that, on how you operate?

RESPONSE: It is a rather straightforward procedure, easy enough to do. We have a nurse technician who does it under medical supervision. Now the way it's done in my unit is, when we first started it, it was a problem of responsibility of one person we call a registrar, a Resident Physician (with other duties) and then as we increased our activities, we got a full-time person. Now it's more routine, is easier, and we have a junior Staff doctor, a group of three people who are on one night in three, and one nurse. There's a machine and it's done in a side room off of our ancient Victorian ward. The major problem we have is vascular access. The rest is simple and there is little to discuss, really.

MODERATOR: You have not had any acute problems during the performance of the procedure?

RESPONSE: We have been very fortunate in that people have been very careful. Other people have had pulmonary edema. You need to be very, very sure you don't overload your patient with priming and that kind of thing. We don't have problems with hypotension which has been reported in this country. Mainly, we are very fortunate in having a very safe protein fraction preparation which is free of hypotensive effects. The problem with plasma exchange is that it is too easy and its use is becoming very widespread under circumstances where the information is not subject to monitoring of a scientific kind or under a process of controlled trial. In Southern England, I know of people having attacks of migraine who occasionally have plasma exchange!

MODERATOR: That is without having the stimulus of making a few bucks which would be so in our Society with private enterprise. We are fortunate in having very responsible physicians in private practice who are most cautious in the use of the few machines available in this community.

RESPONSE: Yes. We don't have those stimuli in England. We just do it for the glory.

MODERATOR: What about the question of immune complexes in the nephrotic syndrome? You touched on the nephrotic syndrome and we are very interested. We have visited and shared information with the group at the Child Institute in London. What is your interpretation of their data and methodology in general for immune complexes?

RESPONSE: It's a difficult question to answer simply. Certain groups find certain immune complexes in patients with steroid responsive nephrotic syndrome. They further show that in patients who've got persistence of circulating immune complexes, after the nephrotic syndrome responded to steroids, the immune complexes decrease when compared to relapse. That seems to be the sort of body of evidence that could be used to argue the case for a role for circulating immune complexes. There is an enormous body of evidence against it. There are patients who have minumum change nephrotic syndrome without immune complexes in the circulation and relapse without immune complexes in the circulation. So, if you are a cynic you might want to agree that immune complexes in the circulation in these patients are some kind of secondary phenomenon and not related in a primary way to the disease of the kidney. My own position is that I just don't know. I don't understand that disorder. I think what you've got to hang on to is that the disease responds to steroids and cyclophosphamide. That seems to me to suggest that it is inherently more likely to be related to a product of a steroid or cyclophosphamide sensitive cell. That's about as far as I would take it.

MODERATOR: It has been suggested that what they measured was not immune complexes or that the different so-called immune complex determinations may measure different substances. Is that logical?

RESPONSE: Yes. That's logical. One measures by all the tests for immune complexes, material which has reactivity that also can be ascribed to immune complexes. C_{1q} dependent reactions, for example, measure C_{1q} binding properties of immune complexes, but substances other than immune complexes bind C_{1q}. This kind of problem underlies all the assays. It's the reactivity you are measuring, not like when you measure zinc, calcium or aluminum; in those cases you are measuring molecules which are defined. With an immune complex, even when it is an immune complex, it is not defined; it's in a state of continuous equilibrium with antigens and antibodies, where the complexes are aggregated and disaggregated and so on. This is the reason why people have received about 20 or 30 different assays because the underlying philosophy has been that when you fail to find immune complexes in the circulation of a patient in whom you feel on certain grounds that there ought to be immune complexes, you conclude that the techniques are wrong. But the techniques are not wrong; they are right and the concept is wrong. The whole position is in limbo, really.

MODERATOR: Changing the subject, what about complications from diuretics. We had the experience a number of years ago (Dr. Mel Grumbach, Dr. Schotland and myself were working with some patients with nephrogenic diabetes insipidus) with a patient on one of the thiazide diuretics who developed bone marrow aplasia. I wonder how often that is present? How would one go about detecting such a severe complication?

RESPONSE: I've not seen a patient with that. It's so rare that I would not advise routine, regular white blood cell count in patients who are on diuretic therapy.

RESPONSE: Going back to a previous question, we've seen a number of children who had not only severe renal osteodystrophy but have had myelofibrosis. This question you brought up, I wonder if you have any experience with that. In response to the question, "Have you ever seen Goodpasture?", we have seen two children with it-one of whom, one morning while we were waiting for the biopsy report to come back, sat up, started having lung hemorrhage, and died in about nine minutes.

COMMENT: We haven't seen any patients with myelofibrosis but we haven't looked for it. In terms of diagnosis, how do you diagnose it apart from bone marrow aspiration?

RESPONSE: These were children who have had persistent thrombocytopenia, neutropenia, who had had bone marrow aspiration routinely.

COMMENT: We absolutely don't do bone marrow routinely. Some of the children tend to run low white counts but we don't see any thrombocytopenia and they are all anemic. But no, I can't say that we have specifically seen it.

MODERATOR: What about other methods short of bone marrow biopsy or bone biopsy to assess osteodystrophy?

RESPONSE: There are methods, such as radioactive techniques to determine bone marrow mineral density, which apparently are much more sensitive than ordinary straight x-rays. However, mineral density does not necessarily indicate correction of osteodystrophy because with calcium alone you can increase bone density. You can increase the mineral but the pattern of the bone is irregular. So it is not as specific. On the other hand, bone biopsy is not that specific either because on different areas of the skeleton there are different stages of alteration and perhaps iliac crest biopsy may not be representative of the total net situation in the body. Anyway, as far as we are concerned, bone biopsy is rather theoretical.

COMMENT: We have quite a number of patients with myelodysplasia and we've had a Research Protocol for the last couple of years to look at the children on hemodialysis or in renal failure to come up with some ideas on the pertinent subjects to clarify the pathology and the etiology of it. Another thing to look at along with what has been mentioned, is the evidence of leukopenia and, of course, anemia; also, extra-medullary hematopoiesis, and radio iron incorporation, over the liver and spleen. Compare this to bone marrow following injection. It's our feeling right now from the data, that there is secondary hyperparathyroidism. It seems to be much more common in those patients who have urological type diseases rather than glomerular diseases. We are now in the process of putting our data together.

QUESTION: Changing the subject, would you go into more detail about the training process that is used with peritoneal dialysis and also if there is any differentiation between the diet requirements of hemodialysis patients as compared to peritoneal dialysis patients.

RESPONSE: We have a training manual put together. What we have done is ask one of our nurses to assume responsibility for all home peritoneal dialysis training; she works with the kid and the family. They have a step-wise procedure including a number of check points with examination, etc.

QUESTION: Is there any difference in diet between the different dialysis procedures?

RESPONSE: We tend to be a little more liberal with the kids on peritoneal dialysis. You also probably remove more albumin during peritoneal dialysis than you do during hemodialysis, so you are able to offer a higher protein diet in terms of trying to deal with the problem of hypoproteinemia. It's interesting, just as an aside, to mention that there are studies trying to use dialysis solution as a way of providing nutrients-putting amino-acids and seeing what happens in terms of moving their metabolism in the other direction.

QUESTION: What preparation would you use in patients with kidney and liver disease when you cannot use a vitamin D metabolite that has not been hydroxylated ?

RESPONSE: I would have to pass that question to someone else because I don't know. You had a child, so you tell us what you did.

COMMENT: We did not succeed in treating him because we gave him Hytacherol and he didn't respond.

RESPONSE: With these end stage kidney diseases, a lot of times we give the 1,25 metabolite, that apparently is the most active metabolite. You cannot give anything that has to go through the liver and 1,25 fulfills that requirement.

COMMENT: Hytacherol supposedly has to be hydroxylated in the liver.

RESPONSE: Hytacherol yes, but not 1,25 dihydroxycholecalciferol. Anything else available has to go through the liver.

MODERATOR: Neither of you was here during another discussion when one of the panelists mentioned that he would add, I believe, the 24,25 compound also.

RESPONSE: I didn't mention it because it was explained so well. Certainly, 1,25 is not the whole answer but it is the only thing we have. Experimentally, the 24,25 compound is available. One may end up giving a combination of the two. The alternative would be, in the absence of glomerular disease, to give a combination of 25 hydroxycalciferol and 1,25 dehydroxycholecalciferol. The 25 may be hydroxylated to the 24,25. But that's all very experimental at this time.

MODERATOR: We will have the answer when our group finishes its study on 24,25 dihydroxycholecalciferol! We must adjourn for now. Thank you.

WORKSHOP:

IMMUNO-CLINICO-PATHOLOGIC CORRELATIONS

Moderator: José Strauss, M.D.

Div. Pediatr. Nephrol., Dept. Pediatr., Univ.
Miami Sch. Med., Miami, Fla. 33152 USA

MODERATOR: The first case will be presented by Dr. Gaston Zilleruelo.

DR. ZILLERUELO: This is an 18 year old black female who has the history of nephrotic syndrome started in September 1972 at the age of 11 years old. At that time she was found to have moderate edema, heavy proteinuria, hematuria and mild hypertension. She had been a well developed and completely healthy child. No history of familiar renal disease except that her father died at 32 years of age due to hypertension and "Chronic Glomerulonephritis".

Laboratory work-up on the first admission included, in blood: Hb 12.9 g/dl, Hct 36.7%, a normal total protein of 4.4 g/dl, albumin 2.0 g/dl, calcium 7.7 mg/dl, phosphorus 4.6 mg/dl, cholesterol 465 mg/dl, BUN 10 mg/dl, serum creatinine 0.6 mg/dl, C_3 normal, ASO and ANA titers negative, LE cell preparation negative, serum immunoglobulins with decreased IgG and increased IgM, protein electrophoresis with a nephrotic pattern (decreased albumin and increased alpha 2 globulins). In urine: protein 3+, blood small, RBC casts +; IVP with enlarged kidneys and left double renal artery.

The patient had a kidney biopsy in October 1972 that showed an acute diffuse exudative and proliferative GN with electron dense deposits and gammaglobulin in the mesangium. She had a second renal biopsy in July 1973 that showed "segmental disseminated mesangial sclerosis (10/10)."

She was started on prednisone therapy, did not respond and also was resistant to a vincristine trial. Because of persisting proteinuria and edema, a three month course therapy with cyclophosphamide and prednisone was instituted from April to June 1975 with some improvement in her condition (edema decreased). Patient received therapy with prednisone until December 1975. Because of serum immunoglobulins with decreased IgG and increased IgM, a trial of transfer factor was done in January 1976, without significant improvement.

During this time, she persisted with heavy proteinuria (ranging from 2 to 4 g/day). Several ANA titers were negative. Also complement was found to be normal except for occasional low level up to our lower normal which is 80 mg/dl for C_3. Her renal function showed at first a slight decrease of the creatinine clearance (Ccr) from 76 ml/min/1.73 m^2 (July 1973) to 68.8 ml/min/ 1.73 m^2 (June 1976). However, in December 1976 her Ccr was normal, 92 ml/min/1.73 m^2, with a serum creatinine of 1 mg/dl. She remained relatively stable with normal renal function and no evidence of edema until November 1977 when she presented a clinical reactivation of her disease with increased proteinuria and reappearance of edema. After then a progressive deterioration of her renal function occurred. In February 1979 her BUN was 28, creatinine 3.5. In March 1979 BUN was 36 and creatinine 4.5. An A-V fistula for hemodialysis was placed on her arm on April 25, 1979. Four months later, her BUN had gone up to 74 and creatinine was over 15 mg/dl.

The patient had to start on chronic hemodialysis on September 8, 1979. Bilateral nephrectomy and splenectomy were performed in November 1979. Finally, on December 21, 1979, she had a successful renal transplant obtained from one of her brothers. At the present time, she is doing well with normal renal function and normal urinalysis.

DR. PARDO: The first biopsy as you see in Figure 1 is from October 1972. The first impression I had when I looked at this biopsy was that there is an increase in nuclei; also, an increase in granulocytes. You can see this on high magnification, the detail of these cells. You get the impression that there is an increased cellularity. There is something I missed when I looked at this slide. You notice that this area here seems to have some small adhesions. I interpreted this initially as displacement of the loops. I was very impressed with the lesions in the loops. I think you can see the increase in granulocytes here and there. This is an exudative component. Again some of the loops seem to approximate the basement membrane of Bowman's capsule but I really didn't pay as much attention to that as I should have done. I was more impressed with the exudative component and perhaps a slight mesangial proliferation but this is not demonstrated. It is very difficult to demonstrate. I think that the main component was the exudation.

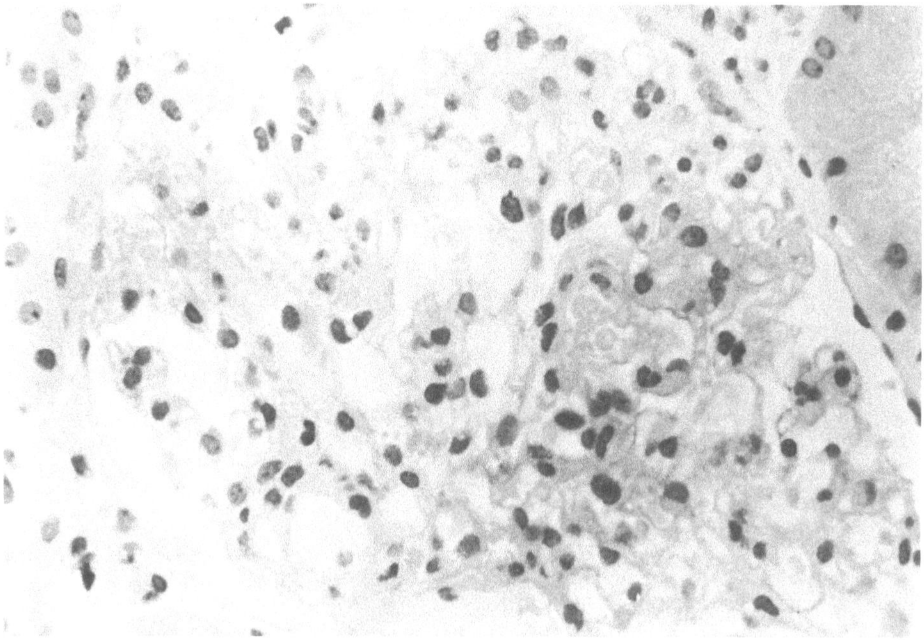

FIGURE 1

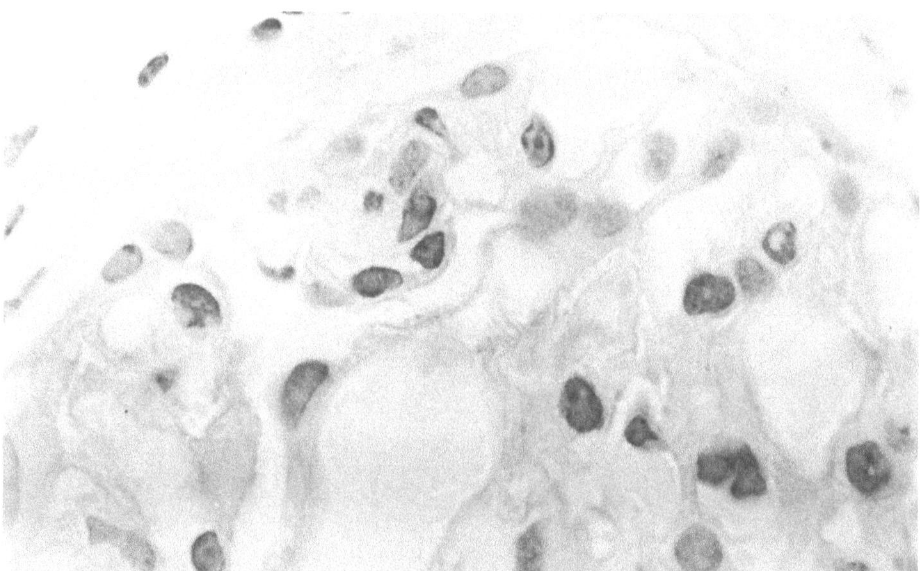

FIGURE 2

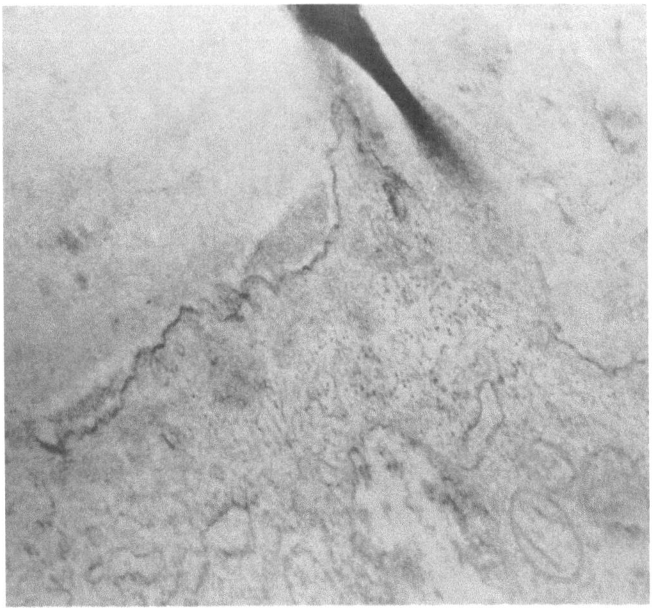

FIGURE 3

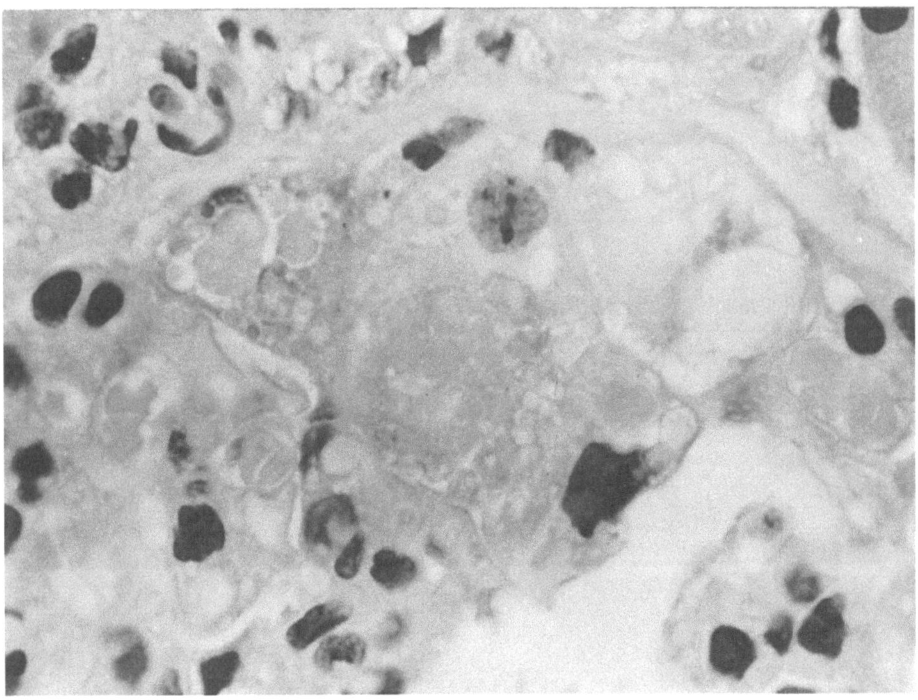

FIGURE 4

On high magnification, look at those areas which seem to be just areas of loops adjacent to the Bowman's capsule (Fig. 2). You can see that there is fusion of the basement membrane of Bowman's capsule with some of the basement membrane of the loops. For example, here you can see the contours of the basement membrane of Bowman's capsule, parietal epithelium and a loop. Very minute lesions. There were no foam cells at this stage. There were no hyaline insudative lesions.

One of the things that threw us off was the electron microscopy study. In Figure 3, we have the lamina densa; this is the endothelial side. Here we have the cytoplasm of the epithelial cells. I think you can see mostly subepithelial electron dense deposits.

The second biopsy, done in July 1973, I think shows now very clearly an adhesion (Fig. 4). There is foamy material in here, probably a foam cell. You can see some hyaline type material in the lumen. The epithelial cells have large granules containing protein that you see quite frequently on the epithelial lesions of focal and segmental glomerular sclerosis.

This is something that appeared now (Fig. 5). On the silver stain you can see that there is initiation of tubular atrophy, basement membrane of many tubules is wrinkled and irregular, and there is increase in interstitial connective tissue. So, there were some patchy areas of interstitial fibrosis and tubular atrophy. The nephrectomy specimen was that of "end stage" and was not helpful in the diagnosis.

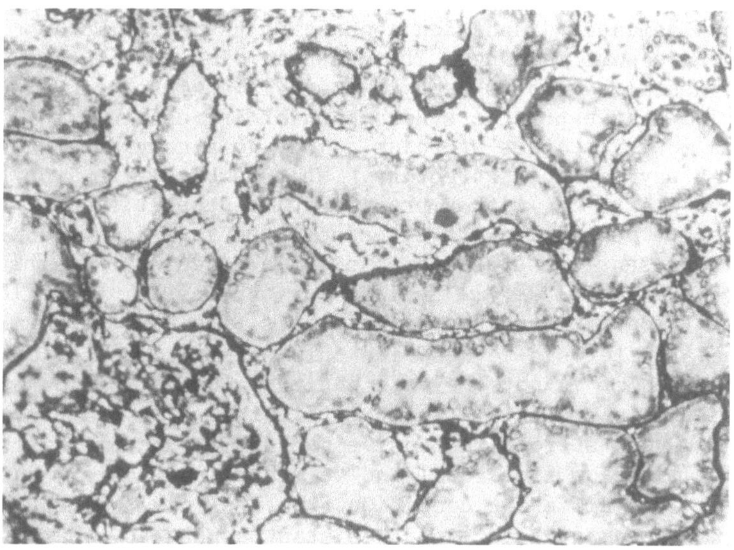

FIGURE 5

MODERATOR: Basically, we are back to a case we presented two or three years ago when the late Dr. McIntosh was with us. There was some confusion; just a few statements suggested that maybe this was a case of focal segmental sclerosis but Dr. Pardo wanted to bring this back to emphasize the difficulty in the diagnosis. Some of the panelists were here, and have helped us diagnose difficult cases in the past. Would you like to comment?

COMMENT: It seems to me clear that it is an idiopathic nephrotic syndrome. The first biopsy was clearly mild mesangial proliferation and there were some adhesions in the glomeruli to Bowman's capsule. In the second biopsy, really the aspect of the adhesion is more apparent. I have not seen the glomerulosclerosis so it is not clear to me. From that point to the end, six years have passed, so anything could happen in that time. It would be very rare if it stopped as a mesangial proliferation. It could develop glomerulosclerosis during these years. It's quite possible. Again, if it was a mild mesangial proliferation, it is not surprising that this is a case that didn't respond to the usual therapy for the nephrotic syndrome. My guess is that maybe it is a case of idiopathic nephrotic syndrome with mesangial proliferation.

MODERATOR: Without focal and segmental glomerulosclerosis?

RESPONSE: Yes. I couldn't see it. But it s just a picture so it is quite possible. If it was mesangial proliferation progressing to glomerulosclerosis, it's quite possible.

COMMENT: I think that there is a great danger of getting involved in a semantic discussion about this patient. Words have got to have some meaning. The understanding that I have of focal segmental sclerosis or hyalinosis is a histology which is accompanied by a nephrotic syndrome which is resistant to treatment-in most instances steroids. That is a core observation. That, you can say, defines an entity. What we have here, you have a patient who starts off with a proliferative nephritis, an acute exhudative nephritis with adhesions, the sort of lesions that could represent the starting point of crescents. Now this inflammatory process, like all inflammatory processes, is followed by a degree of scarring, mesangial sclerosis. To use the term, focal segmental sclerosis to describe this, seems to me to just lead to confusion when it is not the core entity. The definition of focal segmental sclerosis presents a great difficulty. For example, some patients who have a steroid responsive nephrotic syndrome will show on careful examination some focal and segmental sclerosis. But quite clearly, that is a different condition from the focal segmental sclerosis that accompanies steroid resistant nephrotic syndrome. What we are talking about here is one of the difficulties of basing classification of disease on what you see down the microscope at any one time. The thing that has been shown to be very important about focal segmental sclerosis is that that process of scarring is not a consequence of previous inflammation. This sclerotic lesion appears de novo. When the disease recurs in transplants--which it does in an important proportion of transplanted patients--the first lesion that is seen is the sclerotic one. It is not a consequence of previous inflammation. The only way you could reconcile the histology you showed in the beginning with the diagnosis of focal segmental sclerosis which is called the nephrotic syndrome, and then for some reason there was superimposed upon that an acute nephritis which resolved leaving this basic underlying pathology. That is a very messy explanation. I would favor the view that this is a child with a nephrotic syndrome due to a proliferative nephritis with an exudative component that didn't resolve upon treatment and showed the expected natural history. It is not inconceivable that it is even a streptococcal infection although not very likely. The normal ASO titer and C_3 level make a post-streptococcal nephritis unlikely. What you've got is a proliferative nephritis, which is what you had at the beginning.

COMMENT: Whenever you have to invoke two diseases at the same time, you have a big problem. I am in favor of the interpretation that this patient had basically focal segmental sclerosis. She had an acute glomerulonephritis by the early biopsy findings. Let me make a scheme here. We have seen quite a number of focal segmental sclerosis minimal lesions. For example, we had about four or five women who during pregnancy had a nephrotic syndrome. The only thing that showed was lesions similar to these.

COMMENT: There is a great danger of getting entities mixed up. You have to define the disease. How would you define focal segmental sclerosis?

RESPONSE: I would define it morphologically.

COMMENT: If you don't define more positively, then you don't have an entity because focal scarring can result from focal inflammation. It is part of the natural process of inflammation.

COMMENT: But not isolated focal scarring. You get this from focal mesangial proliferation.

COMMENT: I don't accept your views, with respect. What I am saying is, there are two sorts of processes-one in which focal scarring follows focal inflammation. There is another process where this hyalinotic or sclerotic process seems to develop without an increase in inflammatory cells and exudate. I am not saying that you couldn't be right-that somebody with focal sclerosis isn't entitled, just as all the rest of us are, to get an additional focal proliferative glomerulonephritis. But that becomes intellectually untidy.

RESPONSE: In the second biopsy, there is very little mesangial proliferation. I am conservative on that. However, there is an area where you can feel secure that there are more than three nuclei in the mesangium. What you see mainly is an exudative component. The other thing you see in these loops is the picture of post-infectious glomerulonephritis. Probably you have some mesangial increase. This is a pure lesion of peripheral loops. That is the reason I don't see any other possibility except focal segmental glomerulonephritis.

QUESTION: How often do you see adhesions in focal sclerosis?

RESPONSE: Like this? I see them quite frequently.

QUESTION: And polymorphs?

RESPONSE: Polymorphs, no. I think that it was superimposed on a focal segmental sclerosis. You may be right or I may be right. But my working hypothesis is that when an exudative component disappears, in order for the sclerosis to be related to the exudative process, it has to be a completely peripheral lesion without mesangial hyperplasia or mesangial sclerosis. I don't think that this is the usual picture we see in late stages of post-infectious glomerulonephritis.

QUESTION: And the electronmicroscopy findings? How often do you see those?

RESPONSE: That also confused me initially because they were subepithelial. The patient probably had an acute glomerulonephritis and that threw me off completely.

QUESTION: So, two diseases then?

RESPONSE: Yes, that's a valid assumption.

QUESTION: Have you performed immunopathology studies in this biopsy?

RESPONSE: It was a very small biopsy. There was some IgG. I don't think it was too good. There was only one glomerulus for this purpose. Also, at about that time we started our immunofluorescence. The second biopsy had some focal IgM. I think that would favor the diagnosis of focal sclerosis.

COMMENT: It seems to me that with the theory which was set up by the people in Paris, this case is quite easy to explain. In this explanation, idiopathic nephrotic syndrome could have four histological patterns. First, minimal lesions; second, focal sclerosis; third, mesangial proliferation; and, fourth, mesangial proliferation plus focal sclerosis. With this interpretation, this case is possible within the frame of idiopathic nephrotic syndrome with steroid resistance. The fact that focal sclerosis was not obvious on the biopsy is not an evidence that sclerosis did not develop afterwards and reached this stage of destruction of the glomeruli. So, it seems to me that it is an idiopathic nephrotic syndrome with steroid unresponsiveness which did not recur at transplant. But it's one of those patients who evolve to renal failure within more than three years. As you know, there was a study some years ago that showed that the cases which evolved to renal failure within two or three years had recurrence in 3/4 of the cases. If we consider the cases with the longer evolution, the recurrence is rare, but it's possible, too.

COMMENT: Well, I think I tend to agree with one of the earlier comments a little bit. Recently, I was sitting on one side of the microscopy and Dr. Pardo was sitting on the other side. I said "Gee, I can see all these lesions from this side of the microscope as well." I was sitting in his chair at the time. He may see a lot more of the focal segmental sclerosis on his side of the microscope. I think that it is a semantic problem. Dr. Pardo and I agree on most of these logical diagnoses. Maybe to expand the discussion a little more, I'd like to say that it is morphological rather than just a semantic confusion. I don't have a lot of experience with focal segmental sclerosis, but to me, as somebody who deals with inflammation and the treatment of inflammation by immunosuppression, I think that focal segmental sclerosis is a pathological diagnosis which probably has nothing to do with the etiologic entities involved. Depending upon the time that the disease is diagnosed morphologically, is all that the bearing shows in the pathology. What I mean by that is that focal segmental sclerosis, when it recurs in a transplant, recurs because that's the type of response that the transplanted patient is able to produce morphologically. The reason you don't see an exudative proliferative glomerulonephritis in the transplanted patient is because immunosuppression has now made that response aberrant for the most part. What you do see, however, is hyalinization and mesangial proliferation. I think that the other components are inhibited.

COMMENT: If you take anti-GBM disease, you see a very nice, active, acute inflammatory process in the transplant.

COMMENT: Depending upon the stage, if you had an anti-GBM, Goodpasture syndrome, if you hit that patient hard enough and often enough with cortico-steroids, you are not going to see the polys. You might see the deposition of immunoglobulins; certainly you would see that. There was a lot made about polys in transplant patients earlier in the prognosis as to whether there was going to be an acute rejection or not because of an early biopsy that revealed polymorphonuclear cells in the glomeruli. This has come to mean absolutely nothing, depending on how much or how little immunosuppression the patient is given. You can certainly get rid of polys by high dose steroids. The thing that you can't get rid of without killing the patient is humoral immunity. I think that's probably what you are seeing although nobody has demonstrated that this is an immune disease.

COMMENT: One of the great advances these days is that in order to make a good classification we have not only a morphological description but also the immunopathology which helps a great deal- particularly in this case. We have a nephrotic syndrome which persisted with the usual therapy. Then, we have a proliferative glomerulonephritis. We should have immunopathology and if this has the classical deposition of immunoglobulins and complement, then we shouldn't have any difficulty in making the diagnosis. If, on the other hand, we have negative immunofluorescence or just a focal deposit like seems to be in the second biopsy, then we have to be inclined to make the diagnosis of one of the patterns of the idiopathic nephrotic syndrome which is mesangial proliferation. So, the only difficulty that I see is that, if we are not following the exact classification, we get confused because there are many patterns. In this case, there is mesangial proliferation; the adhesions, which are circumstancial, are not going to change the diagnosis. The same applies to the exudative changes and the adhesions to Bowman's capsule. I don't think they are the most important features in this case. So, I would stay with the possibility that this is a mesangial proliferation, a nephrotic syndrome which is resistant to steroid therapy. In many of these cases, we may see progressive renal failure as happened in this case.

QUESTION: What about these lesions; can they be used for classification? I guess the only thing we can say which is clinically valid is whether a patient has a steroid resistant or a steroid sensitive nephrotic syndrome.

MODERATOR: Everybody agrees on that. There is another point we need to touch on; we need to say something about transplantation questions in these patients.

COMMENT: It was alluded to; I think there was some evidence presented. I think he said 30% recurrence.

COMMENT: Depending on duration of the interval prior to transplantation.

COMMENT: Well, I'm not sure also because of my way of thinking about focal segmental sclerosis in that probably it is due to humoral immunity. I think that humoral immunity is quite hard to abolish. The question is whether you can detect humoral immunity or whether you can't detect it, but it still might be there. And whether on immunosuppression it can be inhibited to the point that it will not recur in a transplanted patient. I'm not sure that we know the answer to that and perhaps the prognostic sign of a long-standing disease is a very good one, that we ought to try and transplant the ones who are long-standing. The other question is whether the disease itself can burn out after a period of years and perhaps then be more amenable to transplantation. I'm having several other thoughts about this as far as how to transplant these patients. There has been experimental work in animals and some early work in humans of putting a kidney in and then putting another kidney in to try and absorb the initial factors known or unknown and then using a second kidney from a cadaver donor for the actual transplant. This early work was done in Boston. That's the work I know of anyway. But some of these do recur after transplantation and I am not sure that it is all related to the rapidity of the disease. I think any disease that is rapid and hard is going to recur more frequently. For instance, the transplant that is rejected rapidly has a much greater chance on the second transplant of being rejected rapidly. So, I think this is an immune disease which in some way can recur. The question is whether transplantation is efficacious or not. The answer is not known so we do transplant them because we have no way, really, of classifying the etiology of the disease as it exists in a morphological state.

MODERATOR: Do you think that the patient should not have been transplanted?

RESPONSE: I'm a little bit concerned. I didn't realize this patient had a father who died of what was called glomerulonephritis. Are there any thoughts about the inheritance pattern in diseases like this?

MODERATOR: Nobody present has information in this regard. We shall now go to case number two which will be presented by Dr. Rafael Galindez.

DR. GALINDEZ: This is a fourteen year old white female who presented at Jackson Memorial Hospital Emergency Room on November, 1979 with a three weeks history of weight gain and pedal edema and a one week history of facial edema. She had been in excellent health until approximately four weeks prior to admission. Then she developed an upper respiratory infection with fever which lasted approximately one week. For that she took decongestants and improved. She did well until approximately five days prior to admission when she noted periorbital edema in the morning which slowly decreased throughout the day. She had gained approximately 6 lbs, from 108 to 113 lbs in three weeks. The patient denied other symptoms such as arthralgias, myalgias and skin rash. She never had gross hematuria or any other problems. Past medical history was essentially unremarkable except for asthma. Family history was unremarkable. Physical examination on admission showed the patient in no acute distress, moderately hypertensive (blood pressure was 160/92 mm Hg, weight 114 lbs and she had as remarkable findings in the rest of the physical examination, a systolic murmur grade II/VI, which was heard in the apex area. Laboratory on admission: she was obviously anemic with a hemoglobin of 7.6 g%, hematocrit 23.9%, WBC 9,400/mm^3, platelet count 288,000/mm^3. The urinalysis showed a pH of 6, positive for protein (3+), and there were RBC, hyaline and granular casts. Serum electrolytes showed mildly increased potassium at 6.1 mEq/L; the rest of the electrolytes were within normal limits. BUN was 69 mg/dl and creatinine on admission was 5.3 mg/dl. Calcium was 8.3 mg/dl; liver enzymes (SGOT and SGPT) were both normal, as well as alkaline phosphatase. ANA was negative. C_3 and C_4, repeated several times, were normal. VDRL was nonreactive. ASO titer was negative as well as streptozyme; Coombs test was negative. Sedimentation rates were 78 and 47 mm/hr. Australia antigen was negative; haptoglobin test was normal. CRP was normal. A 24 hour urine collection for protein ranged from 1.7 to 2.8 g throughout the admission. Creatinine clearance on admission was 6 ml/min/1.73 m^2. Cholesterol and triglycerides were normal. Chest X-ray was normal as well as the EKG. KUB showed no signs of obstruction and the kidneys were fully visualized. No calcifications were seen. Diagnosis on admission was acute glomerulonephritis. The patient was treated initially with bed rest, fluid restriction, 2 g sodium for 24 hours, 2.5 g potassium for 24 hours and 50 g protein for 24 hours. Five days after admission a percutaneous renal biopsy was done and showed crescentic glomerulonephritis associated with a microscopic form of polyarteritis nodosa. She was placed on steroids, 80 mg/day; however, since BUN continued to climb, prednisone was decreased to 60 mg/day. After two weeks of steroids, and due to the fact that the patient didn't respond as expected, cyclophosphamide and azathioprine, 50 mg of each, were added. In December, 1979, an A-V fistula was created on her right arm and she was started on hemodialysis. Currently she is scheduled for dialysis three times a week.

DR. PARDO: This case has little difficulty. You can see (Fig. 6) the artery with the fibrinoid changes in the wall and then the extensive inflammatory infiltrate with quite a large number of eosinophils. The arterioles in the vicinity appear to have a thickened media. In Figure 7, a higher magnification shows the transition between the normal wall and the necrotic band with the inflammatory infiltrate with marked predominance of eosinophils.

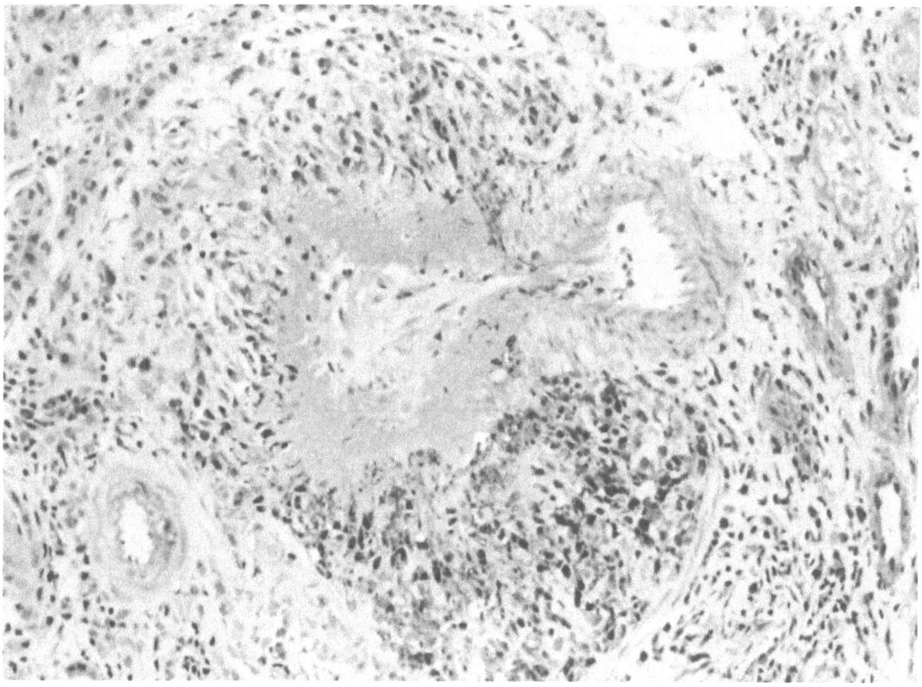

FIGURE 6

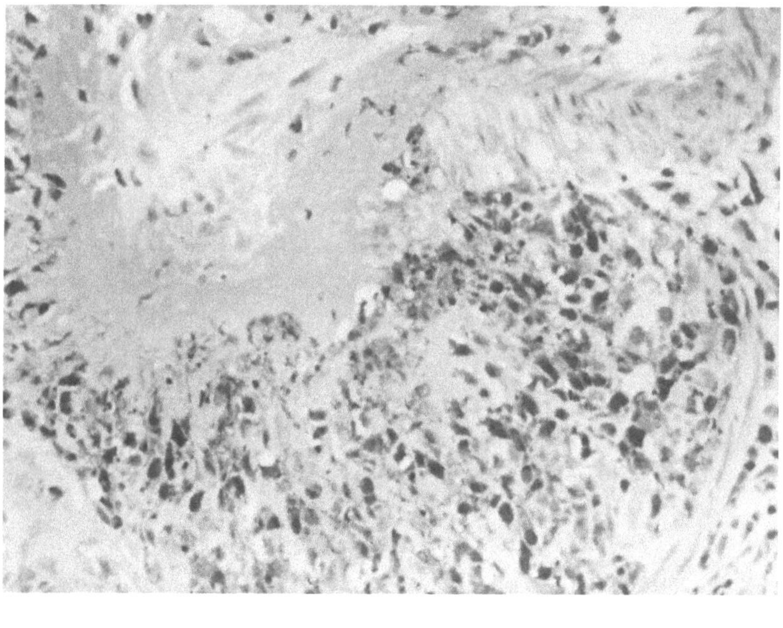

FIGURE 7

Figure 8 shows the thickening of the wall of the arterioles. I asked the clinicians about the possibility of hypertension and they told me she was only mildly hypertensive, but I was very impressed with the involvement of the non-arteritic vessels.

In Figure 9 are the glomeruli with the crescentic reaction with partial collapse of the loops. And here we see another crescent. There is really quite an extensive interstitial infiltrate, fibrosis and tubular atrophy.

By electron microscopy (Fig. 10), we found the classical deposits of fibrin. This is the lamina densa which appears to be normal in thickness. These are the proliferated epithelial cells. This is the fibrin with its fibrillar pattern, and here is a granular type of deposit.

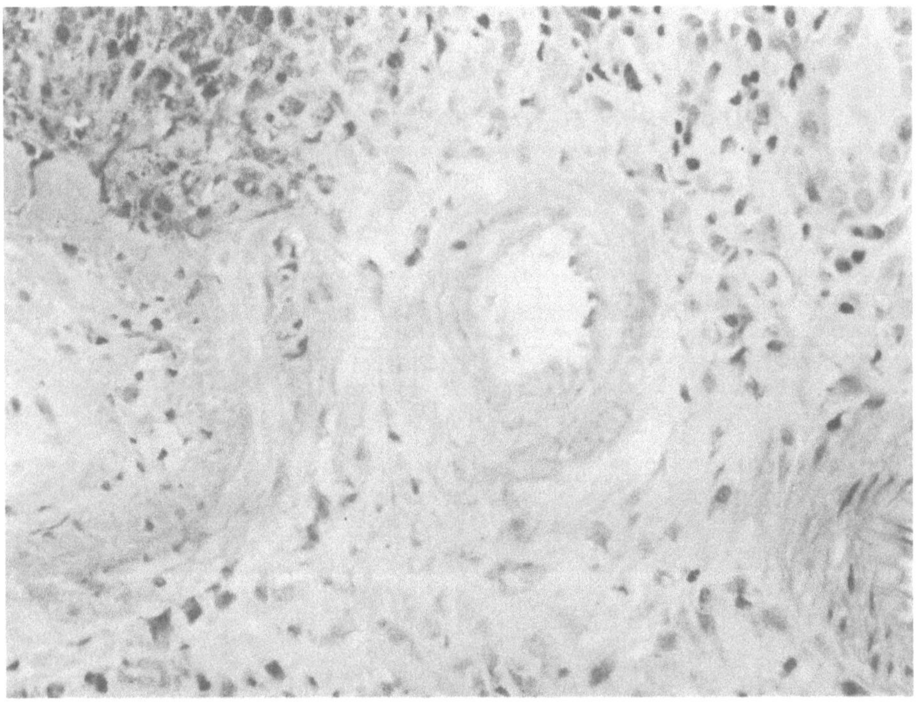

FIGURE 8

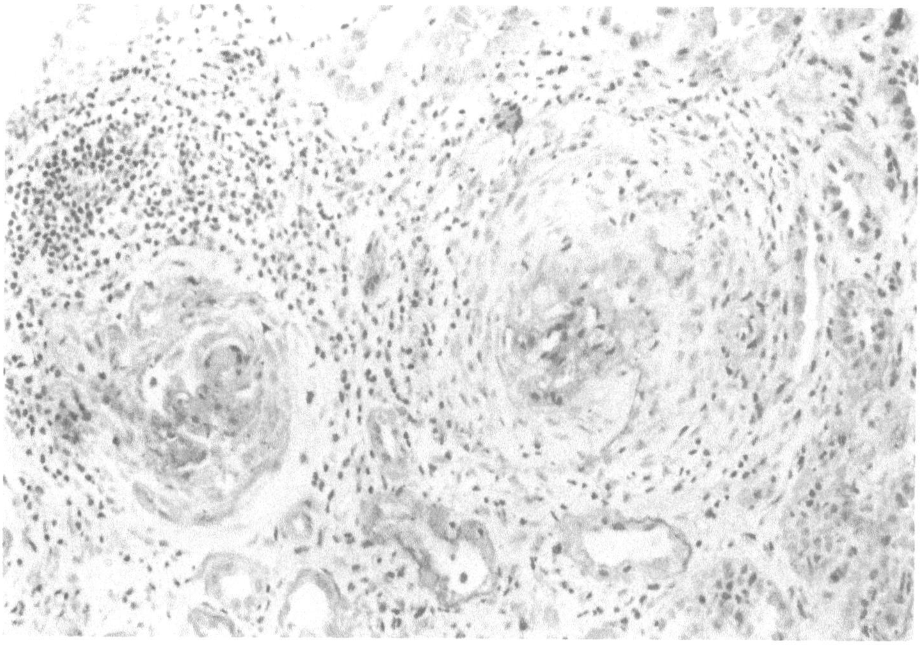

FIGURE 9

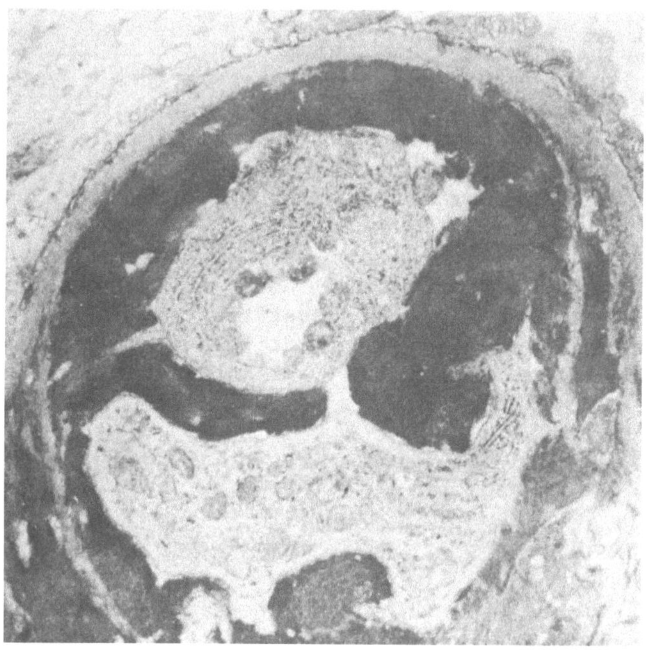

FIGURE 10

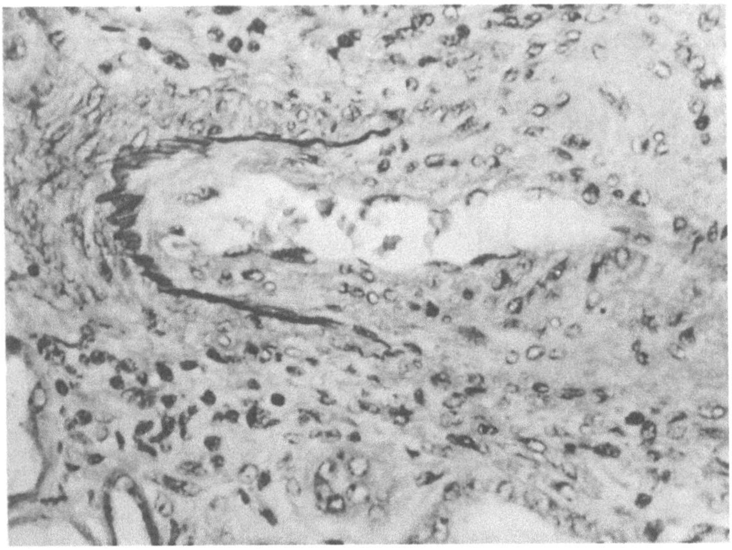

FIGURE 11

Figure 11 (nephrectomy specimen prior to transplantation) shows rupture of the elastica interna as the only remnant of the original lesion. Here is the denuded basement membrane.

There was something a little bit atypical in this case, at least in my limited experience with polyarteritis. It was that the glomeruli showed quite a number of deposits of IgG, also C_3 and some IgM. Other cases I have seen have negative immunofluorescence or just mild changes; in this case, they were strongly positive. I don't know what is the significance.

COMMENT: I am slightly surprised that the patient didn't show more response to treatment. I don't think I can find any doubts about the diagnosis. It's just that patients with polyarteritis who are started on treatment with serum creatinine at about 6 mg/dl, often do reasonably well at least in the short term. It's interesting that this patient didn't respond.

MODERATOR: Would you have started this patient on treatment?

RESPONSE: Yes.

QUESTION: Don't you think that the fact that she has a crescentic glomerulonephritis associated with almost 90% of glomeruli is really the decisive point? When you have a case of polyarteritis with a mild or limited glomerular lesion you may have a better response. This is really a full grown crescent.

RESPONSE: I think that you must be right. The biopsy you showed is, in fact, more representative than the serum creatinine. It's very interesting. We have a very large experience with microscopic polyarteritis and related diseases. You take patients, for example, with anti-GBM disease with crescentic nephritis, if the patient is anuric or oliguric or shows that kind of biopsy, he virtually never shows any improvement. Every now and then, there may be one patient. We have one patient out of 34 with anti-GBM disease who is anuric who has recovered. But, by contrast, this sort of patient can do remarkably well. For example, we had a patient recently with 19 out of 20 glomeruli completely surrounded by crescents, who was oliguric, with a serum creatinine of 1200--that's about 15 mg/dl, I suppose, whose creatinine came down to about two. I don't know why this is, but there does seem to be a distinction in a group of patients--the non anti-IgM patients--who do better. I am not sure why that is. Maybe it has something to do with there being less collapse of the glomerular tufts or something like that. Do you have access to the measurement of circulating immune complexes?

DR. PARDO: We have only anti-glomerular basement membrane immunofluorescence-an indirect method; we don't have any immune complex method.

COMMENT: It is unusual to see much in the way of deposits of immunoglobulins and C_3.

COMMENT: Once the methods are used, they are going to be found to be present in almost every renal disease.

COMMENT: In this type of case that has almost 90% glomeruli affected with crescents, that has such extensive vascular lesions, that if they are going to be cured, they are going to be obliterated, that already has lesions in other vascular beds, that has extensive interstitial fibrosis and tubular atrophy. What is the point of treating the renal disease?

RESPONSE: Well, the point is that some patients like this can, although it's a surprising histology, go back to a creatinine clearance of about 30 to 40 ml/min and may have 3 or 4 or 5 years before the scarring process takes over and they come to renal failure. That's the point. Of course, you've got to be sure you don't kill the patient with immunosuppressant drugs on the way.

MODERATOR: This patient was a very clear example of that problem. She came back with really massive pneumonia. The question came up, should we discontinue the so-called immunosuppression? We really have been worrying and wondering all along whether we were entitled to treating her at the risk of killing her. We felt that there was no clear evidence for or against but that the suggestions seemed to favor treatment. Therefore, we continued treatment because there were some systemic indicators of activity but the questions continued and we now favor tapering off medication.

COMMENT: It's our practice, except in people who got Wegener's Granulomatosis, of not giving cyclophosphamide for more than eight weeks even in patients of this kind. That's one of the ground rules. The other is that the dosage--this doesn't affect pediatric nephrologists, but it's very important in adult nephrology--if you give normal doses to people over the age of 55-of cyclophosphamide, say 3 mg/kg, and if you combine with azathioprine, say 1 mg/kg, you are going to invariably run into serious problems. So, there needs to be dose reduction at the other end. In most of these patients, if you regard cyclophosphamide of value, you should start it early on and if you don't need to continue for too long, you should be all right. The one exception is Wegener's where there is a clear example of not being able to control the disease with azathioprine.

MODERATOR: We administer 1 mg/kg of each one of the two drugs but we are aware of the limitations-the need to limit the period of time, as suggested by the London studies.

COMMENT: This is from the infectious point of view rather than from any other side effect.

QUESTION: I'm unfamiliar with the use of azathioprine and cyclophosphamide simultaneously. Could you make some comments on that?

MODERATOR: We touched on that this morning. Anybody want to summarize that?

COMMENT: I think it is empirical. It just happens in our unit in the treatment of anti-GBM disease. This regimen has been adopted and it seems to be curiously effective with plasma exchange in arresting all antibody synthesis. Then, there are groups around the world--I think one of the first groups to do this probably was people in Singapore--who claimed remarkable results with some histological backing. The argument is that giving cyclophosphamide and azathioprine together you produce a more profound immune suppression, if that is your aim. But, as you know, there are no data on this. It's entirely empirical.

MODERATOR: We shall continue then with case number three. Dr. Helen Gorman will present this case.

DR. GORMAN: The patient is a 4 yr old white girl who was well until March 1978, when she developed anuric acute renal failure, anemia, hypertension, seizures and coma. She was admitted to a Florida University Hospital. Blood smear showed fragmented and helmet-shaped red cells. BUN was 310 mg/dl, C_3 was low and C_4 normal. Peritoneal dialysis was performed. Later, a maculopapular erythematous rash and thrombotic microangiopathy of the left fifth distal digit developed. These gradually resolved.

Three weeks later, renal function began to improve; hematuria and proteinuria were present. The first renal biopsy was obtained and was reported to be consistent with the recovery phase of hemolytic uremic syndrome. Fifty percent of glomeruli were hyalinized. Mesangial deposits of IgM and C_3 were present in a granular pattern.

BUN and creatinine fell to normal, C_3 remained low and the child was well until February 1979 when she was admitted to a hospital in Jacksonville with nephritic - nephrotic syndrome and BUN 45 mg/dl. A second renal biopsy was consistent with membranoproliferative glomerulonephritis type I. Granular deposition of IgM, C_3 and fibrin was observed in the mesangium.

In April 1979, creatinine was 2.2 mg/dl and BUN 59 mg/dl. She was hypertensive and remained edematous. Hematuria and proteinuria continued. She developed diarrhea and vomiting and was admitted to Jackson Memorial Hospital in Miami on April 18, 1979. BUN was 66 mg/dl, creatinine 3.8 mg/dl, C_3 was low and C_4 normal. ESR was 42 mm/hour. Hb was 5.9 g %. She was severely hypertensive and very lethargic. On April 28, a nodular purpuric rash appeared on her limbs. Biopsy of a lesion showed leukocytoclastic vasculitis. Peritoneal dialysis was instituted. By April 29, BUN had risen to 102 and creatinine to 11 mg/dl. Hemodialysis was begun. The rash resolved, and the main management problems were severe hypertension and repeated clotting of her external shunt. On May 10, a third renal biopsy was obtained. The findings were consistent with hemolytic-uremic syndrome; there were mesangial deposits of C_3. After less than a week at home, she was readmitted on May 28, 1979 because of recurrence of nodular purpura on the left arm and shoulder. A skin biopsy was studied by direct immunofluorescence. IgM and C_3 were found in a broad band pattern. C_3 was 37 and C_4 was 24 mg/dl. Coombs, ANA and HBsAg were negative. IgG 1234, A 247 and M 190 mg/dl. Viral cultures were negative. Platelets were normal. Treatment with prednisone, azathioprine and cyclophosphamide, 1 mg/kg/day of each, was begun on June 7, 1979. By June 22, C_3 had risen to 67 mg/dl, and ESR was 20 mm/hour. Pre-dialysis serum creatinine had fallen to 1.3 mg/dl by July 10. During subsequent weeks, however, creatinine gradually rose to a level of about 4.0 mg/dl.

On August 13, bilateral nephrectomy and splenectomy were performed, and hypertension resolved. On September 10, 1979, C_3 was 85 mg/dl. Treatment with prednisone, azathioprine and cyclophosphamide was continued until the patient received a renal transplant donated by her mother on October 3. Immunosuppressive therapy was then changed to methylprednisolone and azathioprine in dosage appropriate for management of transplant recipients. Since then, there has been no recurrence of her rash or of proteinuria, and renal function is normal. No rejection episodes have occurred.

DR. PARDO: These two biopsies were sent to us from an outside hospital. The two light microscopy slides are quite similar, so both biopsies are going to be shown as a single slide of light microscopy (Fig. 12). The number of glomeruli were quite limited. There were only about two or three glomeruli. The slides are a bit pale. If you look at this glomerulus here you can see some areas with "double contour". You can see also that there is a mesangiocapillary component. It is a very early one. I don't think it is very prominent. The mesangium is widened. You have to look carefully to pick out the areas of "splitting" of the basement membrane.

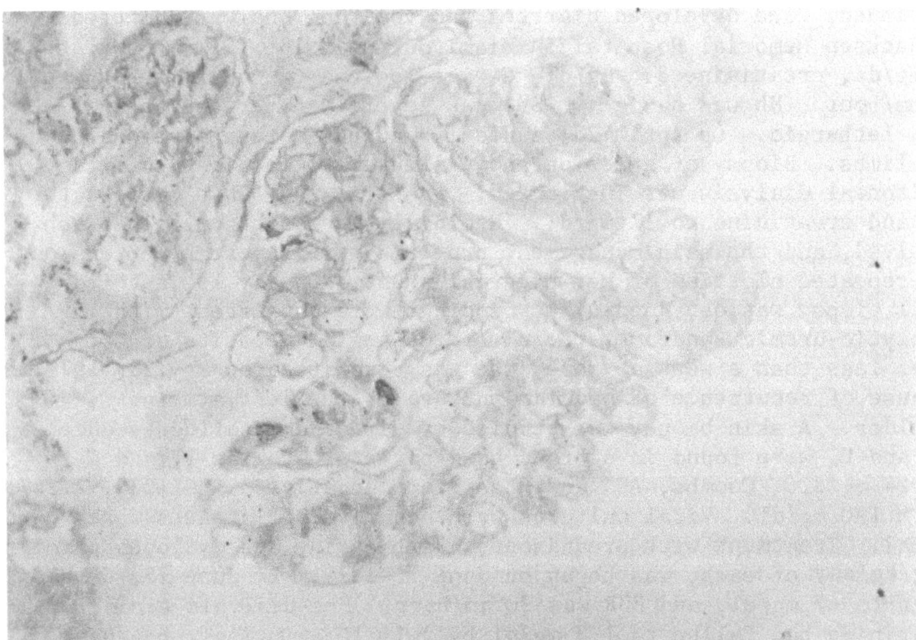

FIGURE 12

Figure 13 is a peripheral blood smear showing the schistocytes. There was positive immunofluorescence for IgM and complement C_3 (Fig. 14). I interpreted this as being predominantly of mesangial distribution. This type of deposits I believe in general are non-specific. They may be deposits of plasma proteins and not due to immunological mechanisms.

Figure 15 is EM. At this magnification, the most we can see is that there is a subendothelial deposit going along the inner portion of the lamina densa. This dense deposit shows some fibrils in it. The deposits are in the inner aspect of the lamina densa. There was another EM picture which showed increase in mesangial cells and matrix.

Figure 16 is a more advanced lesion in which we can see that the mesangium is growing inside the capillary loop. This is typical for the late stages of the fibrin deposit being partially re-absorbed or depolymerized. You can see the lumen of the capillary, the endothelium, the lamina densa, and the epithelium on the side. You can see the type of material which is characteristic of the late stages of fibrin deposition. We know also that secondary to this fibrin deposition, you may have a mesangiocapillary reaction and the lesion may be very similar to mesangiocapillary type I or membranoproliferative GN type I. I think the thing that helps here is the appearance of the deposits. That means it's just a late stage of the hemolytic uremic syndrome or any other process associated with intravascular coagulation and deposits of fibrin in the capillary wall of the glomeruli.

Figure 17 is our biopsy of April, 1979. The lesion, I believe, has advanced a little bit. There is quite an amount of mesangial sclerosis. Once in a while one can see some capillaries opened. One can see some lumina in the peripheral portion of the capillaries which is suggestive also of mesangiocapillary extension. And there are a few granulocytes here and there. So, there is an exudative component here also.

There were some arteriolar lesions (Fig. 18). You can see this arteriole, very similar to the one I showed you in the previous case. I don't think it is obliterated but at the least the lumen is so small that any tangential section produces a lumenless vessel. We have here an old vessel which shows lesions which may be hyaline changes. There is arteriolar nephrosclerosis. These tubules here show some wrinkling of the basement membrane, suggestive of early stages of atrophy.

Figure 19 is a skin biopsy that shows the leukocytoclastic angiitis. I believe here we have the dermis, the vessel coming here, bifurcating probably. You can see an area of fibrinoid necrosis, and the extensive deposition of granulocytes.

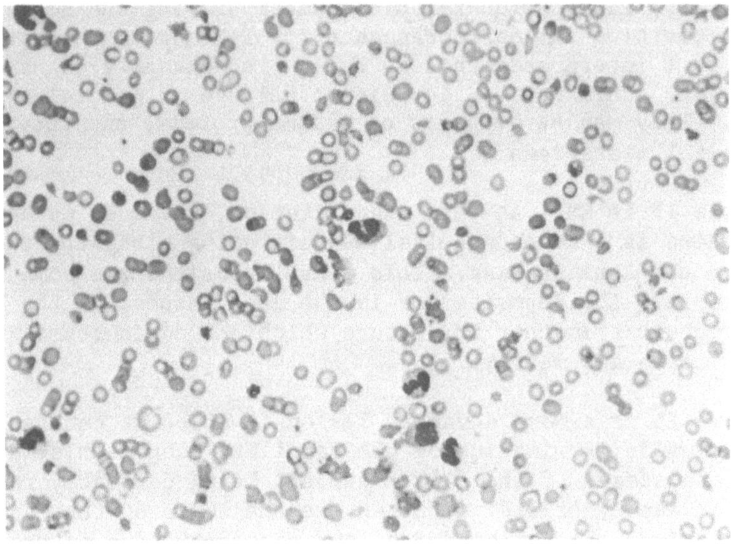

FIGURE 13

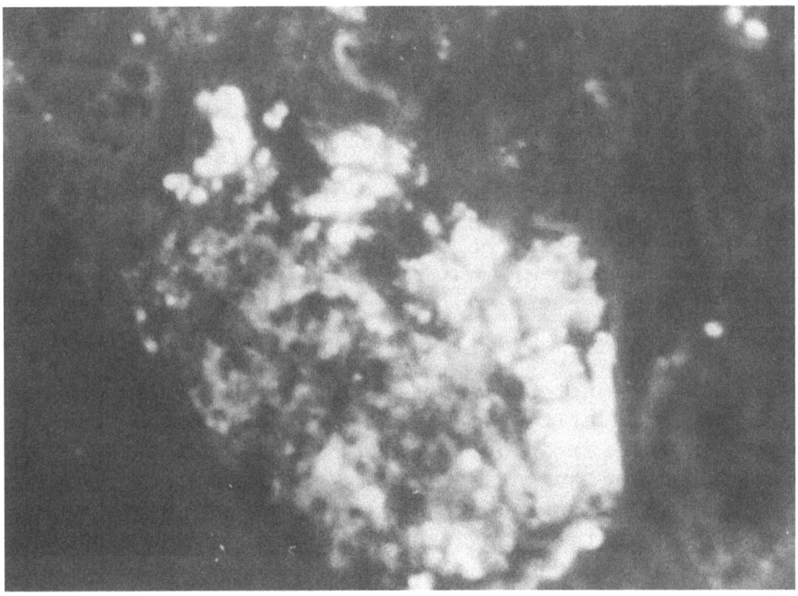

FIGURE 14

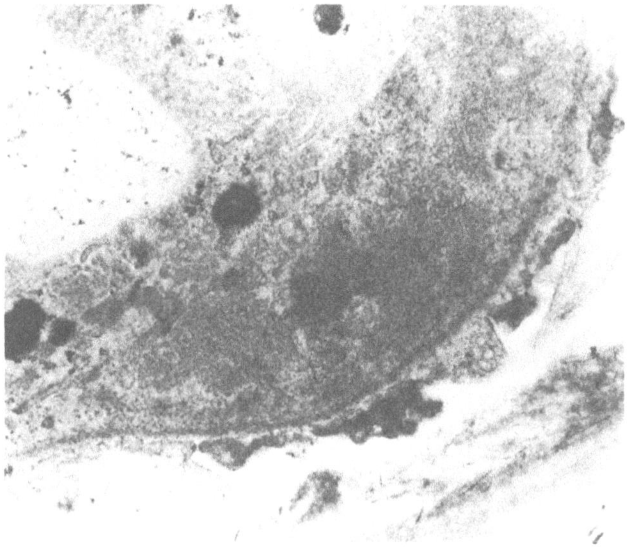

FIGURE 15

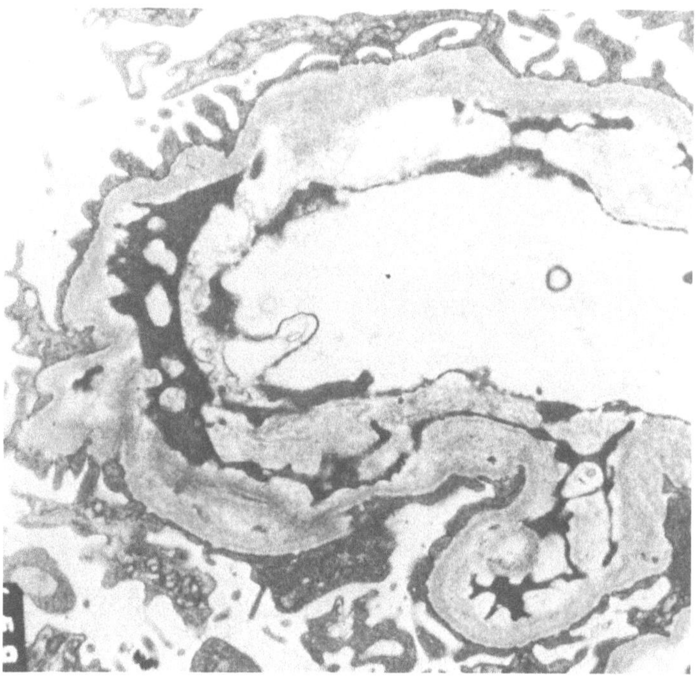

FIGURE 16

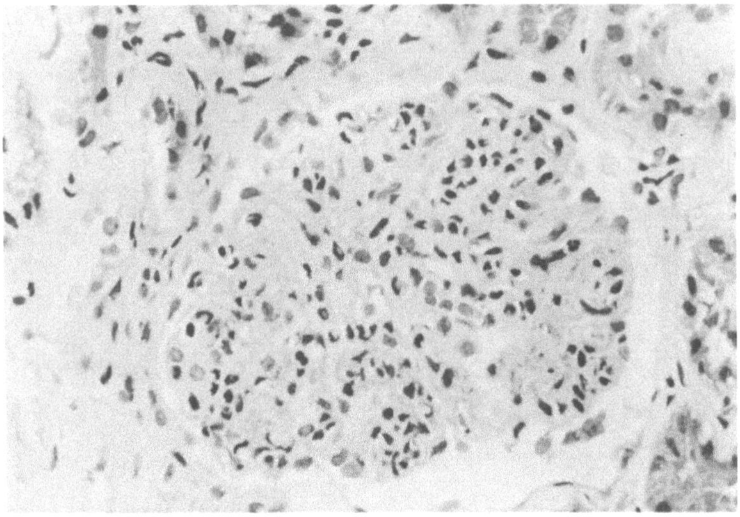

FIGURE 17

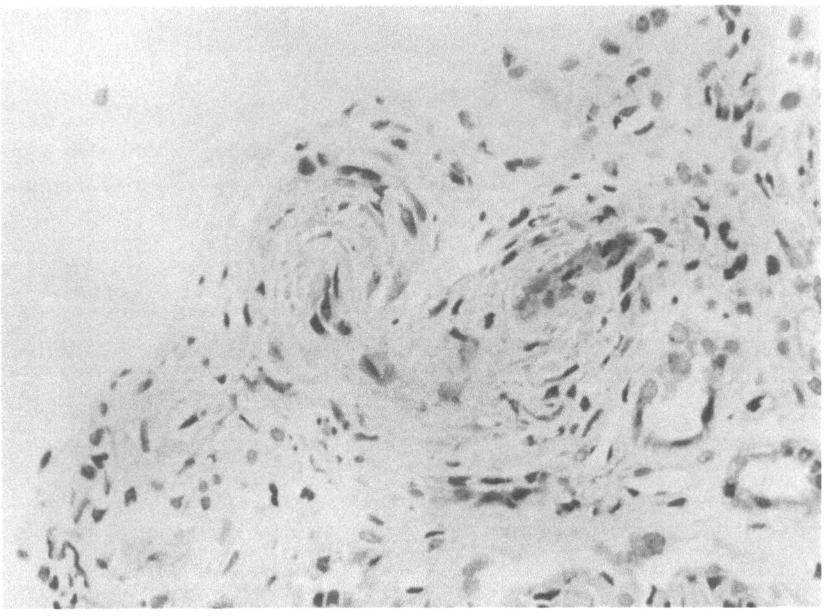

FIGURE 18

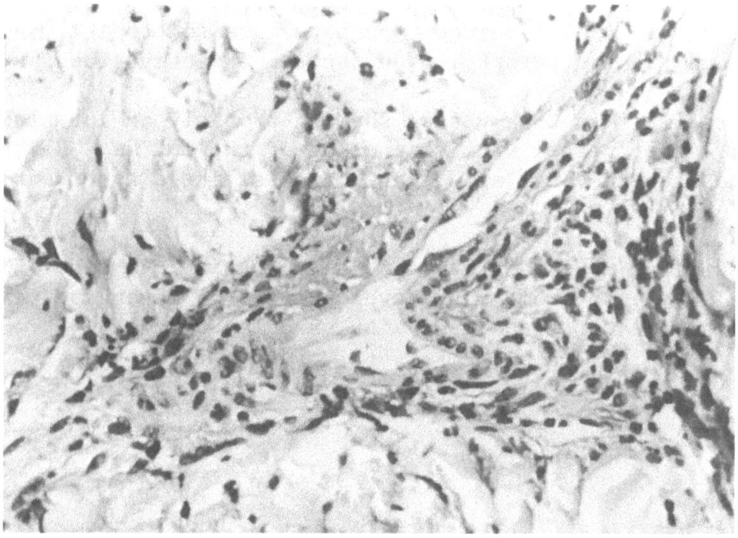

FIGURE 19

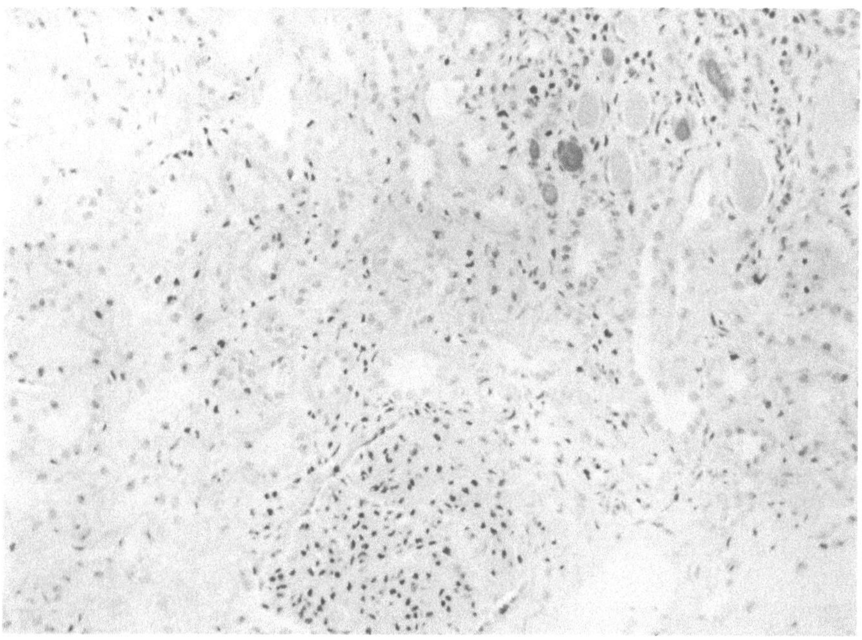

FIGURE 20

Figure 20 is the nephrectomy specimen; it shows essentially the same type of glomerular changes, perhaps more sclerosis , interstitial fibrosis and tubular atrophy. You can see extensive tubular atrophy.

Figure 21 is another vessel showing probably an interlobular vessel, a larger vessel with thickening of the intima. So, the patient has severe vascular disease. Looks like a hypertensive type.

In summary, my interpretation is that this is a case of the hemolytic uremic syndrome with development of a mesangiocapillary type of lesion later associated with vascular changes.

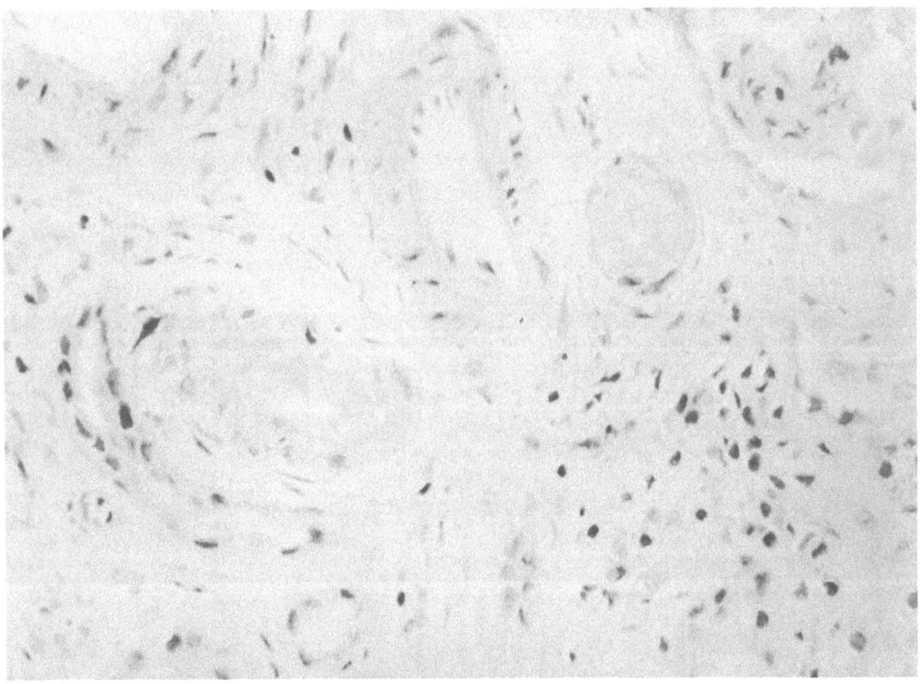

FIGURE 21

MODERATOR: Thank you Dr. Gorman and Dr. Pardo. Any comments? Questions? Diagnostic disagreements? Treatment disagreements?

COMMENT: Somebody said this morning that he thought that some plasma might be beneficial in this entity as in TTP. I wonder if there is any experience with that approach.

MODERATOR: He did mention that during the panel discussion. Anybody want to comment on that?

QUESTION: Not on that question. I would like to know why did you give immunosuppressive therapy to this child. Also, did you check the C_3 level in the family members?

MODERATOR: Who would like to answer that question? It was a combined decision between the Transplantation and Pediatric Nephrology Services.

RESPONSE: In terms of transplantation, this disease has also had a recurrence rate, again unpredictable but there have been a number of different case reports, sometimes very early, sometimes later. It's my philosophy in these patients and in the previous patient that was presented, when there is a humoral component that is suspected most of the time, but can't be clearly demonstrated, we ought to apply immunosuppression and wait as long as possible before transplantation because I think this is the hardest type of disease entity to prevent recurrence or prevent some type of aberrant immune response in the transplant. So, it was our decision to start on immunosuppression even before we took the kidneys out in preparation for a subsequent transplant. Since we had evidence of immune activity by the low complement levels, at least the C_3 level that was done, we felt that we could measure something objectively before we did the transplant and see if we got an improvement. We started the patient on drugs that we thought would be helpful in preventing or affecting humoral immunity such as cyclophosphamide because we are very limited at the present time. Our armamentarium after transplantation primarily affects T-cells and we do a lot of monitoring in the post-transplant period. When humoral immunity is present after a transplant, as we said before, you are really sunk; either in the short or long haul, that kidney is going to be lost. So we do our best to try and treat humoral immunity first. It's interesting that the T-cell has to have a component in most cases of humoral immunity as well. And helper cells are very important in amplifying a humoral immune response. When you start a patient on an immunosuppressive regimen, you are affecting both suppressor cells and helper cells. The question is: how much are you really going to affect the humoral immune component? I really think it's a subjective type of decision but because there was the potential for recurrence of this particular disease, we started on immunosuppression. We did do bilateral nephrectomy and just as in Goodpasture's, we would wait until we had actually objective evidence and long afterwards of defervescence of the process by the lack of glomerular basement membrane antibody directed against the kidney. After nephrectomy, we wait six months longer than that even before we do a transplant. Here we really were forced because of the smallness of the child in that we felt long term dialysis and also the problem of transportation from where she lived was not going to be very effective. We waited two months with immunosuppression raising the C_3 level, and then did the transplant. Of course it remains to be seen whether it's going to work or not.

MODERATOR: The C_3 did normalize and the erythrosedimentation rate which was elevated also came down.

QUESTION: In a child who has a hypocomplemententemic type of glomerulonephritis, would you routinely measure the complement in the potential living related donor? Do you think this would be worthwhile? If the mother were hypocomplemententemic but asymptomatic, what kind of difference would that make?

RESPONSE: Well, I don't know. I think it's an interesting thing to do. Maybe there is a susceptibility and it may even have to do with an inheritance pattern with HLA, not only with the complement level. Maybe we ought to be doing a study like that. Certainly, if there are low complement levels in the recipient, this has been shown not only with this type of hemolytic uremic syndrome but in other types of glomerulonephritis such as rapidly progressive hypocomplementemic glomerulonephritis. In those patients we would like to see evidence of normalization.

MODERATOR: We did not do complements in the family, right?

RESPONSE: No, we did not.

QUESTION: On what basis were you working? Which kind of disease were you talking about because for me it was not so obvious.

RESPONSE: I don't really know too much about renal disease. Again, the morphological entity and how it behaves clinically might not really have much to do with what the etiology of the disease is. All that I could say was that there appeared to be an immune component that perhaps might be modified by immunosuppressors in the very elementary immunosuppressive regimen that we have.

COMMENT: I asked because apparently the treatment of the disease was based only on a low level of complement but if we go to the biopsy, the immunopathology, these findings were not consistent with a membranoproliferative glomerulonephritis.

There were some deposits in the mesangium but the characteristic deposits in the loops, you don't see. I don't think we can make this diagnosis.

MODERATOR: Which diagnosis are you questioning or proposing?

RESPONSE: I'm questioning the diagnosis of membranoproliferative glomerulonephritis.

MODERATOR: Would you accept the hemolytic uremic syndrome?

RESPONSE: I would accept the renal microangiopathy and if we accept this diagnosis, I don't think there is any basis to give this kind of treatment.

COMMENT: To me, hypocomplementemia is usually associated with a humoral immune response. We had systemic manifestations of the disease that are also probably associated with a humoral immune component. That was my only reason.

COMMENT: The low level of C_3 has been described, too, in the hemolytic syndrome. Usually, it is a transient decrease; sometimes it could last for weeks. Another point, I am not aware of any effect of immunosuppressive treatment in hemolytic syndrome. On the contrary, there were some cases of hemolytic syndrome occurring during immunosuppressive treatment. So, I continue not to be satisfied with that answer.

COMMENT: I would like to clarify something that I'm sure most of you have already in your minds. I have limited experience with mesangiocapillary glomerulonephritis, the so-called membranoproliferative glomerulonephritis. But morphologically, by EM, we have thickening of the basement membrane and increase in nuclei. With EM we know that's a peripheral extension of the mesangium. It's a morphological diagnosis. So we can have mesangiocapillary glomerulonephritis that corresponds to the hypocomplementemic variety of membranoproliferative glomerulonephritis type I; we can have a membranoproliferative type II; we can have hemolytic uremic syndrome; we can have sickle cell anemia; we can have a lot of entities which may produce similar morphological changes. But, when you clinicians are talking of membranoproliferative, I think in general, you are talking about this one. So we have to dissect the morphological criteria. I think this case you can call mesangiocapillary because morphologically it is a mesangiocapillary glomerulonephritis.

COMMENT: I agree very much with what has just been said. We've got a morphology and we need more impact from the information before we can make specific assignments. I must say, I join forces with other members of the panel in being concerned about treating this patient the way she was with immunosuppressive drugs. There is no doubt, it seems to me, she is a rather unusual patient with some curious systemic features. You may well be right but I don't think you are right for the reason you put forward. I think to treat hypocomplementemia as some general indication of a disturbance in humoral immunity could be debatable and lead to the most terrible trouble. I can show you populations of patients with lipodystrophy who have C_3 levels about 5% of normal who are absolutely healthy except for the fat problem. I do hope they don't get into your hands if you are going to fill them up with cyclophosphamide.

I think that in this day and age, you need to be able to say something more than "the complement is low". Because we don't understand the process in the kidney, it doesn't have to be due to the humoral arm of immunity. I think that when methods which could seriously affect the patient's life are to be adopted, you do it either because you have an empirical basis, mainly it's been done before and it works but we don't understand why, or because you've got some rational approach based upon hard data. One or the other is OK but I don't think somewhere in between is acceptable.

RESPONSE: I guess I am used to working with witchcraft and we do quite a few assays. I think that the assays for immune complexes are in their infancy. Some of the things that are now being thought to be immune complexes probably are not immune complexes. But, I think that in this individual patient we were very justified. In some of the other patients that we see, in whom we have a suspicion of humoral immunity occurring, we are probably justified. Certainly hypocomplementemia can be due to either a comsumption problem or a production problem. I would agree that if somebody has an inherited hypocomplementemic abnormality due to an HLA link or DR link, in general the problem is an immune deficiency in itself which you would not treat with immunosuppression. On the other hand, we do know that many of the entities that were called glomerulonephritis in the past that were associated with just the elementary disturbance of low C_3, have had their recurrences in transplants. Also, we had a four year old patient here who for all intents and purposes is only a transplant candidate. So what is the best way to treat this patient? I simply don't know the best way to treat this patient but I would tend to err more on the side of more immunosuppression than less immunosuppression. One of the things that we do here which I think is very helpful in our post-transplant period, and we did her actually pre-transplant as well, is follow the T-cell quantitation weekly in the post-transplant period for several months actually. We've found that this is an extremely sensitive index of the degree of immunosuppression. Because T-cells are the most sensitive in terms of being able to affect with immunosuppression, that doesn't mean that the graft isn't going to be rejected. But it does help tell us when we are giving too much immunosuppression. So this is what we did and I would do it again. I'm not sure that we are treating this patient correctly now. I think that if I could follow her a little more closely, I'd probably put her on cyclophosphamide as well as azathioprine and use triple therapy although cyclophosphamide would be a little bit lower.

COMMENT: Well, it seems to me that there is an approach which is somewhat more rational. If you believe that humoral factors are predominately responsible for a particular renal or vasculitic disease, then the technique that makes most sense to me is to carry out plasma exchange and see if there is a response to it. If there is no response to it, then the hypothesis that you have put up is not supported. If there is a response, it is supported-not proven, but supported. You may well be right that immunosuppression was the right treatment for this patient. What I am quarreling with you about is the argument you used to support it. The recurrent disease that has occurred in membranoproliferative glomerulonephritis certainly can't be attributed to hypocomplementemia directly. The fact is that in the hypocomplementemic nephritis, C_3 levels give no guide as to what happens in the kidney. If treatment works, then it works, If that's what you believe, that's fine but you cannot blame complement for it. On the question of monitoring by measuring T-cells, OK. If you say this is a good way of adjusting the dose of steroids, cyclophosphamide, azathioprine, or whatever happens to be your favorite poison, that's alright. That is really gauging the dosimetry of a drug after the transplant takes place. I don't see that as an argument for or against. I am neutral in respect to whether or not the drug might be of value at a time when there is a leucocytoclastic vasculitis of unknown etiology or a low C_3 brought about by the enzymic activation of complement. That has nothing to do with it. If you said, "I believe this; I don't have any evidence but I've done it before and it seems to work", I'd say "OK, fine, that's what doctors are entitled to believe". But that is not the pursuit of science.

COMMENT: I would go further and call it witchcraft. I'm afraid that I must have been misinterpreted because I'm telling you a rationale that I used but I don't think that we have any objective evidence. I hope that the audience did not understand me to say that we had objective evidence of an immune problem other than some peripheral evidence. Also, that this patient is an entity in itself. In similar patients, in patients where we are dealing with either transplant and live or dialysis and perhaps extension of a long or more chronic interval before death, I think that is essentially what we have in most patients of this age and size. I would err on the side of more immunosuppression than less, especially when we have some evidence for a systemic immunologic process and I think we do although we don't have objective, iron clad evidence. I think that most pathologists and individuals involved in these diseases would say that this patient had evidence of some type of immunodeviant state, although we couldn't characterize it, that was giving her systemic manifestations and kidney problems.

QUESTION: In cases of rapidly progressing glomerulonephritis when you have immune complex demonstrated, do you treat the patient with plasmapheresis alone, and you don't have to treat them with immunosuppressant therapy?

RESPONSE: The question is: would you use plasma exchange alone without drugs in treatment of rapidly progressive glomerulonephritis due to immune complexes? The answer is no. We have used plasmapheresis alone in the treatment of peripheral vasculitis where there is no life-threatening condition with some very striking short term results. But in patients with rapidly progressive glomerulonephritis it doesn't make any difference whether you detect any immune complexes in the circulation or not so far as we can discern in respect to plasma exchange. In that sense, I am with what my colleague said earlier. We are at a stage of early development of these assays and it would be wrong if we put too much weight upon them except when they are positive and they do go away with the treatment. Then you can use that as evidence for yourself as you are disposed.

MODERATOR: Shall we go to the next case? Dr. John Richardson has been kind enough to come and present this case.

DR. RICHARDSON: This case is an 8 year old boy admitted to Variety Children's Hospital, Miami, Florida, on November 11, 1979, with history of intermittent, mild abdominal pain for two months. One month before the admission, the family physician found anemia and started oral iron preparation. After failure to improve, he was referred to the pediatrician who arranged for hospitalization. Examination was normal except for pallor.

Urinalysis showed 1-2+ protein, 25-30 WBC and 80-100 RBC/hpf. WBC was 6500 with normal differential. Hemoglobin was 6.8 g/dl, hematocrit 22%, platelets 321,000/mm^3, BUN 19 mg/dl, creatinine 0.6 mg/dl, uric acid 4 mg/dl; total serum protein 6.2 g%, albumin 4.1 g %. Direct and indirect Coombs tests and ASO titer were negative. Total iron binding capacity was 228 and serum iron 25 mcg/dl. Bone marrow changes were consistent with iron deficiency. ANA titer and serum C_3 and C_4 complements were normal.

Chest x-ray films showed borderline cardiomegaly and dense infiltrate in the right middle and lower lung fields and left mid-lung field. Several small nodular densities were seen at the left apex. An infectious etiology was thought most likely. Upper G.I., barium enema and IV pyelogram films were normal.

Several small blood transfusions were given. Secretions from the pharynx showed large number of iron-laden macrophages. Nephrology consultation was requested on November 15, 1979. The urine sediment was loaded with RBC's and casts. Many casts were composed of RBC. A needle biopsy of the kidney was carried out two days later.

DR. PARDO: In Figure 22, you can see in this portion of the biopsy section, that there is a crescent here with the collapsed capillaries in the center. This is a PAS stain. This glomerulus is preserved; it may show some mesangial hyperplasia but no crescents. You look at the parenchyma and there is no inflammatory infiltrate. It's a pure crescentic lesion. Usually one sees more inflammatory infiltrate, plasma cells, and reaction of the parenchyma between the glomeruli.

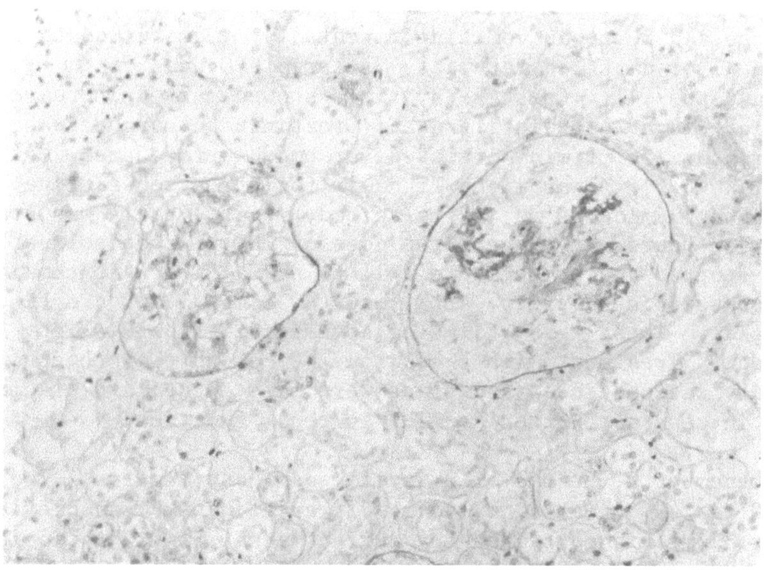

FIGURE 22

Figure 23 shows a great variation in the number of affected glomeruli from section to section. There were about 50% of glomeruli showing crescents.

By electronmicroscopy (Fig. 24), there is increase in intracapillary and epithelial cells. The only thing that is important here is the lamina densa; you can see that it is thinned out in one area, and almost lost in another. This is quite frequent in cases of rapidly progressive glomerulonephritis or crescentic glomerulonephritis of any etiology, seen frequently in lupus and other types of diseases. There seems to be a destruction of the lamina densa. There are no electron dense deposits.

By immunofluorescence (Fig. 25), there were linear deposits of IgG that are demonstrated here. We took the serum of the patient and we obtained a positive reaction incubating the serum with the target kidney and then using antihuman IgG fluorescein conjugated to demonstrate the localization of the antibody (Fig. 26). The patient's serum reacted at up to a dilution of 1 to 5,000. In summary, we thought it was a case of crescentic glomerulonephritis with anti-glomerular basement membrane disease.

DR. RICHARDSON: We felt sure that this was a Goodpasture syndrome.

The child felt well until November 18, 1979 when he developed spiking fever and nonproductive cough. Ampicillin was given. Temperature elevation increased daily until November 21, when it reached 103 degrees and he began vomiting repeatedly. Vomitus contained a great deal of dark red material. Arterial PO_2 was 55 mm Hg, PCO_2 30 Torr and pH 7.41. Chest x-ray films showed marked increase of the right lower lobe infiltrate. Creatinine clearance was 65.8 ml/min or 126 ml/min corrected for body surface area. Methylprednisolone 0.5 g was given IV daily for three consecutive days and cyclophosphamide 50 mg (2 mg/kg body weight) daily was started. Within a few hours after the first dose of methylprednisolone, vomiting stopped and temperature fell to normal where it remained. Cough decreased in severity. BUN rose to 32 mg/dl and creatinine to 1.3 mg/dl. Chest x-ray films on November 25 showed slight improvement. Treatment with prednisone 40 mg and cyclophosphamide 50 mg daily was continued and plans were made to utilize plasmapheresis in case of further decline in renal function.

On December 1, he had mild facial edema and ascites. Two days later BUN was 49, creatinine 1.5 mg/dl, creatinine clearance 16.6 ml/min or 32 ml/min corrected for surface area. Implantation of arterial and venous cannulas was scheduled for the next day with plasmapheresis to follow, but early December 4, hemoptysis recurred, respirations increased to 32/min, and he developed fine rales bilaterally. He was transfused, given oxygen by mask and transferred to ICU.

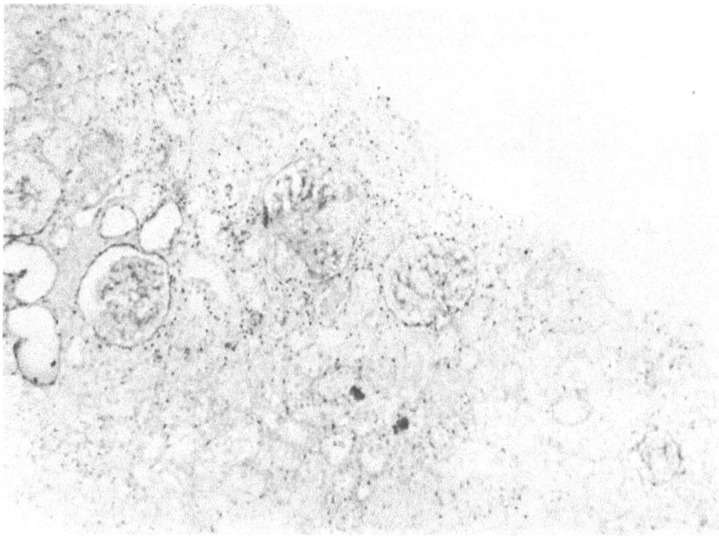

FIGURE 23

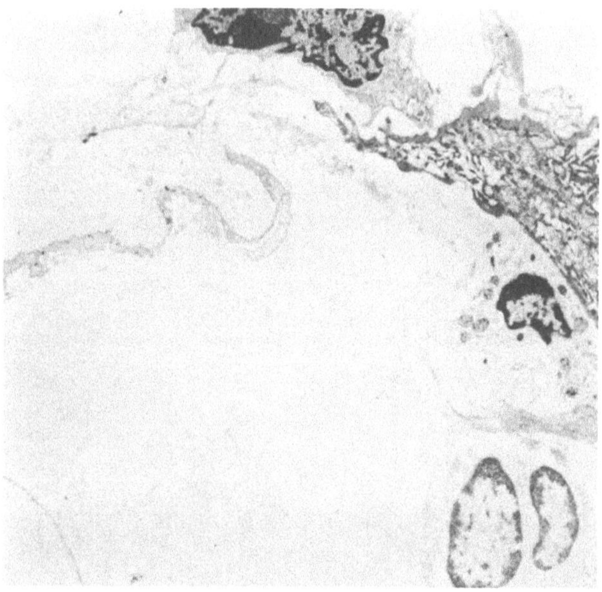

FIGURE 24

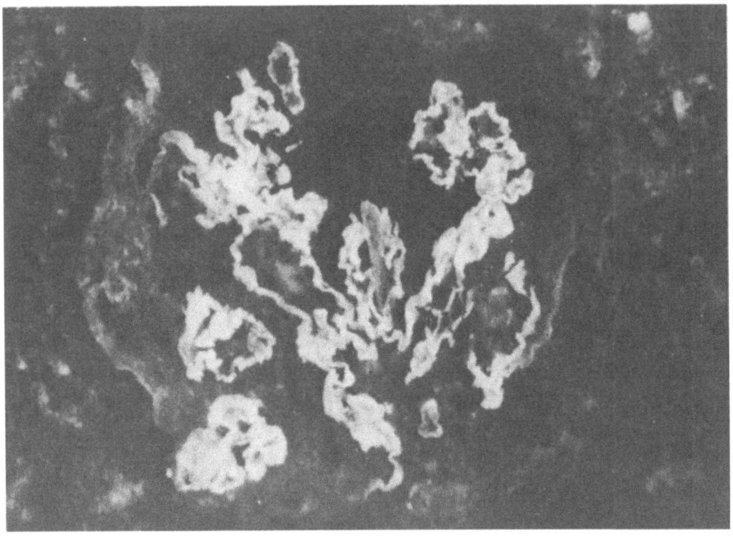

FIGURE 25

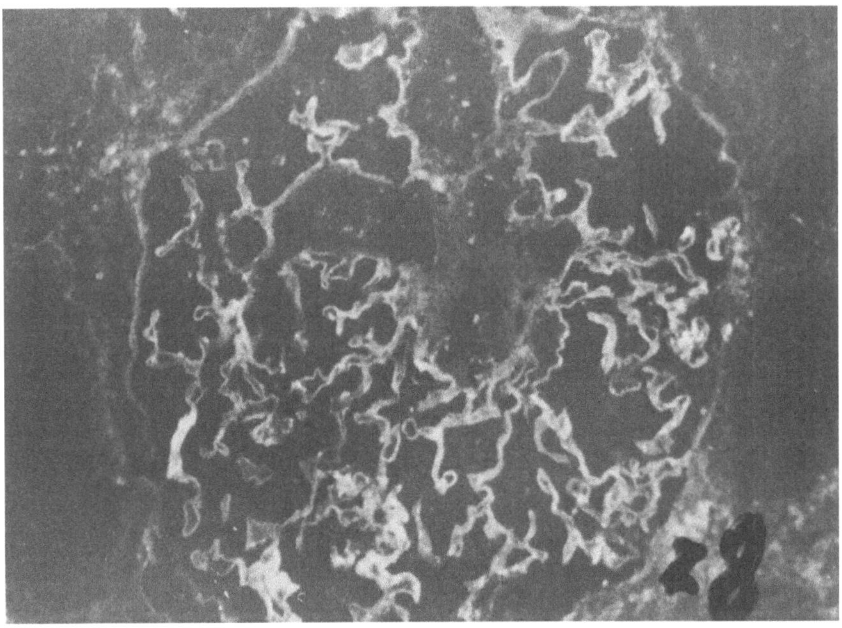

FIGURE 26

PaO_2 was 46 mm Hg. He was given furosemide, methylprednisolone 0.5 g IV and IPPB. Endotrachial intubation was required and PEEP was given. However, pulmonary hemorrhage became massive and he died that evening.

One unusual feature of this case is the young age. Few of this age have been reported.

DR. PARDO. I am going to show now the autopsy material. Figure 27 is the kidney. It was normal in size for this child. The only gross finding is the multiple petechiae. This is the so-called flea bitten kidney, classically described as glomerular hemorrhages. But I wonder if in most instances they are really glomerular hemorrhages or tubular hemorrhages that are seen at the surface. Some of them may be congested stellate veins. So I think that the classical criterion that these petechiae are hemorrhagic glomeruli is questionable.

This is the light microscopy (Fig. 28). Ninety percent of the glomeruli showed crescents. There is extensive tubular hemorrhage.

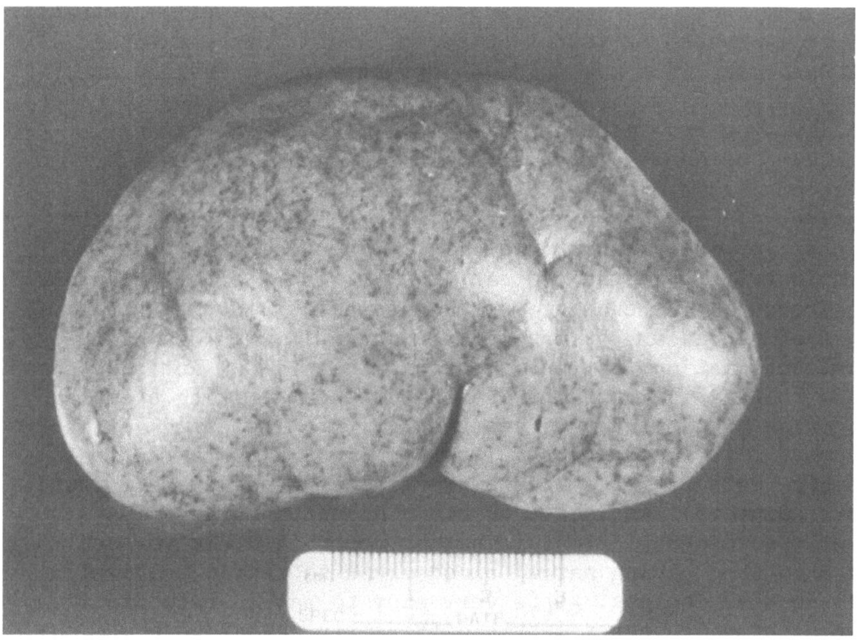

FIGURE 27

Figure 29 is the lung with the massive hemorrhage. I don't have the reticulum stain here, but when you do reticulum stain you can see that some of these areas do not show any alveolar septa. It looks almost like a pulmonary infarction. Massive destruction. When I tried to do electronmicroscopy of many of these areas, I couldn't do much because there was a total destruction of the wall. So, it's going to be a very difficult problem to get an area that shows initial changes by EM.

We also did a second serum determination from the patient ten days after he was first treated. The level was the same: 1 to 5,000.

MODERATOR: I imagine most panelists will have comments. This is presented as an unusual case in pediatric nephrology but your comments on plasmapheresis and related subjects will be appreciated.

COMMENT: The number of children with anti-GBM disease is rapidly increasing. That is known. There have been at least two in England in the past 18 months. One died recently, last summer. And there have been several in France as well. Perhaps with more awareness it is not quite as rare. This patient is very interesting in a number of points that we've learned the hard way as you have. Perhaps I can just take a few of them. Clinically, you have made the diagnosis of anti-GBM disease. The features of anemia, nephritis, and the absence of any evidence of a systemic disorder other than anemia is very suggestive. If you do quite simple things like looking at the protein strip, measuring the total proteins you find that the albumin is 4.1, the total protein is 6.2. There's no hyperglobulinemia. There's an absence of systemic disease which means that in nine out of ten cases you can make a diagnosis with ordinary clinical information, without resorting to anti-GBM antibody assay. The next thing it illustrates is that it is a striking example of infection precipitating disease activity. The child got sick on November 11th and developed fever. I would guarantee that that is the set-off for anti-GBM disease, as it did here. Then, the next point to make is the way this disease can go from apparently quiescence into fulminating nephritis. We've seen patients go from having normal blood ureas to anuria in five days-in no time in fact. It's very easy to say in retrospect that we might do things a little differently. What we would do if this patient had come to us is, back in November, we would presumably have confirmed the high titer of anti-GBM antibodies. The chest x-rays, by the way, are almost certain to give you just pulmonary hemorrhage. You get this low pattern, quite extraordinary. Typical lower pneumonia just due to pulmonary hemorrhage. What we would have done at that stage, on the basis of the evidence

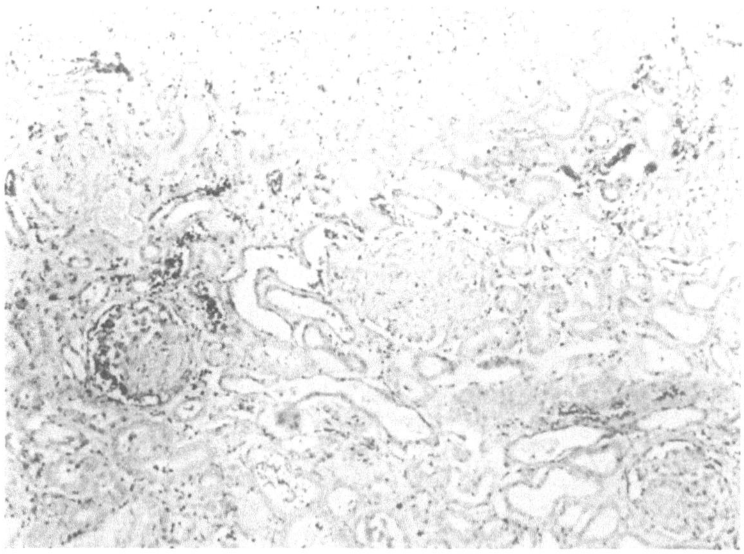

FIGURE 28

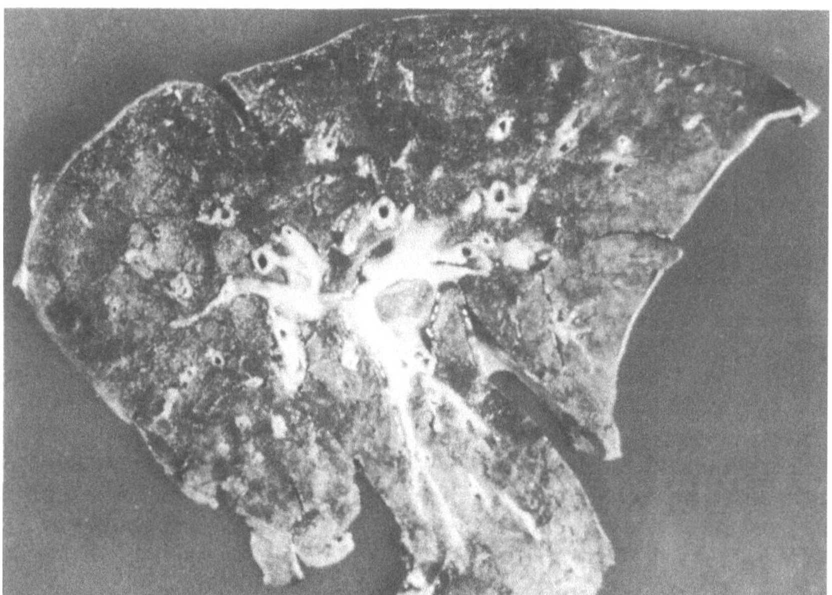

FIGURE 29

of disease activity, namely, the day after urine sediment, is then to start treatment with intensive plasmapheresis. We regard this kind of constellation of things--high titer of antibody and an active deposit--as something requiring immediate action because you never know when the patient is going to get an infection and just go off like this. We've had them from the beginning when we couldn't get plasmapheresis and we couldn't get vascular access and so on, and lost several of them. Nowadays, we don't do a renal biopsy, for example, because if you do renal biopsy you can't do plasma exchange very easily the following day because of problems with anti-coagulants and danger of bleeding and so on. So we make a diagnosis clinically. We get a serum sample off for antibody levels. We make an analysis of disease activity based on urine sediment and decide whether to treat them or not on that basis. This is a very interesting case, very interesting.

MODERATOR: You must realize that we are very back in the woods in terms of having plasmapheresis, plasma exchange facilities. This is a very difficult item for us yet. We have been working and trying to set it up. It's quite hard. We are making progress but we don't have it available yet.

RESPONSE: I appreciate that. This kind of experience, unfortunately, is what happens in most places. One of the problems of any treatment is that in many centers, by the time you get around to plasma exchange, you've lost a lot of glomeruli and it's very difficult to turn the clock back. Our own position at the moment, because we can do it quickly since we've got it all set up, we have not failed to cure--I use the word in the sense of eliminating anti-GBM antibody--anybody like this in the last year or so.

QUESTION: How do you follow the levels? Do you use radioimmunoassay?

RESPONSE: Yes. We do radioimmunoassay which gives us an answer within two hours.

COMMENT: Again, as a backwoodsman, and suicidal, one of the things that we used to do with this disease in the absence of plasmapheresis was an emergency nephrectomy. I just wonder, again using the retrospectroscope and very liberally, whether there was some time during the period between the 18th of November and the time the patient expired, when this was considered. I feel that by then, your back is up against the wall and there is not too much you can do. The question is: when the PO_2 is 55 mm Hg, when pulmonary infiltrates are beginning, it's certainly not the best type of treatment but we have, luckily I guess, pulled some patients through that period. It really does depend upon the rapidity of the disease.

COMMENT: I've been aware of the use of bilateral nephrectomy for a good many years but our review of the information is that it is frequently not effective and to my mind, frequently not effective at all. Certainly it's a very major operation, at that point the kidney function has not been wiped out and I would be more than loathe to take out someones kidneys if they were not truly end stage.

COMMENT: I am playing the devil's advocate but in some of these patients, the kidneys in some of the cases that were mentioned are just gone very rapidly and you don't know whether they are going to come back or not. Certainly, you are on the horns of a dilemma but the pulmonary infiltrations sometimes are more insidious and don't come on as rapidly. I've been involved in a number of these and we have done the bilateral nephrectomy and the disease has undergone remission after that.

MODERATOR: If there are no further comments or questions, we will go to the next case. Dr. Gustavo Gordillo will present the case.

DR. GORDILLO: This is a 16 y/o female with an unremarkable past history. She started her present illness when she was 7 y/o with generalized edema, hematuria and oliguria 2 months prior to admission.

On admission, she was found to have generalized edema, B.P. 130/90 mm Hg, proteinuria 143 mg/hr/m^2, serum creatinine 0.7 mg/dl, serum complement (CH 50%) 30 U (normal > 100 U). A percutaneous renal biopsy revealed type 2 MPGN. The immunofluorescence showed IgG, IgM and C_3 deposits in the mesangium with a slight linear deposit in the loops characteristic of Dense Deposit Disease (DDD) (Fig. 30).

She was in chronic renal failure 2 years later. She was placed in the chronic hemodialysis program within 2 months. She was transplanted from a live related donor (her father) in May, 1973.

Her evolution was excellent until 4 years post-op, when she developed seizures. EEG revealed generalized high voltage and slow waves. She was put on phenilhydantoins (200 mg/day) in divided doses. Because of high blood pressure difficult to control, the original kidneys were removed. The nephrectomy material revealed progression of the lesion already seen in the biopsy. After this procedure, her B.P. was 120/90 mm Hg; diuresis 1500 ml/day, serum creatinine 1.2 mg/dl. Two years later, in September 79 (6 years, 4 months post-transplantation) they noticed polyuria (3 liter/day). Maximal urinary concentrating capacity 244 mOsm/liter, serum creatinine 7 mg/dl. Methylprednisolone 1 g I.V. daily was given for 3 days with no response.

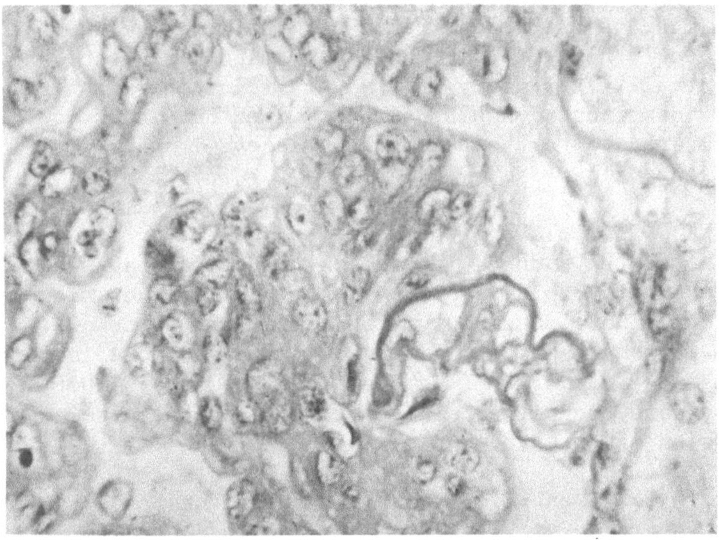

FIGURE 30

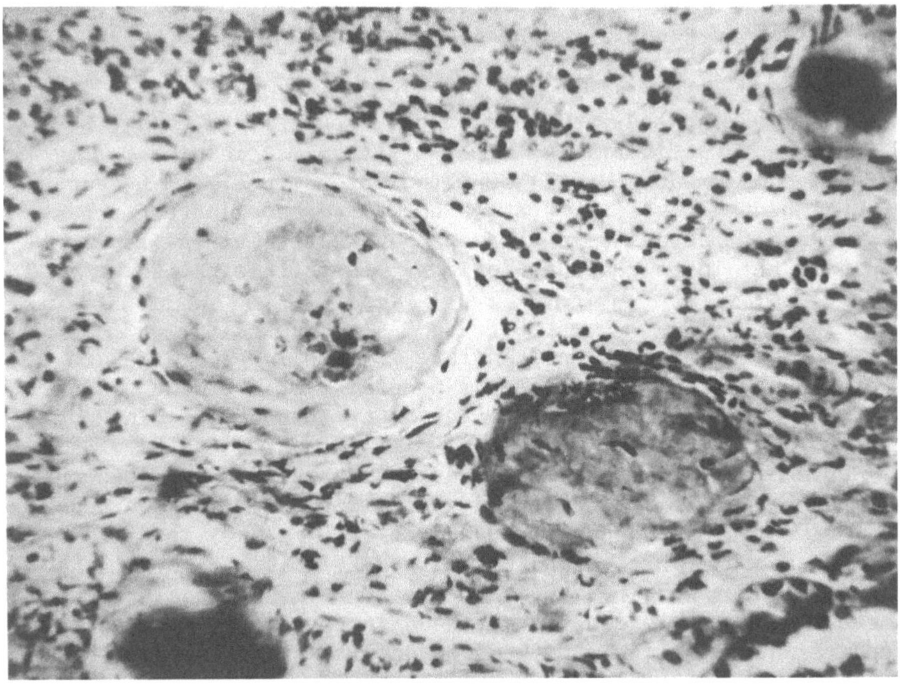

FIGURE 31

Percutaneous graft biopsy was made. Fourteen glomeruli were seen, 2 normal and 12 sclerosed. Findings included interstitial fibrosis with mononuclear cell infiltration (Fig. 31), collapsed tubuli and arteriolar walls hypertrophy with almost obliterated lumen. There were two glomeruli that were preserved in this small area of sclerosis. Immunofluorescence was negative. After seeing the biopsy, phenylhydantoin was discontinued and she was shifted to mysoline.

Four months later she was asymptomatic, B.P. 130/80 mm Hg, with less polyuria, serum creatinine 1.5 mg/dl. She is receiving prednisone 10 mg on alternate days, and azathioprine 25 mg daily. The reason I brought this case was that we would like to have comments about what seemed to be a chronic rejection. But we were in doubt about a possible interstitial nephritis caused by the phenylhydantoin. We stopped this treatment and the patient improved very rapidly.

COMMENT: I don't know if it is interstitial nephritis linked with phenylhydantoin but I can say that use of such medication certainly causes difficulties with steroid therapy because of acceleration of metabolism and elimination of corticosteroids. It was shown some years ago that transplant recipient patients who were on phenobarbital did less well than others and rejected more frequently. So maybe in the discussion of this case, we can include, besides the toxic nephritis, some effect of less effective steroid therapy which after discontinuation of the hydantoin, disappeared.

MODERATOR: What about the possibility of PTH or other hormonal changes? As discussed at one of our previous Seminars, there are some problems with vitamin D at the time of administration of an anti-convulsant.

QUESTION: What was the percentage of normal glomeruli and affected glomeruli on the biopsy?

RESPONSE: Fourteen glomeruli. Two were preserved; twelve were affected.

QUESTION: How much interstitial fibrosis and tubular atrophy?

RESPONSE: In the whole specimen.

COMMENT: There must be some sampling problem. I don't see how a kidney so destroyed can recuperate so well.

RESPONSE: This is not the only case I have seen. I have seen some other cases that are even worse than this one, and they recovered at least functionally. I didn't want to make another biopsy after the improvement.

COMMENT: We rely on the histopathology very heavily. I'd better preface my remarks by saying that on the other hand, rejection is a focal phenomenon and I would have to agree that administration of anticonvulsants, mainly phenobarbital and Dilantin, has been associated in my "objective" experience with increased difficulty with immunosuppressive management. So again, relying on rumbles of our own intestines, we increase our immunosuppressive doses and watch our T-cells very closely.

The other thing-about the biopsy-I found that it is very difficult to correlate in the post-transplant period, the function with the biopsy. It may well be that it is just focal. I think perhaps, getting a little more science into it, we really don't know what those lymphocytes are doing in the kidney. When you don't have glomeruli, that's a different story, but looking at a kidney and seeing a lot of interstitial infiltrate does not necessarily mean that the kidney has a loss of function. Some of those lymphocytes may be other than cytotoxic or killer cells and it's difficult to correlate. Now, when you don't have glomeruli, again, I would look at that biopsy and say: "My God, there's no way it's going to come back". On the other hand, we would have treated it anyway to see if it would.

COMMENT: I've got the wrong sort of memory for this kind of thing. Am I not right in thinking that this type of interstitial nephritis was described when receiving hydantoins in the absence of transplantation?

COMMENT: No, except two years ago in the 4th Seminar of this Series, in one case that turned out to be a carencial rickets, it was stated that the child had a convulsion and received phenylhydantoin. And then, this child went into renal failure. We performed a biopsy and it was a very severe tubulointerstitial nephritis. We just stopped the medication and the child recovered.

QUESTION: I gather that in this case at the moment you are giving very low doses of immunosuppression, aren't you?

RESPONSE: Yes.

QUESTION: Is there a reason why she is on 25 mg of azathioprine rather than the usual dose for what I presume is a reasonably sized child?

RESPONSE: She is 16 years old now. I really don't know why. Probably theoretically it would be indicated to increase the dose, but she is doing quite well on the low dose, so...

MODERATOR: Well, on that cheerful note, we shall adjourn for now. Thanks to all participants.

Participants

Program Chairman

*José Strauss, M.D., Professor of Pediatrics; Director, Division of Pediatric Nephrology, University of Miami School of Medicine, Miami, Florida, USA.

Guest Faculty - Seminar 6

*Giuseppe A. Andres, M.D., Professor of Microbiology, Pathology and Medicine, New York State School of Medicine, Buffalo, New York, USA.

*Jorge de la Cruz, M.D., Director, Division of Pediatric Nephrology, Hospital Infantil Lorencita Villegas de Santos, Bogota, Colombia.

*Gustavo Gordillo-Paniagua, M.D., Professor of Nephrology, Universidad La Salle School of Medicine, Mexico City; Director, Division of Pediatric Nephrology, Hospital Infantil, Mexico City, Mexico.

*Renée Habib, M.D., Director of Research, Institut National de la Sante et de la Recherche Medicale, Hôpital Necker, Enfants-Malades, Paris, France.

*Robert H. Heptinstall, M.D., Baxley Professor, Director, Department of Pathology, Johns Hopkins University School of Medicine; Pathologist-in-Chief, Johns Hopkins Hospital, Baltimore, Maryland, USA.

*John C. Hodson, F.R.C.P., F.R.C.R., Professor of Diagnostic Radiology, Yale University School of Medicine, New Haven, Connecticut, USA.

*Felipe Mota-H., M.D., Division of Pediatric Nephrology, Hospital Infantil, Mexico City, Mexico.

*Ricardo Muñoz-A., M.D., Division of Pediatric Nephrology, Hospital Infantil, Mexico City, Mexico.

Guest Faculty - Seminar 7

*Lewis Barness, M.D., Professor and Chairman, Department of Pediatrics, University of South Florida, Tampa, Florida, USA.

*Michel Broyer, M.D., Associate Professor of Pediatrics, Faculte de Medicine de Paris, Hôpital de Enfantes Malades, Paris, France.

*Gustavo Gordillo-Paniagua, M.D., Professor of Nephrology, Universidad La Salle School of Medicine, Mexico City; Director, Division of Pediatric Nephrology, Hospital Infantil, Mexico City, Mexico.

*Alan Gruskin, M.D., Professor of Pediatrics, Temple University; Director, Department of Nephrology, St. Christopher's Hospital, Philadelphia, Pennsylvania, USA.

*Jack Metcoff, M.D., George Lynn Cross Research Professor, Departments of Pediatrics, Biochemistry & Molecular Biology, University of Oklahoma, Oklahoma City, Oklahoma, USA.

Keith Peters, M.D., Professor and Director, Department of Medicine, Royal Postgraduate Medical School, London, England.

*George Richard, M.D., Professor and Chief, Division of Pediatric Nephrology, University of Florida, Gainesville, Florida, USA.

Miami Faculty

George Abdenour, M.D., Assistant Professor of Radiology and Pediatrics, University of Miami School of Medicine, Miami, Florida, USA.

Rex Baker, M.S., Research Assistant Professor of Pediatrics, Coordinator of Research, Division of Pediatric Nephrology, University of Miami School of Medicine, Miami, Florida, USA.

*Jacques J. Bourgoignie, M.D., Professor of Medicine; Director, Division of Nephrology, University of Miami School of Medicine, Miami, Florida, USA.

Hernan Carrion, M.D., Assistant Professor of Urology, University of Miami School of Medicine, Miami, Florida, USA.

*George Christakis, M.D., Professor of Epidemiology & Public Health; Chief, Nutrition Division, University of Miami School of Medicine, Miami, Florida, USA.

Violet Esquenazi, Ph.D., Research Assistant Professor of Surgery, University of Miami School of Medicine, Miami, Florida, USA.

*Rafael Galindez, M.D., Adjunct Instructor of Pediatrics, Division of Pediatric Nephrology, University of Miami School of Medicine, Miami, Florida, USA.

Carl Goldsmith, M.D., Associate Professor of Medicine, Division of Nephrology, University of Miami School of Medicine; Medical Director, Dialysis Unit, Jackson Memorial Hospital, Miami, Florida, USA.

*Helen M. Gorman, M.B.,B.Ch., Assistant Professor of Pediatrics, Division of Pediatric Nephrology, University of Miami School of Medicine, Miami, Florida, USA.

Michael A. Kaplan, M.D., Clinical Assistant Professor of Medicine, University of Miami School of Medicine, Miami, Florida, USA.

George Kyriakides, M.D., Assistant Professor of Surgery, University of Miami School of Medicine, Miami, Florida, USA.

Joyce Lentz, M.D., Instructor of Radiology, Division of Diagnostic Radiology, University of Miami School of Medicine, Miami, Florida, USA.

Charles M. Lynne, M.D., Associate Professor of Urology, University of Miami School of Medicine, Miami, Florida, USA.

Adolfo Maldonado, M.D., Assistant Professor of Radiology and Orthopedics, University of Miami School of Medicine; Chief, Diagnostic Radiology, University of Miami Hospitals and Clinics, Miami, Florida, USA.

*Barry J. Materson, M.D., Associate Professor of Medicine, University of Miami School of Medicine; Assistant Chief of Medical Services, Veterans Administration Hospital, Miami, Florida, USA.

Joshua Miller, M.D., Professor of Surgery and Microbiology; Chief, Transplantation Division, University of Miami School of Medicine, Miami, Florida, USA.

Gaston Murillo, M.D., Assistant Professor of Radiology and Pediatrics, University of Miami School of Medicine, Miami, Florida, USA.

Victoriano Pardo, M.D., Professor of Pathology, University of Miami School of Medicine; Director, Electron Microscopy Laboratory, Veterans Administration Hospital, Miami, Florida, USA.

J. Philip Pennell, M.D., Assistant Professor of Medicine, Division of Nephrology, University of Miami School of Medicine, Miami, Florida, USA.

*Guido Perez, M.D., Associate Professor of Medicine, University of Miami School of Medicine; Chief, Dialysis Unit, Veterans Administration Hospital, Miami, Florida, USA.

Eliseo Perez-Stable, M.D., Professor of Medicine, University of Miami School of Medicine; Chief, Medical Services, Veterans Administration Hospital, Miami, Florida, USA.

Victor A. Politano, M.D., Professor of Urology; Chairman, Department of Urology, University of Miami School of Medicine, Miami, Florida, USA.

Catherine Poole, M.D., Professor of Radiology and Pediatrics; Chairman, Department of Radiology, University of Miami School of Medicine, Miami, Florida, USA.

Ramon Rodriguez-Torres, M.D., Clinical Professor of Pediatrics, University of Miami School of Medicine; Chairman, Department of Pediatrics and Chief, Section of Pediatric Cardiology, American Hospital, Miami, Florida, USA.

Akram Tamer, M.D., Associate Professor of Pediatrics, University of Miami School of Medicine, Miami, Florida, USA.

*Carlos Vaamonde, M.D., Professor of Medicine, University of Miami School of Medicine; Director, Division of Nephrology, Veterans Administration Hospital, Miami, Florida, USA.

*Adel Yunis, M.D., Professor of Medicine and Biochemistry, Division of Hematology, University of Miami School of Medicine, Miami, Florida, USA.

*Gaston Zilleruelo, M.D., Assistant Professor of Pediatrics, Division of Pediatric Nephrology, University of Miami School of Medicine, Miami, Florida, USA.

Other Contributors

*Jean-Louis Bacri, M.D., Institut National de la Santé et de la Recherche Medicale, Hôpital Necker Enfantes-Malades, Paris, France.

*H. Jorge Baluarte, M.D., Department of Pediatrics, St. Christopher's Hospital for Children and Temple University School of Medicine, Philadelphia, Pennsylvania, USA.

*L. Cathelineau, M.D., Pouponniere de la Croix Rouge, Margency, France.

*A.M. Dartois, M.D., Service de Néphrologie Pédiatrique, Hôpital des Enfants-Malades, Paris, France.

*Abdelaziz Y. Elzouki, M.D., Department of Pediatrics, St. Christopher's Hospital for Children and Temple University School of Medicine, Philadelphia, Pennsylvania, USA.

*Robert S. Fennell, III, M.D., Division of Pediatric Nephrology, College of Medicine, University of Florida, Gainesville, Florida, USA.

*Eduardo H. Garin, M.D., Division of Pediatric Nephrology, College of Medicine, University of Florida, Gainesville, Florida, USA.

*Ricardo Gastelbondo-Amaya, M.D., Hospital Infantil de Mexico, Mexico City, Mexico.

*Francoise Gros, M.D., Service de Néphrologie Pédiatrique, Hôpital des Enfants-Malades, Paris, France.

*M. Guillot, M.D., Service de Néphrologie Pédiatrique, Hôpital des Enfants-Malades, Paris, France.

*M. Guimbaud, M.D., Pouponniere de la Croix Rouge, Margency, France.

*Sung Lan Hsia, M.D., Professor, Department of Dermatology, University of Miami School of Medicine, Miami, Florida, USA.

*Abdollah Iravani, M.D., Division of Pediatric Nephrology, College of Medicine, University of Florida, Gainesville, Florida, USA.

*Genevieve Jean, M.D., Service de Néphrologie Pédiatrique, Hôpital des Enfants-Malades, Paris, France.

*Anthony Kafatos, M.D., Nutrition Division, Department of Epidemiology and Public Health, University of Miami School of Medicine, Miami, Florida, USA.

*Claire Kleinknecht, M.D., Service de Néphrologie Pédiatrique, Hôpital des Enfants-Malades, Paris, France.

*Micheline Levy, M.D., Institut National de la Santé et de la Recherche Medicale, Hôpital Necker Enfantes-Malades, Paris, France.

*Felipe Mota-Hernandez, M.D., Hospital Infantil de Mexico, Mexico City, Mexico.

*Ricardo Muñoz-Arizpe, M.D., Hospital Infantil de Mexico, Mexico City, Mexico.

*Bernice Noble, Ph.D., Department of Microbiology, State University of New York at Buffalo, School of Medicine, Buffalo, New York, USA.

*John K. Orak, M.D., Division of Pediatric Nephrology, College of Medicine, University of Florida, Gainesville, Florida, USA.

*Martin S. Polinsky, M.D., Department of Pediatrics, St. Christopher's Hospital for Children and Temple University School of Medicine, Philadelphia, Pennsylvania, USA.

*James W. Prebis, M.D., Department of Pediatrics, St. Christopher's Hospital for Children and Temple University School of Medicine, Philadelphia, Pennsylvania, USA.

*Authors

AUTHOR INDEX

SUBJECT INDEX

MIX
Papier aus verantwortungsvollen Quellen
Paper from responsible sources
FSC® C105338

If you have any concerns about our products,
you can contact us on
ProductSafety@springernature.com

In case Publisher is established outside the EU,
the EU authorized representative is:
Springer Nature Customer Service Center GmbH
Europaplatz 3, 69115 Heidelberg, Germany

Printed by Libri Plureos GmbH
in Hamburg, Germany